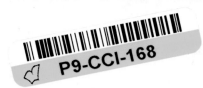
Guide to
Clinical Documentation

Second Edition

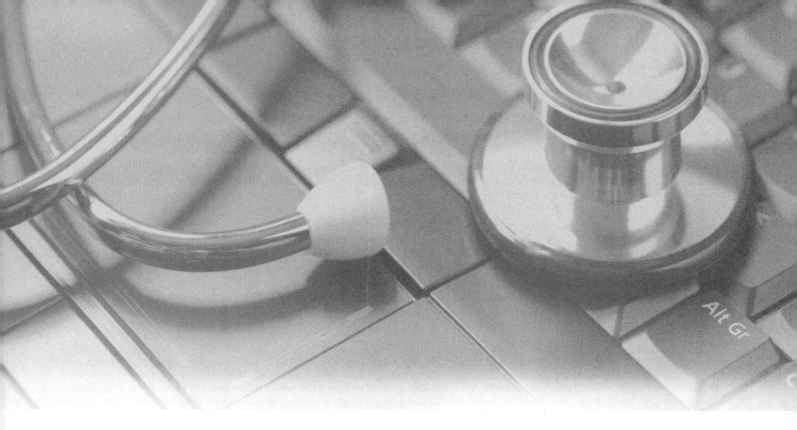

Guide to
Clinical Documentation

Second Edition

Debra D. Sullivan, PhD, RN, PA-C

Nurse Consultant, Risk Management
Banner Health
Phoenix, AZ

Clinical Adjunct Faculty, Associate Professor
Midwestern University
Arizona College of Osteopathic Medicine
Glendale, AZ

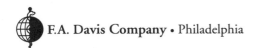 F.A. Davis Company • Philadelphia

F. A. Davis Company
1915 Arch Street
Philadelphia, PA 19103
www.fadavis.com

Printed in the United States of America

Last digit indicates print number: 10 9 8 7 6

Senior Acquisitions Editor: Andy McPhee
Manager of Content Development: George W. Lang
Developmental Editor: Nancy Hoffman
Design and Illustration Manager: Carolyn O'Brien

As new scientific information becomes available through basic and clinical research, recommended treatments and drug therapies undergo changes. The author(s) and publisher have done everything possible to make this book accurate, up to date, and in accord with accepted standards at the time of publication. The author(s), editors, and publisher are not responsible for errors or omissions or for consequences from application of the book, and make no warranty, expressed or implied, in regard to the contents of the book. Any practice described in this book should be applied by the reader in accordance with professional standards of care used in regard to the unique circumstances that may apply in each situation. The reader is advised always to check product information (package inserts) for changes and new information regarding dose and contraindications before administering any drug. Caution is especially urged when using new or infrequently ordered drugs.

Library of Congress Cataloging-in-Publication Data
Sullivan, Debra D.
   Guide to clinical documentation / Debra D. Sullivan. — 2nd ed.
      p. ; cm.
   Rev. ed. of: Documentation for physician assistants / Debra D. Sullivan, Lynnette J. Mattingly. c2004.
   Includes bibliographical references and index.
   ISBN-13: 978-0-8036-2583-9
   ISBN-10: 0-8036-2583-9
   1. Physicians' assistants. 2. Medical records. 3. Medical protocols. I. Sullivan, Debra D. Documentation for physician assistants. II. Title.
   [DNLM: 1. Forms and Records Control—methods. 2. Medical Records—standards. W 80]
   R697.P45S85 2012
   651.5'04261—dc22

                            2011014762

Dedication

It is an honor to dedicate this book to two very special women. First, to Dr. Tracy O. Middleton, who embodies professionalism, caring, compassion, and the ability to multitask. The sheer number of SOAP notes, histories and physicals, and other forms of documentation Tracy has read over the years in her roles of teacher, physician, colleague, mentor, and friend would stagger us all. Dr. Middleton has positively affected literally hundreds of health-care professionals, and I am fortunate to be one of them.

There is a saying that you can't pick your parents; if I could have chosen, I would still choose the ones God chose for me. I'm blessed beyond measure to have Louise Howard Dover as my mother. As a nurse, she has helped me with this book in several ways, and I'm always grateful for help. As a woman, she is the epitome of selflessness, humility, and compassion. As a mother, she has always encouraged me and challenged me to be my best. Thanks for everything, Mom.

Reviewers

GILBERT A. BOISSONNEAULT, PhD, PA-C
Professor
Clinical Sciences
University of Kentucky
Lexington, Kentucky

CHRISTOPHER K. COOPER, MPAS, PA-C
Instructor
Medical Education
University of North Texas Health Science Center
Fort Worth, Texas

ERICH A. FOGG, PA-C, MMSc
Program Director
Physician Assistant Department
University of New England
Portland, Maine

SARA HADDOW, MSA, PA-C
Education Director, Assistant Professor
Physician Assistant Department
Medical College of Georgia
Augusta, Georgia

JOANNE HAEFFELE, PhD
Assistant Professor
Nurse Practitioner Faculty
University of Utah College of Nursing
Salt Lake City, Utah

JOELLEN W. HAWKINS, RNC, PhD, FAAN, FAANP
Professor Emerita
William F. Connell School of Nursing
Boston College
Chestnut Hill, Massachusetts

PAT KENNEY-MOORE, MS, PA-C
Associate Professor, Associate Director,
   Academic Coordinator
Division of Physician Assistant Education
Oregon Health & Science University
Portland, Oregon

PETER D. KUEMMEL, MS, RPA-C
Clinical Associate Professor, Vice Chair
Physician Assistant Education
Stony Brook University
Stony Brook, New York

MARY ANN LAXEN, MAB, FNP, PA-C
Program Director, Retired
Physician Assistant Department
University of North Dakota
Grand Forks, North Dakota

NORA LOWRY, MPA, PA-C
Program Director
Physician Assistant Department
Wagner College
Staten Island, New York

CHERYL MOREDICH, RN, MS, WHNP-BC
Associate Professor
Nursing
Purdue University
West Lafayette, Indiana

DIANE E. NUÑEZ, RN, MS, ANP, BC
Clinical Associate Professor
College of Nursing & Healthcare Innovation
Arizona State University
Tempe, Arizona

MICHELE ROTH-KAUFFMAN, JD, MPAS, PA-C
Associate Dean & Chair
Physician Assistant Department
Gannon University
Erie, PA

BARBARA L. SAULS, EdD, PA-C
Clinical Professor
Physician Assistant Studies
King's College
Wilkes-Barre, Pennsylvania

Emily K. Sheff, CMSRN, FNP, BC
Family Nurse Practitioner
School of Nursing
MGH Institute of Health Professions
Boston, Massachusetts

Chika Ugorji, MD
Community Pediatrics
University of Florida
Jacksonville, Florida

Acknowledgments

From the very beginning stages of the first edition through every page of the second, I've had the unwavering support of my husband, Greg. Not only did he take on dish duty, grocery shopping, and other miscellaneous chores, but he has also pitched in as proofreader, cheerleader, advisor, and sounding board.

I've spent many years in my life being a student. From nursing school, to PA school, and through my master's and doctorate programs, I have been fortunate to learn from some of the best. So, I take this opportunity to say a heartfelt thanks to them, and to teachers everywhere, for the amazing work they do. I've also known and worked with so many bright, caring, and truly gifted medical professionals over the years and several careers. They deserve far more thanks than I can express here. There are too many to mention by name, but I must acknowledge Kristin Neal, MPH, PA-C and Lynnette Mattingly, MHPE, PA-C for their work as contributing authors, their years of friendship, and the laughter of girls night out!

I'm also grateful to Sheila Carvalho for lending fresh eyes to the proofreading process. I'm indebted to Maritza Santamaria-Hoffman, RN, JD, not only for reviewing sections of the text, but for being a tremendous encourager and fantastic boss, and for introducing me to the world of risk management. These strong and capable women have blessed me beyond measure

There are so many people at F. A. Davis who were a part of this project. First and foremost, thanks to Andy McPhee, for having a vision and helping to make it reality. I appreciate Nancy Hoffman and her work as developmental editor, and all the help and guidance along the way to keep things moving forward. I extend my gratitude to George Lang, Manager of Content Development at F. A. Davis, for his work on the manuscript, and to Sharon Lee, Production Manager. This is truly a team effort!

—DEBBIE SULLIVAN

Contents

Introduction

I was honored when Andy McPhee of F. A. Davis approached me about writing a second edition of this book. I have always known that good documentation is important; however, over the past few years, I have developed an even greater appreciation for it. My renewed sense of the importance of documenting clinical encounters is related to my work as a nurse consultant within the Risk Management Department of a large health-care system. I have had the opportunity to read hundreds of charting entries. I've seen really good documentation and extremely poor documentation. I have a working theory that if there are any problems associated with a health-care encounter, the documentation about that encounter either will make those problems appear less significant or, as seems more often the case, will magnify the problems because of the lack of good documentation.

Documentation used to be mostly a memory aid for the provider—a quick note of his or her thoughts about a patient's presentation, a likely diagnosis, maybe a few words about the treatment plan. Over the past few decades, however, documentation has become a more complex task. This is due, in part, to the ever-increasing number of medications and treatment modalities available to health-care providers. Another reason is that patients live longer with a greater number of comorbid conditions, adding to the complexity of caring for them and reflecting that complexity when authoring a medical record. The fact that our society is so litigious certainly adds more weight to clinical documentation and puts a greater burden on the providers to capture their thoughts and actions for others to read and interpret years after the event.

Dr. Mitchell Cohen wrote about this evolution of documentation in an article that appeared in *Family Practice Management*.* Dr. Cohen explains:

> From time to time I'll stumble upon an old chart in my office that goes back 40 years. My predecessors charted office visits on sheets of lined manila card stock, which would suffice for at least 15 to 20 visits. Clearly, these charts were only intended for the physicians as a way to refresh their memory of what happened from one visit to the next. For example, the documentation for one visit read simply, "1/20/67: pharyngitis » penicillin."

These days chart notes are primarily not for the physician or patient, but for all the others who aren't in the exam room and yet feel they have a stake in what takes place in this once confidential arena. To satisfy coders and insurers, my documentation for a 99213 sore throat visit must contain one to three elements of the history of present illness, a pertinent review of systems, six to eleven elements of the physical exam, and low-complexity medical decision-making. My malpractice carrier and my future defense attorney would also like me to explain my clinical rationale for why the patient has strep throat and not a retropharyngeal abscess or meningitis. A table with a McIsaac score calculating the likelihood that this patient does indeed have strep throat might be nice as well. If I prescribe a weak narcotic for a really nasty case of strep, the state medical board would be pleased if I addressed what other medication has been tried and whether the patient has any history of addiction. I'll also need to document that I explained the proper use of any medications and the need for follow up if the patient doesn't get better.

When I'm finally done with my note, it looks like this:

CC: Sore throat x 2d

HPI: 17 y/o F with 2d h/o sore throat. Has an associated headache and fever to 101°. No significant cough. Patient has noticed some swollen lumps in neck. Having significant pain despite use of Tylenol, ibuprofen and salt water gargles.

Social history: No history of substance abuse or addiction.

ROS: Denies neck stiffness or back pain, no rash. No difficulty speaking.

PE: VS: AF, VSS.
Gen: Alert, pleasant female in NAD.
HEENT: NC/AT, PERRLA, EOMI, TM clear b/l,
OP notable for tonsillar enlargement with exudates.
No asymmetry or uvular deviation present.
Neck: + tender anterior cervical adenopathy, no
nuchal rigidity or meningismus.
CV: RRR S1/S2 without murmurs.
C/L: CTAB.
Abd: Soft, nondistended, nontender, no
hepatosplenomegaly.
McIsaac's score = 4; Rapid strep: +
A: Streptococcal pharyngitis
P: 1. PenVK 500mg PO TID x 10 days. Discussed
risks of medication including allergic reaction and
complications of not taking full course of antibiotics
including rheumatic fever and valvular heart disease.
2. Hydrocodone elixir QHS to help relieve pain par-
ticularly when trying to rest. Has already tried aceta-
minophen and NSAID and will continue salt water
gargles. Follow up if no improvement in one week.

Have discussed other potential diagnoses and re-
viewed warning signs of retropharyngeal abscess and
meningitis. Patient agrees and understands plan.
Like I said, "pharyngitis » penicillin."
(*Used with permission of the American
Academy of Family Physicians)

You may be feeling overwhelmed or a little intim-
idated by documentation at this point. Trust me,
you're not alone and not without help. The goal of
this book is to give you a good foundation on which
to build your skills. You will develop your own style of
documentation as you learn more and more about
medicine, about patients, and about the importance
of communicating through the medical record. This
book should be considered a "guide," not a mandate.
It is a basic road map to help you start on your journey.
I hope you enjoy it along the way.

Debbie Sullivan
Phoenix, Arizona

Chapter 1

Medicolegal Principles of Documentation

OBJECTIVES

- Discuss medical and legal considerations of documentation.
- Identify groups of people who may access medical records.
- Identify general principles of documentation.
- Discuss medical billing and coding.
- Identify benefits of using electronic medical records.
- Identify challenges and barriers to using electronic medical records.
- Define the terms *electronic medical records*, *meaningful use*, and *interoperability*.
- Identify components of the Health Insurance Portability and Accountability Act.
- Discuss principles of confidentiality.

Medical Considerations of Documentation

You might be asking, "Why a book on documentation?" Documentation is one of the most important skills a health-care provider can learn. You might feel tempted to focus considerably more time and energy on learning other skills, such as physical examination, suturing, or pharmacotherapeutics. These are essential skills, but documentation is likewise extremely important. State licensure laws and regulations, accrediting bodies, professional organizations, and federal reimbursement programs all require that health-care providers maintain a record for each of their patients.

Good documentation is critical for many reasons. The medical record chronologically documents the care of the patient and is an important element in contributing to high-quality care. The medical record is the primary means of communication between members of the health-care team and facilitates continuity of care and communication among the professionals involved in a patient's care.

The patient's medical record establishes your credibility as a health-care provider. It is important to remember that you are creating a record that other professionals will read; therefore, you should use professional language and include appropriate content. Other health-care providers will assume, rightly or wrongly, that you practice medicine much in the same manner in which you document. If your documentation is sloppy, full of errors, or incomplete, others will assume that is the way you practice. Conversely, thorough, legible, and complete documentation will infer that you provide care in the same way, thus establishing your credibility. Some excellent providers simply do not have good documentation skills. However, this is the exception rather than the rule. It is very difficult to persuade those who read sloppy documentation that the person who wrote that way can, and did, provide good care.

Legal Considerations of Documentation

All medical records are legal documents and are important for both the health-care provider and the patient, regardless of where the patient care takes place. The most important legal functions of medical records are to provide evidence that appropriate care was given and to document the patient's response to that care. An often-quoted principle of documentation, which every health-care provider has probably heard, is that if it is not documented, it was not done. This is a fallacy because it is impossible to capture with documentation every nuance of a patient-provider encounter, and it is impossible to create a perfect record of every encounter. However, the principle behind the quote is important in a legal context; there is a considerable time lapse between when events occur (and are documented) and when litigation occurs. It may be anywhere from 2 to 7 years from the occurrence of an event until you are called to give a sworn account of the event. The medical record is usually the only detailed record of what actually occurred, and only what is written is considered to have occurred. You will not remember the details of an event that happened 6 years ago; your only memory aid will be the medical record. As a legal document, plaintiff attorneys, defense attorneys, malpractice carriers, jurors, judges, and most likely the patient will have access to the medical records you author. You should keep this in mind at all times when documenting.

Other Purposes of Documentation

Reviewers from various organizations can obtain access to a medical record for a variety of purposes. Representatives from insurance companies or state or federal payers can review the record for purposes of deciding on payment or looking for evidence of fraud and abuse. Peer review organizations might read the record to determine whether the care reflected in your documentation is consistent with the standard of care. Researchers often obtain access to medical records for purposes of conducting scientific studies. Although it is important to remember that these audiences may have access to your records, you should keep in mind that the primary audience of the medical records will be medical professionals involved in direct patient care.

Throughout this book, you will analyze examples of documentation. You may also complete the worksheets, which will help you apply the information you have just read. The purpose of this book is to teach documentation skills and critical analysis of medical records. Our intent is not to instruct on the practice of medicine or to teach medical decision making. The content of a medical record—or learning *what* to document—varies greatly, depending on the patient's presenting problem or condition. The principles of *how* to document and *why* documentation is important do not vary as much and thus are the focus throughout this book.

General Principles of Documentation

The Centers for Medicare and Medicaid Services (CMS) is one agency of the U.S. Department of Health and Human Services (HHS). As one of the nation's largest payers for health-care services, CMS has established specific guidelines for documentation that we reference several times throughout this book. There are two sets of documentation guidelines currently in use: the 1995 and the 1997 guidelines. CMS published an evaluation and management guide in 2009; however, it was offered as a reference tool and did not replace the content found in the 1995 and 1997 guidelines. There are minor differences between the two guidelines, and it is recommended that health-care providers refer to the 1995 guidelines to identify those differences. Additional information may be found at www.cms.gov. Both sets of guidelines recognize the following general principles of documentation:

1. The medical record should be complete and legible.
2. The documentation of each patient encounter should include the following:
    • Reason for the encounter and relevant history, physical examination findings, and diagnostic test results
    • Assessment, clinical impression, or diagnosis
    • Plan for care
    • Date and legible identity of the observer
3. If not documented, the rationale for ordering diagnostic and other ancillary services should be easily inferred.
4. Past and present diagnoses should be accessible to the treating and consulting providers.
5. Appropriate health risk factors should be identified.
6. The patient's progress, response to and changes in treatment, and revision of diagnoses should be documented.
7. The *Current Procedural Terminology* (CPT) and *International Classification of Diseases*, 9th revision (ICD-9) codes reported on the health insurance claim form or billing statement should be supported by the documentation in the medical records. (More discussion of billing and coding is included later in this chapter.)

There are other generally accepted principles of documentation, such as that each entry should include the date and time the record was created and should identify the person creating the record. In settings in which care is provided around the clock, military time is often used to avoid confusion between a.m. and p.m. One o'clock in the afternoon is 1300, 10:30 at night is 2230, and so forth. A patient's record should never be charted in advance of seeing the patient. A patient's medical record may be amended, but should never be altered. At times, it will be necessary to make corrections to a record. When making a correction, you should draw a single line through the text that is erroneous, initial and date the entry, and label it as an error. If there is room, you may enter the correct text in the same area of the note. You should not write in the margins of a page; if there is no room to enter the correct text, use an addendum to record the information. You should never obliterate an original note, nor should you use correction fluid or tape. When using a ruled sheet such as an order sheet or progress note, there should not be any blank lines. If a record is dictated and then transcribed, the author should read the transcription before signing, correcting any errors in the process. You should not stamp a record "signed but not read"—doing so will call attention to the fact that you did not verify the content of the record.

We assume that you already have some knowledge of commonly used medical abbreviations; therefore, we have used abbreviations throughout the book and have incorporated them into the chapter worksheets. We offer one caution about using abbreviations: always be clear about your intended meaning. For example, if you use the abbreviation "CP," one person could read that as "chest pain" and another as "cerebral palsy." Of course, the rest of the entry should make clear which term the abbreviation is being used for. Some hospitals and other health-care entities have a published list of abbreviations that should not be used at all. The health-care provider is responsible for complying with the institution's policies regarding use of abbreviations.

Medical Billing and Coding

Concise medical record documentation is critical to providing patients with quality care and to ensuring accurate and timely reimbursement. Medical records are subject to review by payers to validate that the services provided were medically necessary and were consistent with the individual's insurance coverage. Guidelines for coding evaluation and management (E/M) services were developed by CMS to assist health-care providers and may be found at www.cms .gov/MLNEdWebGuide/25_EMDOC.asp.

For billing purposes, a procedure code must be selected that reflects the level of service provided. The American Medical Association (AMA) created and maintains the CPT code set used for insurance billing and other reporting requirements. CPT is a listing of descriptive terms and identifying codes for reporting medical services and procedures and is the uniform language for claims processing, medical care review, medical education, and research.

Evaluation and Management Services

When a patient presents for care, a provider evaluates the patient and then proceeds to manage the presenting complaint. The encounter between patient and health-care provider may vary from brief to comprehensive depending on the patient's chief complaint. For example, the time required for evaluation of a child who presents with a sore throat is typically brief, and the management options are fairly straightforward. Conversely, more time is required for evaluating an elderly person who has several chronic conditions and a new complaint of chest pain, and the medical decision-making and management process is more complex.

CPT codes assigned for E/M services are determined by several factors. One factor is whether the patient is new, established, or seen for consultation services, and another is the type of facility where care is provided. Level of service is another factor and is determined by three key elements: history, physical examination, and medical decision making. Factors that modify the level of service are time spent on counseling and coordination of care, the nature of the presenting problem, and time spent face to face with the patient, family, or both. The complexity of medical decision making takes into account the presenting complaint, coexisting medical problems, amount of data to be reviewed (i.e., tests and old records), amount of time spent with the patient, number of diagnoses and treatment options, and risk for significant complications. Table 1-1 provides examples of CPT coding for a new outpatient visit.

International Classification of Diseases Coding

Whereas E/M codes indicate what services and procedures were provided, ICD codes explain the reason for the services. The ICD code is a diagnostic coding system that classifies diseases and injuries and is used to track mortality and morbidity statistics. These standardized codes are used by national and international agencies and organizations to forecast health-care needs, evaluate facilities and services, review costs, and conduct studies of trends in diseases over the years. Either a 9 or 10, referring to either the 9th or 10th Revision, usually follows ICD.

ICD-9 was published in 1979. It is a numerical set of codes used to identify a specific condition; for

Table 1-1 Examples of *Current Procedural Terminology* Coding for a New Patient Visit

99201—Usually the presenting problems are self-limited or minor, and the physician typically spends 10 minutes face to face with the patient, family, or both. E/M requires the following three key components:
- Problem-focused history
- Problem-focused examination
- Straightforward medical decision making

99202—Usually the presenting problems are of low to moderate severity, and the physician typically spends 20 minutes face to face with the patient, family, or both. E/M requires the following three key components:
- Expanded problem-focused history
- Expanded problem-focused examination
- Straightforward medical decision making

99203—Usually the presenting problems are of moderate severity, and the physician typically spends 30 minutes face to face with the patient, family, or both. E/M requires the following three key components:
- Detailed history
- Detailed examination
- Medical decision making of low complexity

99204—Usually the presenting problems are of moderate to high severity, and the physician typically spends 45 minutes face to face with the patient, family, or both. E/M requires the following three key components:
- Comprehensive history
- Comprehensive examination
- Medical decision making of moderate complexity

99205—Usually the presenting problems are of moderate to high severity, and the physician typically spends 60 minutes face to face with the patient, family, or both. E/M requires the following three key components:
- Comprehensive history
- Comprehensive examination
- Medical decision making of high complexity

example, 401 is the code for essential hypertension, and 530.81 is the code for gastroesophageal reflux. To improve disease tracking and speed transition to an electronic health-care environment, the HHS proposed that the ICD-9 code set be replaced by an expanded ICD-10 (10th revision) that is alphanumerically based. ICD-9 contains only 17,000 codes, whereas the ICD-10 code sets have more than 155,000 codes along with the capacity to accommodate new diagnoses and procedures, expand descriptions of some diagnoses, and allow more detailed tracking of mortality and morbidity. Although the ICD-10 codes are now available for public viewing, they are not currently valid for any purpose or use. The effective implementation date is October 1, 2014. After this date, ICD-10 codes must be used on all Health Insurance Portability and Accountability Act (HIPAA) transactions; otherwise, the claims may be rejected or cause delay in reimbursements.

An appropriate code is assigned to identify the diagnosis, symptom, condition, problem, complaint, or other reason for the encounter. ICD-9 codes are numbered 001.0 to V84.8 and consist of three, four, or five digits. "V" codes are used to identify encounters for reasons other than illness or injury, such as immunizations and preventive health services

(e.g., V70.0, routine adult health checkup). "E" codes are used to identify causes of external injury and poisoning (e.g., E970, gunshot wound). The first three digits of a code indicate the disease category (e.g., codes 290 to 319 are used for mental disorders). The fourth and fifth digits provide greater detail. For example, the code for acute myocardial infarction (AMI) is 410. If the AMI involved the posterolateral wall, the code would be 410.5, indicating the location of the infarct. A fifth digit "1" is used to specify initial treatment (410.51), such as in the emergency department, whereas a "2" indicates all subsequent treatment (410.52) within 8 weeks of the AMI.

Although it is common for health-care providers to do their own coding, they may have others carry out the coding and billing functions, such as an office manager or an outside service. The documentation must be as accurate and detailed as the CPT code assigned. *Downcoding* is the process by which an insurance company reduces the value of a procedure or encounter and resulting reimbursement because either (1) there is a mismatch of CPT code and description, or (2) the ICD-9 code does not justify the procedure or level of service. The medical record must include documentation that supports the assessment. The quality and accuracy of the medical record are vital to the reimbursement process, which in turn is vital to the delivery of health care.

MEDICOLEGAL ALERT !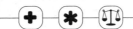

Although getting paid is a very important issue for physicians' offices, they should never code for reimbursement purposes only. This can be construed as fraud. Remember, your documentation must support the diagnoses reported.

Good documentation is absolutely essential to support the level of E/M services and facilitate assignment of correct CPT and ICD codes. The following are some key concepts showing the interrelatedness of documentation and codes and an illustrative example of each concept:

1. Any tests ordered must correlate with an ICD code assigned to the visit.
   • If a urine pregnancy test is performed in the office, a reason for obtaining that test must be associated with a diagnosis such as amenorrhea (626.0), menometrorrhagia (626.2), or abdominal pain (789.9).

2. Assign an ICD code that reflects the most specific diagnosis that is known at the time.
   • The patient's diagnosis is gastroenteritis (558.9). If it is reasonably certain that it is viral, use the code for viral gastroenteritis, 008.8. Suppose that the patient's original complaint was diarrhea (787.91). The result of a stool culture is positive for shigella. When the patient returns for a follow-up visit, the diagnosis would then be enteritis, shigella (004.9).

3. The primary code should reflect the patient's chief complaint or the reason for the encounter.
   • Example: the patient's diagnoses for an office visit are abdominal pain, depression, and diabetes mellitus (DM). The patient presented with abdominal pain. The primary code would be abdominal pain (789.0).

4. Secondary codes are listed after the primary code and expand on the primary code or define the need for a higher level of service.
   • Example: the patient with abdominal pain is late for her menses. A secondary code would be amenorrhea (626.0).

5. Code a chronic condition as often as applicable to the patient's condition.
   • Using example 3, DM is a chronic condition that may pertain to the abdominal pain. Listing it in the assessment portion of your notes points out this fact.

6. Code coexisting conditions that may have an influence on the outcome.
   • In example 3, depression is a coexisting condition that may alter a patient's perception of abdominal pain. The patient may take antidepressant medication, which could cause the pain. Coding both the chronic condition (DM) and coexisting condition (depression) demonstrates the higher level of care needed to manage the patient.

7. Do not use "rule out..." as a diagnosis.
   • There is no code for this. Instead, use a diagnosis, symptom, condition, or problem. You may use "rule out" when documenting the assessment to guide you in your plan of care, although it is not necessary.

8. Signs and symptoms that are routinely associated with a disease process should not be coded separately.
   • An upper respiratory infection (URI) is typically associated with pharyngitis, rhinitis, and cough. The latter should not be coded if URI (465) is used.

9. When the same condition is described as both acute and chronic, code both and use the acute code first.
   • A patient may have chronic sinusitis (473.9) with an acute exacerbation (461.9).

Nomenclature for Diagnoses

Diagnostic terminology can be broad or specific. It is preferable to be as descriptive as the data allow. In general, you should use the medical term for a diagnosis, symptom, condition, or problem rather than lay terminology. Instead of "runny nose," you should use "rhinorrhea." This does not work in every situation. There is no medical term for "chest pain" when used as a diagnosis, unless you know what is causing the chest pain. Consider the following examples:

EXAMPLE 1.1 ⎯⎯⎯

Broad	Specific
Neck pain	Acute cervical sprain
Upper respiratory infection	Sinusitis
Chest pain	Myocardial infarction
Cough	Pneumonia
Arthralgia	Osteoarthritis

EXAMPLE 1.2 ⎯⎯⎯

Lay Term	Medical Term
Joint pain	Arthralgia
Difficulty swallowing	Dysphagia

Menstrual cramps	Dysmenorrhea
Blood in urine	Hematuria
Yeast infection	Candidiasis

For more practice using medical terminology and abbreviations, see the worksheets at the end of this chapter.

Electronic Medical Records

Paper-based medical records have been in existence for decades; replacement by computer-based records has been slowly underway for more than 20 years. The electronic medical record (EMR) lies at the center of any computerized health system. The EMR is a longitudinal electronic record of patient health information generated by one or more encounters in any care delivery setting. Several interchangeable terms may be used for EMR, such as *electronic health record* (EHR), *electronic patient record* (EPR), and *computer-based patient record* (CPR). A more comprehensive definition of EMR is provided by the 1997 Institute of Medicine report, *The Computer-Based Patient Record: An Essential Technology for Health Care*:

A patient record system is a type of clinical information system, which is dedicated to collecting, storing, manipulating, and making available clinical information important to the delivery of patient care. The central focus of such systems is clinical data and not financial or billing information. Such systems may be limited in their scope to a single area of clinical information (e.g., dedicated to laboratory data), or they may be comprehensive and cover virtually every facet of clinical information pertinent to patient care (e.g., computer-based patient records systems).

Much of the stimulus for adoption of EMRs is the increasing evidence that current systems are not delivering sufficiently safe, high-quality, efficient, and cost-effective health care.

The electronic storage of clinical information will create the potential for computer-based tools to help providers significantly enhance the quality of medical care and increase the efficiency of medical practice. These tools may include reminder systems that identify patients who are due for preventive care interventions, alerting systems that detect contraindications among prescribed medications, and coding systems that facilitate the selection of correct billing codes for patient encounters. Numerous other decision-support tools have been developed and may soon facilitate the practice of clinical medicine. The potential of such tools will not be realized, however, if the EMR is just a set of textual documents stored in a computer, that is, a "word-processed" patient chart. To support intelligent and useful tools, the EMR must have a systematic internal model of the information it contains and must support the efficient capture of clinical information in a manner consistent with this model.

Benefits of Electronic Medical Records

A 2003 report by the Institute of Medicine, *Key Capabilities of an Electronic Health Record System*, identified a set of eight core health-care delivery functions that an electronic medical records system should be capable of performing: (1) health information and data; (2) result management; (3) order management; (4) decision support; (5) electronic communication and connectivity; (6) patient support; (7) administrative processes; and (8) reporting.

A closer look at the intended functionality in each of these eight areas identifies some of the perceived benefits of EMRs. An electronic system would provide immediate access to key information, such as diagnoses, allergies, laboratory test results, and medications, that would improve the provider's ability to make sound clinical decisions in a timely manner. Result management would ensure that all providers participating in the care of a patient would have quick access to new and past test results, regardless of who ordered the tests, the geographic location of the ordering provider, or when the tests were ordered or performed. Order management would include the ability to enter and store orders for prescriptions, tests, and other services in a computer-based system that would enhance legibility, reduce duplication, reduce fragmentation, and improve the speed with which orders are executed. Using reminders, prompts, and alerts, computerized decision-support systems would improve compliance with best clinical practices, ensure regular screenings and other preventive practices, identify possible drug interactions, and facilitate diagnoses and treatments. Electronic communication and connectivity would provide efficient and secure communication among providers and patients that would improve the continuity of care, increase the timeliness of diagnoses and treatments, and reduce the frequency of adverse events. Patients would be provided tools that give them access to their health records and interactive patient education and that would help them carry out home-monitoring and self-testing to improve control of chronic conditions. Computerized administrative tools, such as scheduling systems, would improve hospitals' and clinics' efficiency and provide more timely service to patients. Electronic data storage that employs uniform data standards will enable health-care providers and organizations to respond more quickly to federal, state, and private reporting requirements, including those that support patient safety and epidemiological and disease surveillance. Such data could be readily analyzed for medical audit, research, and quality assurance and could provide support for continuing medical education.

Electronic prescribing, or e-prescribing, is a specialized function within a computerized medical record system. Specific legislation and regulations exist that dictate the use of electronic prescribing. This is discussed in detail in Chapter 10.

Barriers to Electronic Medical Records

Many perceived barriers have hampered widespread implementation of EMRs. Although numerous studies have shown that most health-care providers believe that use of EMRs will improve quality of care, reduce errors, improve quality of practice, and increase practice productivity, there is resistance to adopting EMRs. A number of factors contribute to this, including well-publicized EMR failures; limited computer literacy on the part of providers; concerns over productivity, patient satisfaction, and unreliable technology; and the absence of reputable research substantiating the benefits of EMR. Market and economic factors are a concern. Apart from the costs of hardware and software, there is a tremendous cost in staff time and revenue when switching from paper to electronic charts. Ethical and legal issues abound with concerns about safety and security of systems and the ability to protect and keep private confidential health information. There is even disagreement over who "owns" the data entered into any system, as well as debate about accessibility to the data. Technical matters, such as functionality, ease of use, and customer support from vendors are other barriers. It is challenging enough to find an EMR system that works for a single-provider ambulatory care–based practice; it is another challenge altogether to find a system that will work for large institutions and serve the needs of diverse departments.

Interoperability

Perhaps the biggest barrier to widespread adoption of EMR is lack of interoperability. A basic definition for *interoperability* is the ability of two or more systems or their components to exchange information and to use the information that has been exchanged. As it relates specifically to EMRs, the Healthcare Information and Management Systems Society (HIMSS) defines interoperability as "the ability of health information systems to work together within and across organizational boundaries in order to advance the effective delivery of health care for individuals and communities."

Without interoperability, fundamental data and information, such as patient records, cannot easily be shared across and sometimes within enterprises. There are significant barriers to achieving interoperability. There is no standard technical language shared between systems; hence, there is little or no integration with other applications, nor is there the ability of different systems to communicate in a meaningful way with one another. Information technologies were not initially designed with interoperability in mind, so structures are rarely in place to support it. Currently used data storage systems are often proprietary, and access to these systems is difficult. Implementation of interoperable health information systems may require a high degree of technical expertise not readily available to individual providers or smaller health-care organizations. Standards of interoperability are only just being developed—after many health information technology systems have already been installed and implemented. Meeting standards of operability will be an important criterion for the certification of EMR systems that are being developed at this time.

Meaningful Use

In February 2009, President Obama signed into law the American Recovery and Reinvestment Act (ARRA) of 2009, which includes more than $48 billion for health-care information technology for the adoption and effective use of EMR and for regional health information exchange. The Health Information Technology portion of ARRA contains information related to the Health Information Technology for Economic and Clinical Health Act (HITECH); the HITECH Act offers financial incentives for health-care providers and hospitals that comply with the standards of "meaningful use." Full definition and requirements for certification and reporting were ongoing at the time this text was published; however, information in the HITECH act suggests that systems will have to meet at least four criteria: (1) certification, (2) electronic prescribing, (3) quality reporting, and (4) exchange of information with other systems.

Health Insurance Portability and Accountability Act

Confidentiality of medical records has always been a concern for health-care providers. Regardless of the medium of storage, confidentiality of data contained in the records will continue to be of utmost importance. With the emphasis on interoperability and the criteria that define how EMR systems must be able to exchange confidential medical information securely, a discussion of HIPAA (or the Act) is warranted.

Enacted by Congress in 1996 to address a number of issues affecting national health care, HIPAA is a large and complex law continually subject to revisions and amendments by legislative actions. The Act establishes standards, and timetables for adoption of the standards, for electronic transfers of health data, addressing growing public concern about privacy and security of personal health data. The primary goals of the standards are (1) to combat fraud and abuse; (2) to make health insurance more affordable and accessible; (3) to simplify administration of health insurance claims by requiring all entities to bill electronically using one format; (4) to give patients more control of and access to their health-care information; and (5) to protect medical records and individually identifiable medical information from unauthorized use or disclosure, especially in the burgeoning electronic age.

Health Insurance Portability

The Health Insurance Portability provision of the Act (Title I) improves the portability and continuity of health insurance coverage for workers and their families when they change or lose their jobs by limiting the restrictions a group health plan can place on benefits pertaining to a preexisting condition. A preexisting condition is a condition for which medical advice, diagnosis, care, or treatment was recommended or received within the 6 months before the enrollment date for a new health insurance plan. Preexisting conditions can only be excluded from health benefits for 12 months. A person who did not enroll during the initial or open enrollment period is considered a late enrollee, and benefits for preexisting conditions may be excluded for 18 months. If a person had health insurance coverage before enrolling in a new health plan, the exclusion period may be reduced by the number of months a person was insured, as long as there were no significant breaks of 63 or more days of coverage.

Title I has additional important provisions. Preexisting conditions do not apply to pregnancy or to a child enrolled within 30 days of birth or adoption. Insurers are required to renew coverage to all groups regardless of the health status of any group member. Insurers may not establish any rule that discriminates based on the health status of an individual or their dependent, nor may they charge higher premiums or alter the level of benefits. For those individuals with their own private health insurance plan, renewability is guaranteed. Coverage cannot be terminated unless the premiums are not paid, fraud is committed against an insurer, the policy is terminated by the insured, the insured person moves outside the service area of a network plan, or membership in an association is ended if the insurance is only available to members of that association. If the insurance company stops selling the policy, it must offer the insured another policy it sells in the same state. Further details may be found at the CMS website page Health Insurance Reform for Consumers at https://www.cms.gov/HealthInsReformforConsume/ 02_WhatHIPAADoesandDoesNotDo.asp.

Electronic Health-Care Transactions

In 2009, it was estimated that about 400 different formats were being used to process health claims online. Billing and other administrative procedures were inconsistent and varied among health insurers, the government, and other entities. This made it difficult for providers, hospitals, health plans, and health-care clearinghouses to process claims and perform other transactions electronically. In an effort to lower costs and improve efficiency, standards were developed to simplify the administration of health insurance claims by requiring that a common format and data structure be used when exchanging specific transaction types (e.g., billing, mandatory reporting), code sets (e.g., diagnostic, procedural), and identifiers (e.g., for health insurers, providers, employers) electronically. The standards require that the same format is used to transmit the following health-related information: claims and equivalent encounter information, claim status, payment and remittance advice, enrollment and disenrollment in a plan, eligibility for a plan, premium payment, referral certification and authorization, and coordination of benefits. HHS finalized these standards in 2003 and projected that their use would result in a net savings to the health-care industry of $29.9 billion over the next 10 years.

The Privacy Rule

Providers have an ethical and legal obligation to safeguard patients' privacy. Because of the requirements of transmitting sensitive health information electronically, the Privacy Rule was written to protect the confidentiality of individually identifiable health information. The rule limits the use and disclosure of certain individually identifiable health information; gives patients the right to access their medical records; restricts most disclosures of health information to the minimum needed for the intended purpose; and establishes safeguards and restrictions regarding the use and disclosure of records for certain public responsibilities such as public health, research, and law enforcement. Under the rule, improper uses or disclosures may be subject to criminal or civil sanctions prescribed in HIPAA. Federal

HIPAA regulations do not preempt any state laws that are stronger or more protective of consumers' security and privacy.

Protected Health Information and Covered Entities

Protected health information (PHI) relates to the past, present, or future physical or mental health or condition of an individual; the provision of health care to an individual; past, present, or future payment for the provision of health care to an individual; and information that identifies or could reasonably be used to identify a protected individual. This information may be oral, electronic, paper, or any other form. Individually identifiable health information includes such data as name, Social Security number, patient identification number (such as a medical record number), address, demographic data, or any other information that could reasonably allow a person to be identified.

The Privacy Rule applies only to covered entities (CEs) who transmit medical information electronically. There are three categories of CEs: (1) health-care providers, such as doctors, clinics, psychologists, dentists, chiropractors, nursing homes, and pharmacies; (2) health plans, including health maintenance organizations (HMOs), health insurance companies, and government programs that pay for health care, such as Medicare, Medicaid, and the military and veterans' health-care programs; and (3) clearinghouses that electronically transmit medical information, such as billing, claims, enrollment, or eligibility verification.

Use and Disclosure of Protected Health Information

HIPAA has very prescriptive language for the use and disclosure of PHI. A CE may use or disclose PHI without patient authorization for purposes of treatment, payment, or its health-care operations. This includes disclosures to its agents or to another CE, such as another health-care provider. Agents are business associates who perform a function for the CE, such as dictation, legal services, billing, and accounting, and are not subject to the Privacy Rule. When a CE discloses PHI to a business associate, there must be an agreement that the PHI will be handled according to federal and state privacy laws. Additionally, a CE may disclose PHI as required by law, such as reporting child abuse to state child welfare agencies. Treatment covers a wide array of patient-related activities, including providing health care, coordinating services, referring patients, and consulting among providers. Communication between CEs may take place using any method, including oral, written, electronic mail, or facsimile, as long as "reasonable and appropriate safeguards" are used to protect the information. Payment includes activities relating to financial aspects of health care. PHI can be used for billing and claim processing to obtain reimbursement and for utilization review. Health-care operations include a wide range of administrative and management activities in which CEs engage. These include case management and patient care, risk management, legal services, credentialing, quality assessments and outcomes development, guidelines and protocol development, and training students. *Sensitive PHI* includes information about certain conditions or their associated treatment, such as human immunodeficiency virus (HIV) status, substance abuse, or mental health conditions. *Use of PHI* refers to internal use by the CE; *disclosure* refers to sharing of PHI for external purposes. Sensitive PHI may not be disclosed without a patient's written authorization, except in certain circumstances, such as to a consultant who needs this information to assist in the patient's health care.

Consent Versus Authorization

Consent must be obtained from the patient at the first visit, before any services are provided. Patients must sign a consent form stating that they have been notified of the practice's privacy policy, which explains that the practice may use and disclose PHI for treatment, payment, and health-care operations. Consent only needs to be obtained once and is valid until revoked by the patient in writing. In an emergency situation, treatment may be rendered without consent, but consent should be obtained as soon as possible afterward.

For all other uses and disclosures, unless required by law, specific authorization must be obtained from the patient detailing what PHI may be disclosed, to whom it may be disclosed, and an expiration date. An authorization is needed to release PHI to life insurance companies and patients' legal counsel. A CE may not give or sell patients' names for commercial or marketing purposes. For example, a CE may not give or sell names of allergy sufferers to pharmaceutical companies that market allergy products.

Individual Rights

Patients have the right to review and obtain a copy of their medical records, except in certain circumstances. Exceptions to the rule are psychotherapy notes, information compiled for lawsuits, and information that, in the opinion of the health-care provider, may cause harm to the individual or another. A reasonable, cost-based fee may be charged to cover copying and postage expenses. If a medical summary of the record is requested, the fee should be agreed on beforehand.

Patients also have the right to request an amendment or correction if they feel the record is inaccurate or incomplete and may submit a written supplement to be included in their record. If the health-care provider declines the request, the provider must do so in writing and allow the patient to submit a statement of disagreement for inclusion in the record. However, the health-care provider must allow the patient to submit a correction to be placed in the medical record. The CE may also include its own rebuttal. A health-care provider may require a patient to come into the office during normal business hours to access and inspect the record. The provider may also arrange to have someone present who can answer any patient questions or concerns.

Patients have a right to an accounting of certain PHI disclosures by a CE. The CE must be able to report who the recipient was, when the disclosure was made, and for what purpose the disclosure was made. The maximal accounting disclosure period is the 6 years preceding the request. Exceptions to this rule include disclosures for treatment, payment, or health-care operations; to the individual or their representative; pursuant to an authorization; and for national security purposes.

CEs must take reasonable steps to ensure the confidentiality of communications with the patient. The record should demonstrate how the patient would prefer to be contacted regarding PHI, including test results, appointment reminders, or discussions regarding their medical care. The patient may request to be contacted at an alternative address or phone number.

A health-care provider may share relevant information with family, friends, or caretakers involved in a patient's health care as long as the patient does not object and the provider feels it is in the patient's best interest. Information may not be disclosed to a person not involved in the patient's health care, if disclosure is judged to be inappropriate by the provider, or if the patient requests nondisclosure. When disclosing PHI, only the minimal information needed by that particular person should be disclosed; for example, a caregiver needs to know which medications are to be taken, what activity and dietary instructions are prescribed, and what changes in condition to report. Details about the patient's diagnosis and prognosis may not be necessary and should not be disclosed unless requested by the patient or the patient's personal representative. A family member or friend who is not involved in the patient's care may be told of the patient's condition—stable, guarded, critical—but additional information may not be disclosed unless the health-care provider judges it to be in the patient's best interest and as long as the patient has not restricted the release of information to that person.

Minors

The Privacy Rule defers to state or other applicable laws that address the ability of a parent or guardian to obtain health information about a minor child. In most cases, the parent represents the child and has the authority to make health-care decisions about the child; however, the Privacy Rule specifies three circumstances when certain minors may obtain specified health care without parental consent:

• When state or other law does not require the consent of a parent before a minor can obtain a particular health-care service, and when the minor consents to the health-care service. Example: A state law provides an adolescent the right to obtain mental health treatment without the consent of the parent, and the adolescent agrees to such treatment without the parent's consent.
• When a court determines, or other law authorizes, someone other than the parent to make treatment decisions for a minor. Example: A court may grant authority to an adult other than the parent to make health-care decisions for the minor, such as a stepparent or guardian.
• When a parent agrees to a confidential relationship between the minor and the physician. Example: A physician asks the parent of a 16-year-old if the physician can talk with the child confidentially about a medical condition, and the parent agrees.

Even in these circumstances, the Privacy Rule defers to state or other laws that require, permit, or prohibit the CE to disclose to a parent, or provide the parent access to, a minor child's PHI. When the laws are unclear, a licensed health-care professional may exercise professional judgment on whether to provide or deny parental access.

When a health-care provider reasonably believes that disclosure of PHI to the personal representative who is authorized to make health-care decisions for an individual may not be in the patient's best interest, the provider may choose not to disclose, especially in situations in which abuse, neglect, and endangerment are suspected. For example, if a physician reasonably believes that disclosing information about an incompetent elderly individual to the individual's personal representative would endanger the patient, the Privacy Rule permits the physician to decline to make such disclosures.

Notice of Privacy Practices

Covered entities are required to develop a privacy program detailing how their practice complies with the Privacy Rule. The notice must be provided to patients at or before their first encounter, or as soon as feasibly possible in an emergency situation. It must be posted in a clear and prominent location at the practice site and on its website, and a written copy should be furnished to patients at their request. Written acknowledgment of receipt of the Notice of Privacy Practices by the patient is desirable; however, a patient may refuse to sign it (often in the mistaken belief that signing it means the patient agrees with it), in which case the CE must document the reason for failure to obtain acknowledgment by the patient. Each practice should have a HIPAA Privacy Officer or a designated person who is knowledgeable in the standards and rules. A HIPAA attorney may be consulted in questionable matters when disclosure is a concern. Table 1-2 shows the elements that should be included in a privacy policy.

Privacy Violations and Penalties

CEs should have policies and procedures in place that describe sanctions for employees who commit violations, such as accessing a medical record for any purpose outside of treatment, payment, or health-care operations; discussing PHI in public; failing to log off or leaving a computer monitor on and unsecured; or copying or compiling PHI with the intent to sell or use it for personal or financial gain. Depending on the violation, disciplinary actions may range from a letter in the employee's file, to requiring additional training on the privacy rule, to termination. If an

employee does not report observed or suspected violations to a supervisor or HIPAA officer, that employee may be subject to disciplinary action for failure to report.

Although an individual may not sue anyone over a HIPAA violation, a CE may be liable for civil penalties at the state level. A CE's failure to follow the rules and standards of the HIPAA regulations can result in civil penalties of up to $100 per violation, with a cap of $25,000 per year. Criminal penalties for violations by individuals or CEs range from a $50,000 fine and up to 1 year of imprisonment for knowingly obtaining or disclosing PHI to a $250,000 fine and up to 10 years imprisonment if the offense is committed with intent to sell, transfer, or use PHI for commercial purposes, personal gain, or malicious harm.

Security Rule

Security standards were promulgated to protect electronic health information systems from improper access or alteration. The confidentiality, integrity, and availability of electronic PHI must be protected when it is stored, maintained, or transmitted. CEs are required to develop and implement administrative, physical, and technical safeguards to protect against reasonably anticipated threats of loss or disclosure by implementing appropriate policies and procedures. Periodic security awareness and training of workforce members is required. Administrative safeguards must be in place to ensure the following:

- Properly authorized personnel have access only to the PHI they need to perform their job.
- Prevention, detection, containment, and correction of security violations are undertaken, including sanctions against an employee who violates the privacy and security of PHI.
- A disaster recovery plan is outlined.
- A process is in place to develop contracts with business associates that ensure they will safeguard PHI appropriately.

Physical safeguards include measures that accomplish the following:

- Limit physical access to PHI systems while ensuring properly authorized access, such as keeping computers, printers, and fax machines out of patient and high-traffic areas and installing locking doors and alarm systems
- Provide secure access to workstations, including guidelines on use of home systems, laptops, cell phones, and other portable or handheld electronic devices
- Establish procedures for receipt and removal of hardware and electronic media containing PHI

Table 1-2 Elements of a Privacy Policy

The policy should outline the following:
1. Describe how PHI is used and disclosed.
2. State the covered entity's duty to protect PHI, to provide a notice of its privacy practices, and to abide by the terms in its notices.
3. Describe patients' rights to:
   - Inspect and copy their PHI
   - Request a restriction of their PHI by stating the specific restriction and to whom it applies
   - Request confidential communications from the covered entity by alternative means or at an alternative location
   - Request an amendment to their PHI
   - Receive an accounting of certain disclosures the covered entity has made
   - Obtain a paper copy of the Notice of Patient Privacy on their request
   - Complain to the covered entity or to the Secretary of Health and Human Services (HHS) if they believe their privacy rights have been violated
4. Provide a point of contact for further information and for submitting complaints to:
   - A practice's designated HIPAA officer
   - The secretary of HHS

Technical safeguards must be in place that protect and control access to PHI, such as the following:

- Verifying identity of a person or entity
- Allowing access only to persons or software programs that have access rights (e.g., using passwords, electronic signatures)
- Auditing records and examining activity in information systems that contain or use PHI
- Protecting PHI from improper modification or destruction
- Preventing unauthorized access to PHI being transmitted over an electronic communications network (e.g., the Internet)
- Installing and regularly updating antivirus, anti-spyware, and firewall software

Summary of the Act

A CE has the responsibility to develop and track a wide variety of privacy and security processes and establish policies and procedures to address all of the HIPAA standards. Employees must undergo periodic training in privacy and security rules. Risk analysis, monitoring, and testing of information systems' security are essential to ensure the confidentiality and integrity of data. Practices may be audited for HIPAA compliance with or without notice. New rules and policies are frequently written, and CEs must be aware of and comply with these. HHS and CMS websites should be monitored regularly for updates.

To reinforce the content in this chapter, please complete the worksheets that follow.

General and Medicolegal Principles

1. In addition to other health-care providers, list five different types or groups of people who could read medical records you create.

_____

_____

_____

_____

2. List at least 5 general principles of documentation that are based on CMS guidelines.

_____

_____

_____

_____

3. Describe how to make a correction in a medical record.

_____

_____

_____

_____

4. Beside each of the following, indicate whether the statement is acceptable (A) or unacceptable (U) according to generally accepted documentation guidelines.

_____ Use of either the 1995 or 1997 CMS guidelines

_____ Making a late entry in a chart or medical record

_____ Using correction fluid or tape to obliterate an entry in a record

_____ Making an entry in a record before seeing a patient

_____ Altering an entry in a medical record

_____ Stamping a record "signed but not read"

Medical Billing and Coding

1. Indicate whether the following statements are true (T) or false (F).

_____ CPT codes reflect the level of evaluation and management services provided.

_____ The three key elements of determining the level of service are history, review of systems, and physical examination.

_____ Time spent counseling the patient and the nature of the presenting problem are two factors that affect the level of service provided.

_____ ICD codes indicate the reason for patient services.

_____ ICD-9 codes are used to track mortality and morbidity statistics internationally.

_____ ICD-10 code sets have more than 155,000 codes, but do not have the capacity to accommodate new diagnoses and procedures.

_____ "V" codes are used for reasons other than illness or disease.

_____ The medical record must include documentation that supports the assessment.

_____ Assignment of appropriate CPT and ICD codes that support the level of E/M services provided is only dependent on adequate documentation of the history and physical examination.

_____ An ICD-9 code should be as broad and encompassing as possible.

_____ There is no code for "rule out."

_____ The complexity of medical decision making takes into account the number of treatment options.

2. ICD-9 codes are used to identify which of the following? (underline all that apply)

HPI	Diagnosis	Treatment
Physical exam findings	Treating facility	Symptoms
Surgical history	Complaints	Tests ordered
Reason for office visit	Level of service	Conditions

3. For each lay term given below, provide an alternative medical term.

flu	_____	tiredness	_____
rash	_____	stomach	_____
navel	_____	tennis elbow	_____
heartburn	_____	heel	_____
stroke	_____	heart attack	_____
kidney stone	_____	pink eye	_____
flat feet	_____	emphysema	_____
B$_{12}$ deficiency	_____	light intolerance	_____
sugar diabetes	_____	tubal pregnancy	_____
ear drum	_____	blood thinner	_____

Electronic Medical Records

1. List at least five functions that an EMR system should be able to perform.

_____

_____

_____

_____

_____

_____

2. Identify at least five perceived benefits of an EMR system.

_____

_____

_____

_____

_____

3. Identify at least five potential barriers to implementing an EMR system.

_____

_____

_____

_____

_____

4. List at least two criteria required to meet "meaningful" use standards.

_____

_____

_____

_____

_____

HIPAA

I. Indicate whether each statement about the Health Insurance Portability and Accountability Act is true (T) or false (F).

_____ Establishes standards for the electronic transfers of health data

_____ Provides health care for everyone

_____ Limits exclusion of preexisting medical conditions to 24 months

_____ Gives patients more access to their medical records

_____ Protects medical records from improper uses and disclosures

_____ Federal HIPAA regulations preempt state laws.

_____ The Privacy Rule only applies to covered entities that transmit medical information electronically.

_____ Protected Health Information is data that could be used to identify an individual.

_____ Covered entities include doctors, clinics, dentists, nursing homes, chiropractors, psychologists, pharmacies, and insurance companies.

_____ A covered entity may disclose PHI without patient authorization for purposes of treatment, payment, or its health-care operations.

_____ PHI cannot be transmitted between covered entities by e-mail.

_____ Patients are entitled to a list of everyone with whom their health-care provider has shared PHI.

_____ PHI may be disclosed to someone involved in the patient's health care without written authorization.

_____ The Privacy Rule allows certain minors access to specified health care, such as mental health counseling, without parental consent.

_____ A Notice of Privacy Practice explains how patients' PHI is used and disclosed.

_____ An employee cannot be terminated for violating the Privacy Rule.

_____ An individual may not sue their insurance company over a HIPAA violation.

_____ Criminal penalties for HIPAA violations can result in fines and imprisonment.

_____ The confidentiality, integrity, and availability of PHI only need to be protected when the PHI is transmitted, not when it is stored.

_____ Employees are required to attend periodic security awareness and training.

_____ The Security Rule requires covered entities to install and regularly update antivirus, anti-spyware, and firewall software.

_____ Physical and technical safeguards must be in place to prevent PHI from being transmitted over the Internet.

_____ A process to develop contracts with business associates that will ensure they will safeguard PHI is required by HIPAA.

_____ HIPAA may not audit a practice for compliance without notice.

2. From the list below, underline each that would be considered a covered entity according to HIPAA.

chiropractor	social worker	psychologist
nurse practitioner	medical assistant	nursing home
doctor	HMO	lawyer
office manager	PPO	VA hospital
Medicare	Medicaid	employer
hospital		

3. Identify at least two conditions that are considered *sensitive PHI*.

_____

_____

4. Patients have the right to review and obtain copies of their medical records except in certain circumstances. List two.

_____

_____

5. Indicate by yes (Y) or no (N) whether disclosure of PHI to the specific entity would require patient authorization.

_____ Specialist/consultant

_____ Patient's health plan

_____ Life insurance company

_____ Hospital accounting department

_____ Patient's employer

_____ Pharmaceutical companies

_____ Reporting a gunshot wound to police

_____ Reporting names of patients with a communicable disease to a county health department

_____ Reporting suspected child abuse to a child protection agency

_____ Medical billing and coding department

_____ Friends and family involved in a patient's health care

Abbreviations

These abbreviations were introduced in Chapter 1. Beside each, write the meaning as indicated by the context of this chapter.

AMA _____

AMI _____

ARRA _____

CE _____

CMS _____

CPR _____

CPT _____

DM _____

EHR _____

E/M _____

EMR _____

EPR _____

HHS _____

HIMSS _____

HIPAA _____

HITECH _____

HIV _____

HMO _____

ICD-9 _____

ICD-10 _____

PHI _____

URI _____

Chapter 2

The Comprehensive History and Physical Examination

OBJECTIVES

- Discuss the importance of a well-documented comprehensive history and physical examination.
- Describe how the comprehensive history and physical examination may be adapted for various medical disciplines and practice settings.
- Identify components of a comprehensive history and physical examination.
- Analyze sample comprehensive histories and physical examinations.

The comprehensive history and physical examination (complete H&P or H&P) is the vehicle used to document not only the patient's medical history but also the physical examination findings, diagnoses or medical problems, diagnostic studies to be performed, and initial plan of care implemented to address any problems identified. Although obtaining a thorough history and performing a detailed physical examination are critically important, the documentation of the H&P is equally important. This record is often used as the basis for the entire course of medical management for a patient. Failure to take an adequate history or to perform a detailed physical examination—or failure to recognize important findings—may lead to inadequate care of the patient. Failure to document the comprehensive H&P adequately could have the same result.

The comprehensive H&P is typically obtained when a provider sees a patient for the first time in a general medical setting, or when a patient is admitted to the hospital. One exception is when the patient presents with an emergent complaint and initiating treatment is a higher priority than obtaining a detailed history or performing a thorough physical examination. Almost all other types of documentation, including SOAP (*s*ubjective, *o*bjective, *a*ssessment, and *p*lan; discussed in Chapter 5) notes and admission H&Ps (as discussed in Chapter 7), are variations of the comprehensive H&P.

Multiple providers are likely to read this document and use it to guide their management of the patient; this is one reason it is so important that the documented H&P accurately reflects the patient's past and current health status and even documents anticipated problems. Providers in different medical disciplines usually tailor the H&P to their specialty. An H&P conducted and documented by a cardiologist, for example, may differ from an H&P completed by an orthopedist.

Components of a Comprehensive History and Physical Examination

The components of a comprehensive H&P are shown in Table 2-1. The discussion in this chapter is geared to adult patients. Information for pediatric patients is presented in Chapter 4. Specific information that should be documented in each section follows.

History

Identification

The content of the identification section will vary somewhat depending on where the patient presents. If in an office setting, this would include the patient's name, date of birth, race, age, and gender. In a hospital

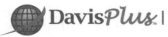 **DavisPlus** | Visit **http://davisplus.fadavis.com** for complete learning activities on actual EMR software at, Keyword: Sullivan

| **Table 2-1** | Components of a Comprehensive History and Physical Examination[1] |

HISTORY

Identification

Chief Complaint (CC)

History of the Present Illness (HPI) or History of the Chief Complaint (HCC)

- Location
- Quality
- Severity
- Duration
- Timing
- Context
- Modifying factors
- Associated signs and symptoms

Past Medical History (PMH)

- Current and past medical problems unrelated to the CC
- Surgeries and other hospitalizations
- Current medications, including prescription and over the counter
- Drug allergies, including how manifested
- Health maintenance and immunizations

Family History

- Age and status of blood relatives
- Medical problems of blood relatives

Psychosocial or Social History

- Patient profile
- Lifestyle risk factors
- Employment
- Education
- Religion, beliefs
- Cultural history
- Support system
- Stressors

Review of Systems (ROS)

- General
- Eyes
- Ears, nose, and throat/mouth
- Cardiovascular
- Respiratory
- Gastrointestinal
- Genitourinary
- Musculoskeletal

- Neurological
- Psychiatric
- Endocrine
- Hematologic/lymphatic
- Allergic/immunological

PHYSICAL EXAMINATION

General

Vital signs

Skin

Head, eyes, ears, nose, throat (HEENT)

Neck

Respiratory

Cardiovascular

Breast

Abdomen

Male genitalia or gynecological (breast examination sometimes documented here)

Rectal

Musculoskeletal

Neurological

- Mental status
- Cranial nerves
- Motor
- Cerebellum
- Sensory
- Reflexes

LABORATORY DATA

- Results of laboratory tests, radiographs, etc.

PROBLEM LIST, ASSESSMENTS, AND DIFFERENTIAL DIAGNOSES

- Most severe to least severe initially
- Other problems added chronologically
- Indicate if active or inactive

TREATMENT PLAN

- Additional laboratory and diagnostic tests
- Medical treatment
- Consults
- Disposition, such as admit, follow as outpatient, etc.

[1] History and Physical Examination headings used by CMS 1997 *Guidelines of Documentation for Evaluation and Management.*

setting, the information would be included as well as the medical record number, attending or referring physician, and consulting physicians. You should document the patient's reliability, that is, the patient's ability to provide historical information accurately. If an interpreter is used to conduct the H&P, this should be documented as well.

Chief Complaint

Document the current problem for which the patient is seeking care. This is best stated in the patient's own words, identified by quotation marks. At times, a patient may present without a specific complaint, such as presenting to establish care or for an annual physical.

Try to avoid vague terms, such as *checkup*, and do not document "no problems" in the chief complaint.

History of the Present Illness or History of the Chief Complaint

The history of the present illness (HPI) or history of the chief complaint (HCC) is a chronological description of the development of the patient's present illness from the first sign or symptom of the presenting problems. The Centers for Medicare and Medicaid Services (CMS) published the 1995 and 1997 *Documentation Guidelines for Evaluation and Management of Services*, identifying these elements of the HPI: location, quality, severity, duration, timing, context, modifying factors, and associated signs and symptoms. Several mnemonics may be used to help you remember the attributes of the HPI that should be elicited; these are shown in Table 2-2. A word of caution: these mnemonics are helpful when the patient presents with a complaint of pain, but may not be as helpful when a patient presents with a vague complaint like fatigue or when the patient presents for monitoring of a chronic condition. The approach to obtaining and documenting the HPI will differ in these situations.

Table 2-2	History of Present Illness Mnemonics
Mnemonic	**Explanation**
PQRST	P—palliative or provocative factors Q—quality of pain R—region affected S—severity of pain T—timing
LOCATES	L—location O—onset C—character A—associated signs and symptoms T—timing E—exacerbating/relieving factors S—severity
OLD CHARTS	O—onset L—location D—duration CH—character A—alleviating/aggravating R—radiation T—temporal pattern S—symptoms associated
COLDERAS	C—character O—onset L—location D—duration E—exacerbating factors R—relieving factors A—associated signs and symptoms S—severity
LIQORAAA	L—location I—intensity Q—quality O—onset R—radiation A—associated signs and symptoms A—alleviating factors A—aggravating factors
QFLORIDAA	Q—quality F—frequency L—location O—onset R—radiation I—intensity D—duration A—alleviating/aggravating A—associated signs and symptoms

Past Medical History

The past medical history (PMH) section is used to document the patient's past and current health. Document when each condition was diagnosed and indicate its present status, such as stable, uncontrolled, or resolved. Information in the PMH may be subdivided into past medical history, past surgical history or other hospitalizations, medications, drug allergies, and health maintenance and immunizations. Using subheadings within the PMH, as shown in Table 2-3, makes it easier to locate information and identify the change from one topic to another.

If the patient has multiple medical problems, it may be helpful to document them as an enumerated list rather than in paragraph format. If the patient has had any surgery or hospitalizations for major trauma or other reasons, the type of operation, date of the surgery, and name of the doctor who performed the surgery should be included.

A medication list is documented as part of the PMH. This includes both prescription and over-the-counter medications, such as herbal supplements, vitamins, minerals, and food supplements. The name of the drug, the dose, how frequently it is taken, and ideally, why the patient takes the medication should be included. This list of medications should be reviewed with the patient at every visit to ensure accuracy.

It is extremely important to document any drug allergies the patient has. Food allergies may also be documented in this section. You should document the specific reaction the patient experiences when the food or drug is ingested. In most settings, there will be a specific way to indicate a drug allergy, such as a special sticker affixed to the front of the patient's chart, so that it is not overlooked.

It is critically important to inquire specifically about and document an allergy to latex. A patient with a latex allergy will need special equipment. Environmental allergies, such as an allergy to cats that results in allergic rhinitis, may also be documented in the PMH. If the patient is treated regularly for allergy-related conditions, these conditions may be documented under the heading of Medical Conditions rather than Allergies.

The health maintenance and immunization section of the PMH will vary according to the patient's age and gender. Chapters 3 and 4 discuss documentation

Table 2-3	Subheadings Used for Past Medical History

Past Medical History
Medical
Surgical/hospitalizations
Medications
Allergies
Health maintenance

of health maintenance activities and immunizations in the adult and pediatric patient, respectively.

Family History

The medical history of first-degree relatives is typically documented. This includes parents, grandparents, and siblings. Remember that a spouse's medical history is not considered part of the patient's family history; although it may be applicable in situations in which a couple presents because of infertility or genetic counseling. Document the age and status (living, deceased, health status) of the first-degree relatives. If deceased, include the age at time of death and cause of death. If the relatives are still living, document their current age and medical conditions, paying particular attention to those conditions that have a familial tendency, such as cardiovascular disease, diabetes, and certain cancers, osteoporosis, and sleep apnea. Also determine whether any first-degree relatives have or had the condition with which the patient is presenting. In addition to medical conditions, inquire about any substance abuse, addictions, depression, or other mental health conditions of family members.

Psychosocial History

One of the main goals of documenting the psychosocial history of the patient is to identify factors outside of past or current medical conditions that may influence the patient's overall health or behaviors that create risk factors for specific conditions. You will often see the heading Social History (SH) instead of Psychosocial. We prefer the latter when documenting the comprehensive history because it serves as a reminder to consider the *whole patient* and the psychological factors that can affect the patient's health rather than just social health habits. Age-specific psychosocial history will also be discussed in other chapters.

Information about the patient's sexual orientation, marital status, and children is included in the patient's profile. Documentation of the patient's past and current employment may help identify potential occupational hazards. Include any military service and where stationed (stateside or overseas) and any possible exposures. If the patient has lived or traveled abroad, document locations and potential exposures, if any. It is important to document the patient's educational level and ability to read and write. If the patient speaks more than one language, you should document which language the patient prefers. If an interpreter is required, this should also be documented. Some state laws and federal initiatives regulate the use of interpreters. In August 2000, the Office for Civil Rights for the Department of Health and Human Services (HHS) issued an extensive Policy Guidance to providers who receive federal funds on how to comply with Title VI of the Civil Rights Act of 1964, which has been widely interpreted as ensuring equal access to health care for the person with limited English proficiency. Especially in the hospital setting, documenting that an interpreter assisted the provider in conducting the H&P helps to meet these legal requirements. To comply with federal requirements, a professional interpreter should be used rather than family members, friends, or even bilingual staff members.

Religion and religious and cultural beliefs may have an impact on a patient's overall health. It can be difficult to determine the difference between a religious belief and a cultural belief, although typically it is not necessary to do so. Specific documentation of the religious and cultural history includes beliefs related to health and illness, family, symbols, nutrition, special events, spirituality, and taboos. Table 2-4 shows questions that can be asked as part of the religious and cultural history.

Another important aspect of the psychosocial history is documentation of the presence or absence of personal habits that would constitute risk factors for developing certain medical conditions or complications from known conditions. These risk factors include tobacco, alcohol, and drug use. If these risk factors are present, document quantity of use and how long the use has occurred. Smoking history should include number of packs per day and the number of years the patient has smoked. If the patient formerly smoked or used smokeless tobacco, the details of the tobacco use should still be documented, with the addition of how long it has been since the patient quit. Avoid ambiguous terms such as *social drinker* that do not assist you or other readers in determining whether there is a risk factor associated with substance use. Typically, the use of illegal substances is documented as drug use, but also determine whether the patient is taking substances prescribed for someone else or misusing prescription medication. If a risk factor is identified, be sure to include it in the problem list and assessment and plan.

Nutritional information is also documented in terms of type of diet the patient follows, caffeine intake, and food allergies or avoidances. If there are questions or concerns about a patient's diet, it may be helpful to record a "typical day" or "last 24 hours" of food intake. Sedentary lifestyle is a risk factor for certain diseases, so document whether the patient exercises. If the patient exercises, include the type, frequency, and duration of exercise.

One basic consideration of a patient's ability to access health care is whether the patient has health care insurance or some other form of payment, such as Social Security or workers' compensation. Although financial records should generally be kept separate from the medical records, you should document whether the

Table 2-4 Questions to Ask for Cultural and Religious History

Communication

- Is a translator needed?
- Primary oral language
- Primary written language

Beliefs Affecting Health and Illness

- What do you think caused your illness or condition?
- How does it affect your life?
- Have you seen anyone else about this problem?
- If yes, who?
- Have you used folk or home remedies for your problem?
- If yes, what?
- Are you willing to take prescription medications?
- Are you willing to take alternative therapies, such as herbal medicine?

Family

- Definition of family
- Roles within family
- Who has authority for decision making related to your health care?

Symbols

- Special clothing
- Ritualistic and religious articles

Nutrition

- Specific food rituals
- Specific food avoidances
- Major foods
- Preparation practices

Special Events

- Prenatal care
- Death and burial rituals
- Beliefs of afterlife
- Willing to accept blood transfusions?
- Willing to accept organ transplantation?
- Organ, blood, or tissue donor?

Spirituality

- Dominant religion
- Active participant?
- Prayer and meditation
- Special activities
- Relationship between spiritual beliefs and health practices

Taboos

- Describe any taboos that would affect health care

patient is insured or uninsured. If uninsured, information about income or ability to self-pay becomes essential psychosocial information. The provision or lack of insurance will guide many health care choices, especially related to prescribing medications. Using generic instead of brand-name medications will result in cost savings for the patient and is often medically neutral, meaning the patient should get the same benefit from generic as from brand-name medications.

Review of Systems

The review of systems (ROS) is an inventory of specific body systems designed to document any symptoms the patient may be experiencing or has experienced. Typically, both positive symptoms (those the patient has experienced) and negative symptoms (those the patient denies having experienced) are documented. A positive response from a patient about any symptom should prompt the provider to explore the same factors as HPI (location, quality, severity, duration, timing, context, modifying factors, and associated signs and symptoms). Rather than asking whether the patient has ever experienced any of the symptoms listed, it is appropriate to limit the review to a specific time frame. That time frame might change depending on the patient's chief complaint and HPI; if you are seeing a patient for the first time, it is usually sufficient to ask about the past year.

We identify 14 systems, consistent with the 1995 and 1997 CMS guidelines, and provide specific symptoms that should be explored in each system. How many symptoms are explored within each system is up to the discretion of the provider and as indicated by the patient's presenting complaint.

- Constitutional: these symptoms do not fit specifically with one system but often affect the general well-being or overall status of a patient. Specific symptoms include weight loss, weight gain, fatigue, weakness, fever, chills, and night sweats.
- Eyes: change in vision, date of last visual examination, glasses or contact lenses, history of eye surgery, eye pain, photophobia, diplopia, spots or floaters, discharge, excessive tearing, itching, cataracts, or glaucoma.
- Ears, nose, and mouth/throat (ENT):
  - Ears: change in or loss of hearing, date of last auditory evaluation, hearing aids, history of ear surgery, ear pain, tinnitus, drainage from the ear, history of ear infections.
  - Nose: changes in or loss of sense of smell, epistaxis, obstruction, polyps, rhinorrhea, itching, sneezing, sinus problems.
  - Mouth/throat: date of last dental examination, ulcerations or other lesions of tongue or mucosa, bleeding gums, gingivitis, dentures or any dental appliances.
- Cardiovascular (CV): chest pain, orthopnea, murmurs, palpitations, arrhythmias, dyspnea on

exertion, paroxysmal nocturnal dyspnea, peripheral edema, claudication, date of last electrocardiogram or other cardiovascular studies
• Respiratory: dyspnea, cough, amount and color of sputum, hemoptysis, history of pneumonia, date of last chest radiograph, date and result of last tuberculosis testing.
• Gastrointestinal (GI): abdominal pain; dysphagia; heartburn; nausea; vomiting; usual bowel habits and any change in bowel habits; use of aids such as fiber, laxatives, or stool softeners; melena; hematochezia; hematemesis; hemorrhoids; jaundice.
• Genitourinary (GU): frequency, urgency, dysuria, hematuria, polyuria, incontinence, sexual orientation, number of partners, history of sexually transmitted infections, infertility.
  • Males: hesitancy, change in urine stream, nocturia, penile discharge, erectile dysfunction, date of last testicular examination, date of last prostate examination, date and result of last prostate-specific antigen (PSA) test.
  • Females: GU symptoms as above and gynecologic symptoms; age at menarche; gravida, para, abortions; frequency, duration, and flow of menstrual periods; date of last menstrual period; dysmenorrhea; type of contraception used; ability to achieve orgasm; dyspareunia; vaginal dryness, menopause; breast lesions, date of last breast examination; breast self-examination; date and result of last Papanicolaou smear, date of last pelvic examination.
• Musculoskeletal (MSK): arthralgias, arthritis, gout, joint swelling, trauma, limitations in range of motion, back pain. (Note that numbness, tingling, and weakness are typically not included in musculoskeletal but in neurological system.)
• Integumentary: rashes, pruritus, bruising, dryness, skin cancer or other lesions.
• Neurological: syncope, seizures, numbness, tingling, weakness, gait disturbances, coordination problems, altered sensation, alteration in memory, difficulty concentrating, headaches, head trauma, or brain injury. (Headache, head trauma, or brain injury may also be listed under head, as part of Head, Eyes, Ears, Nose, Mouth/Throat, or HEENT.)
• Psychiatric: emotional disturbances, sleep disturbances, substance abuse disorders, hallucinations, illusions, delusions, affective or personality disorders, nervousness or irritability, suicidal ideation or past suicide attempts.
• Endocrine: polyuria, polydipsia, polyphagia, temperature intolerance, hormone therapy, changes in hair or skin texture.

• Hematologic/lymphatic: easy bruising, bleeding tendency, anemia, blood transfusions, thromboembolic disorders, lymphadenopathy.
• Allergic/immunologic: allergic rhinitis, asthma, atopy, food allergies, immunotherapy, frequent or chronic infections, HIV status; if HIV positive, date and result of last CD4 count.

Physical Examination

The rationale for physical examination rests on a basic assumption that there is such a thing as normality of bodily structure and function corresponding to a state of health and that departures from this norm consistently result from or correlate with specific abnormal states or disease. It is helpful to think about a "range of normal" when it comes to physical examination findings, rather than a single "normal" for every part of the examination. The physical examination may confirm or refute a diagnosis suspected from the history, and by adding this information to the database, you will be able to construct a more accurate problem list. Like the history, the physical examination is structured to record both positive and negative findings in detail. It is sometimes easier to document the absence of a finding, such as "no cyanosis," rather than try to describe a finding.

Generally, the examination will proceed in a head-to-toe fashion. In some instances, it may be necessary to deviate from this order, such as performing an invasive component at the end of the examination or examining an area of pain last. Regardless of the order in which the examination is performed, documentation of the physical examination should follow the order that follows and in Table 2-5. We recommend that you consult textbooks for instruction on how to perform the physical examination and a discussion on the importance of any findings; here we emphasize the documentation of a comprehensive examination.

Table 2-5 Order in Which to Document Physical Examination

General assessment

Vital signs: temperature, pulse, respiration, blood pressure, height, weight, body mass index (BMI)
Skin
HEENT
Neck
Cardiovascular
Respiratory
Abdomen
Genitourinary or gynecological
Musculoskeletal
Neurological

- General: age, race, gender, general appearance. Documentation of general appearance could include alertness, orientation, mood, affect, gait, how a patient sits on the examination table or chair, grooming, and the patient's reliability to provide an adequate history. Document whether the patient is in any distress or whether the patient appears markedly older or younger than the stated age.
- Vital signs: temperature, blood pressure, pulse, respiratory rate, height, weight, and body mass index (BMI)
- Skin: presence and description of any lesions, scars, tattoos, moles, texture, turgor, temperature; hair texture, distribution pattern; nail texture, nail base angle, ridging, pitting.
- HEENT:
  - Head (including face): size and contour of head, symmetry of facial features, characteristic facies, tenderness or bruits of temporal arteries.
  - Eyes: conjunctivae; sclera; lids; pupil size, shape, and reactivity; extraocular movement (EOM); nystagmus; visual acuity. Ophthalmoscopic findings of cornea, lens, retina, red reflex, optic disc color and size, cupping, spontaneous venous pulsations, hemorrhages, exudates, nicking, arteriovenous crossings.
  - Ears: integrity, color, landmarks, and mobility of the tympanic membranes; tenderness, discharge, external canal, tenderness of auricles, nodules.
  - Nose: symmetry, alignment of septum, nasal patency, appearance of turbinates, presence of discharge, polyps, palpation of frontal and maxillary sinuses.
  - Mouth/throat: lips, teeth, gums, tongue, buccal mucosa, tonsillar size, exudate, erythema.
- Neck: range of motion, cervical and clavicular lymph nodes, thyroid examination, position and mobility of the trachea.
- Respiratory: effort of breathing, breath sounds, adventitious sounds, chest wall expansion, symmetry of breathing, diaphragmatic excursion.
- Cardiovascular: heart sounds, murmurs or extra sounds, rhythm, point of maximal impulse, peripheral edema, central and peripheral pulses, varicosities, venous hums, bruits.
- Breast: symmetry, inspection for dimpling of skin, nipple discharge, palpation for tenderness, cyst or masses, axillary nodes, gynecomastia in males.
- Abdomen: shape (flat, scaphoid, distended, obese), bowel sounds, masses, organomegaly, tenderness, inguinal nodes.
- Male genitalia or gynecological (breast examination sometimes documented here).
- Male genitalia: hair distribution, nits, testes, scrotum, penis, circumcised or uncircumcised, varicocele, masses, tenderness.
- Gynecological: External—inspection of the perineum for lesions, nits, hair distribution, areas of swelling or tenderness, labia and labial folds, Skene's and Bartholin's glands, vaginal introitus; noting any discharge or cystocele if present. Internal—inspect vaginal walls and cervix for color, discharge, lesions, bleeding, atrophy; inspect cervical os for size and shape; bimanual examination for size, shape, consistency and mobility of the cervix; cervical motion tenderness, uterine or ovarian enlargement, masses, tenderness, adnexal masses or tenderness.
- Rectal: hemorrhoids, fissures, sphincter tone, masses, rectocele; if stool is present, color and consistency of stool, test stool for occult blood; prostate examination for males, noting size, uniformity, nodules, tenderness.
- Musculoskeletal: symmetry of upper and lower extremities, range of motion of joints, joint swelling, redness or tenderness, amputations; inspection and palpation of spine for kyphosis, lordosis, scoliosis, musculature, range of motion, muscles for spasm, or tenderness.
- Neurological
  - Mental status: level of alertness, orientation to person, time, place, and circumstances; psychiatric mental status or mini–mental state examinations if indicated.
  - Cranial nerves: see Table 2-6 for details of the 12 cranial nerves and their functions.
  - Motor: strength testing of upper and lower extremity muscle groups proximally and distally graded on a scale of 0 to 5 as shown in Table 2-7.
  - Cerebellum: Romberg test, heel to shin, finger to nose, heel-and-toe walking, rapid alternating movements.
  - Sensory: sharp/dull discrimination, temperature, stereognosis, graphesthesia, vibration, proprioception.
  - Reflexes: brachioradialis, biceps, triceps, quadriceps (knee), and ankle graded on a scale of 0 to 4+ as shown in Table 2-8.

Laboratory and Diagnostic Studies

Following documentation of the history and physical examination, document the results of any studies such as laboratory tests, radiographs, or other imaging

Table 2-6	Cranial Nerves and Their Function	
Number	**Name**	**Major Function**
I	Olfactory	Smell
II	Optic	Visual acuity, visual fields, fundi; afferent limb of pupillary response
III, IV, VI	Oculomotor, trochlear, abducens	Efferent limb of pupillary response, eye movements
V	Trigeminal	Afferent corneal reflex, facial sensation, masseter and temporalis muscle testing by biting down
VII	Facial	Raise eyebrows, close eyes tight, show teeth, smile or whistle, efferent corneal reflex
VIII	Acoustic	Hearing
IX, X	Glossopharyngeal and vagus	Palate moves in midline, gag reflex, speech
XI	Spinal accessory	Shoulder shrug, push head against resistance
XII	Hypoglossal	Stick out tongue

Table 2-7	Muscle Strength Grading
Grade	**Meaning**
0	No motion or muscular contraction detected
1	Barely detectable motion
2	Active motion with gravity eliminated
3	Active motion against gravity
4	Active motion against some resistance
5	Active motion against full resistance

Table 2-8	Grading Reflexes
Grade	**Meaning**
0	Absent
1+	Decreased or less than normal
2+	Normal or average
3+	Brisker than usual
4+	Hyperactive with clonus

studies. All results should be specifically recorded. For instance, rather than documenting, "the complete blood count (CBC) is normal," document the value for each part of the CBC. This is done for several reasons. First, it presents the actual values and allows readers of the H&P to formulate their own conclusions regarding the meaning of the values. Second, it documents the baseline values that the patient has as a reference point. Third, it saves time for other readers to have the values listed rather than having to look them up.

Problem List, Assessment, and Differential Diagnosis

Once all the elements of the history and physical examination and results of diagnostic studies are documented, the clinician evaluates all the information to identify the patient's problems. A numbered list is often used and includes the date of onset and whether active or inactive. The most severe problems are listed first. After the initial list is generated, new problems are listed chronologically.

An assessment of each current problem is made. This entails a brief evaluation of the problem with differential diagnosis. This is a very important component of the comprehensive H&P because it demonstrates the clinician's judgment and documents the medical decision making that took place regarding each problem.

Plan of Care

Document any additional studies or workup needed, referrals or consultations needed, pharmacological management, nonpharmacological or other management, patient education, and disposition, such as "return to clinic" or "admit to the hospital."

Sample Comprehensive History and Physical Examination

A sample comprehensive history and physical examination for Mr. William Jensen is shown in Figure 2-1. Mr. Jensen is a new patient to the practice of Dr. Vernon Scott, and we will follow his medical course through the documentation of his encounters with a surgeon, his admission to the hospital, surgery, hospital course, and discharge. In addition to documentation related to Mr. Jensen, you will have the opportunity to evaluate other documentation.

To reinforce the content of this chapter, please complete the worksheets that follow.

Comprehensive History and Patient Examination

PATIENT NAME: William R. Jensen AGE: 67

SEX: Male DOB: March 30, 19XX

CHIEF COMPLAINT: "I've been feeling tired and I have lost some weight."

HISTORY OF PRESENT ILLNESS: This is a 67-year-old Caucasian male who is a new patient to this practice, having recently moved to the area. Mr. Jensen complains of "feeling tired." He states this has been going on for several months. He first noticed this when he and his wife went on a short hike that he had previously completed without difficulty. Initially, he thought he had a mild "flu-like illness" that would account for his fatigue. The fatigue is worsened with exertional activity. Other than rest, he has not identified any alleviating factors. Mr. Jensen states that he has lost approximately 10 pounds in the past 2 months without any change in his diet or activity level. His appetite is good, and he has not intentionally decreased his food intake or avoided any type of food. Other than these two complaints, he feels well.

PAST MEDICAL HISTORY:
    Medical:
        1. Hypertension: diagnosed at age 53
        2. Dyslipidemia: diagnosed at age 58

    Surgical:
        1. Repair of a torn rotator cuff, right shoulder (Dr. Rodriquez, Grand Rapids, MI), age 45.
        2. Left inguinal herniorrhaphy (Dr. Simmons, Grand Rapids, MI) at age 38.

    Medications:
        1. Lotensin HCT 20/12.5 once daily in the morning
        2. Mevacor 20 mg once daily in the afternoon
        3. Multivitamin once daily (One A Day for men)
        4. Fish oil supplement twice daily, morning and evening
           Over-the-counter medications include occasional acetaminophen for mild headache or pain.

    Allergies: Mr. Jensen states an allergy to PENICILLIN DRUGS that causes him to break out in a rash.

    Health Maintenance: Last complete physical 2 years ago. He had a screening colonoscopy at age 52 but has not had one since. He believes his PSA level was checked at the physical 2 years ago but does not recall the result. He has not had any routine blood work since his physical 2 years ago. That physical was done by Dr. Susan Maxwell in Michigan, where he previously resided.

    Immunizations: Mr. Jensen did get a flu vaccine September 20XX, and his last tetanus immunization was in 20XX. He has never had the pneumonia vaccine.

FAMILY HISTORY: Father is deceased, age 74, complications of COPD and alcoholism. Mother deceased, age 70, breast cancer. One sibling, age 71, who also has hypertension. One sibling, deceased, age 20, secondary to gunshot wound sustained in combat. Three children, alive and well, no significant medical history. Negative family history of diabetes, myocardial infarction. Positive family history of cancer (breast), hypertension/CAD, and COPD.

PSYCHOSOCIAL HISTORY: Mr. Jensen is married and lives in a single-story home with his wife. They have three adult children who all live nearby. Mr. Jensen is sexually active with his wife as his only partner. All sexual encounters have been heterosexual. Mr. Jensen smokes a pipe about 3 times a week and has done so for approximately 26 years. He does not use any smokeless tobacco, drink alcohol, or use any recreational drugs. He is still active and walks approximately 2 miles 4 of 7 days per week. He also bicycles and hikes occasionally. Current symptoms have affected his exercise tolerance. He does not follow a prescribed diet consistently. He limits salt intake and avoids fried foods. He eats fish twice a week, but does not eat many fresh fruits or vegetables. He estimates three or fewer servings of fruits and vegetables daily. He does not have much fiber intake. His caffeine intake includes 2-3 cups of coffee daily and 1-2 soft drinks daily. He does not have any food intolerances or food allergies. Mr. Jensen's primary language is English. He completed an undergraduate degree and trade school. He is a retired electrician. Mr. Jensen occasionally attends a Methodist church. He states prayer is important to him, and he believes that God can heal people because of prayer. He likes to include his wife in decision-making about his health care, as she is a retired nurse and has medical power of attorney for him. Mr. Jensen has a living will. He is willing to accept blood transfusions and would accept organ transplantation if needed. He is an organ donor. In addition to Medicare, he has a supplemental insurance plan that covers hospitalization and some outpatient treatment.

REVIEW OF SYSTEMS:
    Constitutional: Easily fatigued, feels weak. Denies any near-syncope or lightheadedness. He denies any fever or chills. No sleep disturbances.

    Eyes: He has worn glasses since 1985. Denies loss of vision, double vision, or history of cataracts.

(Continued)

ENT: No hearing loss, no prior ear surgery, no recent infections. Denies nasal drainage. Denies chronic sinus infections or epistaxis. Denies chronic or recurrent sore throat. No dentures or dental appliances. Last dental visit was 3 months ago.

Cardiovascular: Specifically denies chest pain, angina, and pleuritic pain. Denies any heart palpitations or irregularities in rhythm. No history of heart murmur. Denies peripheral edema and claudication. Last ECG was 2 years ago at his physical.

Respiratory: He denies SOB, DOE, or hemoptysis. Last chest x-ray was 2 years ago. He does not recall ever having testing for TB.

Gastrointestinal: He has experienced a 10-pound unintentional weight loss over the past 2 months. He denies any change in appetite, any difficulty swallowing or chewing. Some "indigestion" self-treated with liquid antacid. Rarely occurs more than twice per week, and has always been relieved with antacid. His bowel movements are solid, and he has not noticed any frank blood. He states that in the past month, his stool is sometimes "tarry." No constipation or diarrhea. No change in bowel habits. No hemorrhoids.

Genitourinary: Denies any penile discharge or erectile dysfunction. No nocturia, dribbling, incontinence, or loss of force of stream.

Musculoskeletal: Denies any joint swelling or loss of range of motion. No history of arthritis or any joint pain.

Integumentary: Denies rashes or moles. No skin lesions he is concerned about. He sees a dermatologist once a year for full skin examination.

Neurologic: Denies recurrent headaches. No syncope or seizures. Denies any problems with balance or coordination.

Psychiatric: Denies any depression or mood swings. Denies any history of mental illness, drug, or alcohol abuse.

Endocrine: Denies heat or cold intolerance, excessive thirst or urination, or tremors.

Hematologic/Lymphatic: Denies easy bruising or bleeding from gums. Denies any swollen glands. No history of anemia. He has never had a blood transfusion.

Allergic/Immunologic: No asthma or atopy. Denies frequent or recurrent infections. Has never had HIV testing.

PHYSICAL EXAMINATION:
General: Mr. Jensen is a well-developed, well-nourished Caucasian male who is alert and cooperative. He is a good historian and answers questions appropriately.

Vital Signs: BP 142/80; P 86 and regular, R 16 and regular; Temp 97.8 orally. His current weight is 174 pounds. Height is 5'10". BMI is 25.

Skin: Intact, no lesions or rashes noted. Turgor is good. There is no cyanosis, pallor, or jaundice.

HEENT: Head normocephalic, atraumatic. Pupils equal and reactive to light. Wearing glasses. No AV nicking, hemorrhage, or exudate seen on fundoscopic exam. Disc margins are sharp, no cupping or edema. TMs intact bilaterally without erythema or effusion. External auditory canal is patent, no swelling. Nares patent bilaterally. No polyps noted. Nasal mucosa pink without rhinorrhea. No sinus tenderness. Oropharynx without erythema or exudate. Buccal mucosa intact without lesions. Dentition is good, and gums are pink, not inflamed.

Neck: Supple, full range of motion. No thyromegaly. No carotid bruits. No masses palpated. No tracheal deviation noted.

Respiratory: Breath sounds clear to auscultation in all lung fields. Chest wall expansion and diaphragmatic excursion symmetrical, no increased effort of breathing.

Cardiovascular: Heart regular rate and rhythm. No murmurs, gallops, or rubs. No bruit of abdominal aorta. Distal pulses are 3+ and symmetrical bilaterally. No peripheral edema.

Breasts: No gynecomastia, no masses.

Abdomen: Soft, nontender. No distention, masses, or organomegaly. No dullness to percussion. Bowel sounds physiologic in all four quadrants. There is no guarding or rebound noted.

Genitalia: External genitalia exam reveals a circumcised male, both testes descended. No testicular or scrotal masses noted.

Rectal: Prostate nontender, not enlarged. Firm dark stool noted in rectal vault. Good sphincter tone. Stool is positive for blood.

Musculoskeletal: Fully weight-bearing. Full ROM all extremities. Well-healed surgical scars noted right anterior shoulder and left inguinal canal. No joint effusions, clubbing, cyanosis, or edema.

Neurological: Alert and oriented x 3, cooperative. Mood and affect appropriate to situation. CN II–XII grossly intact. Motor: 5/5 upper and lower extremities. Sensory intact to pinprick. DTRs 2+ bilaterally and symmetrical.

(Continued)

Laboratory Data:
    CBC: WBC 5800; Hct 46; Hgb 13, differential unremarkable. Peripheral smear shows normochromic, normocytic cells
    Chemistry: triglycerides 178; LDL 208; total cholesterol 267; otherwise WNL.
    UA: negative for blood, nitrite, leukocytes.
    ECG: normal sinus rhythm, no ectopic beats, no ischemia.

PROBLEM LIST/ASSESSMENT:
    1. Fatigue
    2. Occult blood in stool
       These symptoms, along with anemia and weight loss, suggestive of colon cancer. Pt will need to undergo colonoscopy
       for biopsy. Will call Dr. Michael Bennett's office to schedule as soon as possible.
    3. Hypertension, well controlled.
    4. Dyslipidemia, fairly well controlled.

PLAN:
    1. Refer to Dr. Michael Bennett for colonoscopy and biopsy.
    2. Chest x-ray for baseline.
    3. Continue present medications for hypertension, dyslipidemia.
    4. OK to continue vitamin and fish oil supplements.

Dictated by Vernon Scott, MD

Date dictated:

Date transcribed:

Figure 2-1 Sample Comprehensive History and Physical Examination.

Worksheet 2.1

Tyler Martin, a third-year medical student on a family practice clerkship, was directed to obtain a comprehensive history and physical examination of a new patient: Denise Andrews. Ms. Andrews recently moved to your city and has never been seen at this practice. She comes in today to establish care, and she is complaining of a cough. Following is the student's documentation of the comprehensive H&P. As you read it, keep in mind the requirements set forth in the 1997 *Guidelines of Documentation for Evaluation and Management* by CMS for information that should be included in a medical record. Refer to the H&P to answer the questions that follow.

1. Does this document meet the CMS guidelines for documentation of a comprehensive history and physical? Why or why not?
2. Critically analyze the H&P and list any errors.
3. Did any questions come to mind that you are unable to answer after reading the H&P?
4. Are the diagnoses listed in the assessment section reasonably supported by the history? Why or why not?
5. Did you identify other differential diagnoses or conditions that could be included in the assessment? If so, list.
6. Is the plan reasonable based on the assessments listed? Why or why not?

DavisPlus | Visit **http://davisplus.fadavis.com** for complete learning activities on actual EMR software at, Keyword: Sullivan

PATIENT NAME: Denise Andrews

AGE: 39

DOB: May 11, 19XX

CHIEF COMPLAINT: Cough

HISTORY OF PRESENT ILLNESS: Ms. Andrews presents with a persistent nonproductive cough. She denies trauma. She states the pain lasts all day long. Food and liquids do not make a difference in the cough. Pain is 6/10. Emesis, no fever.

PAST MEDICAL HISTORY: Usual childhood illnesses. UTD on immunizations. Tonsillectomy in 1980. Last physical 2 years ago and was normal.

Medications: Drixoral, Robitussin

Allergies: Penicillin. Seasonal allergies each spring and fall with mild symptoms. She does not take any medications.

Denies alcohol or drug use presently.

FAMILY HISTORY: Both parents were killed in a car accident. Father 56 and mother 49 at time of death.

SOCIAL HISTORY: Homemaker. Lives in house with spouse and children. She has a bachelor's degree.

REVIEW OF SYMPTOMS:
General: Blood pressure is 130/86; pulse is 84, respirations are 16 and nonlabored while at rest, temperature is 98.6ºF. While seen in the clinic, she coughs about every 5 minutes; the cough is dry, coarse, and nonproductive.

CV: Patient denies palpitations, edema, or swelling of the extremities, dizziness, hypertension. Pt states that she has SOB with exertion, orthopnea while going to bed that is relieved with sitting up, nocturnal dyspnea, no SOB at rest, and no chest pain.

Respiration: Pt states she has SOB with activity and when lying down at night; TB test 5 years ago was negative; no SOB at rest, cough present every 5 minutes during the day and worse at night, but denies sputum production, hemoptysis, dizziness, and asthma.

HEENT: Pt denies head or nasal congestion, headache, discharge from the nose, dizziness, otalgia, vertigo, but states she does have occasional sneezing, rhinitis, and allergy symptoms in the spring.

PHYSICAL EXAMINATION:
General: White female in acute distress, coughs several times a minute. Good hygiene.

Skin: Warm and slightly moist, erythema, and moles. No scars, rashes, bruises, tattoos; hair with fine consistency, no nail pitting.

HEENT: Atraumatic, no lesions. Glasses, PEARL, EOMs intact, no conjunctival injection, no papilledema, no lesions. Ears symmetrical, no tenderness or discharge. No turbinate inflammation, no frontal or maxillary sinus tenderness. Patient has watery discharge from nose, but mucosa was pink and moist. No dentures, no exudates, good hygiene.

Neck: No masses, full ROM. Thyroid size WNL.

CV: RRR, no murmurs or rubs.

Respirations: Chest asymmetrical with respirations, no wheezes, no crackles.

Abdomen: No scars, soft, tender to palpation in upper quadrants bilaterally. No masses, no guarding, no rebound. Bowel sounds present, liver and spleen are within normal limits.

Neurological: CN II–XII intact, sensation intact, strength 5/5 and equal bilaterally. Reflexes 2+ and equal bilaterally, no cerebellar dysfunction, no limp or foot drop.

A: 1. Pneumonia
   2. S/P tonsillectomy

P: 1. Z-pak 250 mg as directed
   2. Follow-up; call if any acute breathing problems
   3. CBC, CMP

Tyler Martin, MS-III July 22, 2009

A comprehensive H&P for patient Consuela Gordon is shown. Ms. Gordon is a new patient presenting to an internal medicine office–based practice. Suzette Barnes, an experienced nurse practitioner, authored the H&P. As you read it, keep in mind the requirements set forth in the 1997 *Guidelines of Documentation for Evaluation and Management* by CMS for information that should be included in a medical record. Refer to the H&P to answer the questions that follow.

1. Does this document meet the CMS guidelines for documentation of a comprehensive history and physical? Why or why not?
2. Critically analyze the H&P and list any errors. Identify the strengths of the H&P.
3. Did any questions come to mind that you are unable to answer after reading the H&P?
4. Are the conditions listed in the assessment section reasonably supported by the history? Why or why not?
5. Did you identify other differential diagnoses or conditions that could be included in the assessment? If so, list.
6. List the ICD-9 code for each of the following.
   Weight loss: _____
   Graves' disease: _____
   Migraine headache: _____
   Anxiety: _____
7. Would it be appropriate to include the ICD-9 code for Graves' disease when billing for this visit? Why or why not?
8. Is the plan reasonable based on the assessments listed? Why or why not?

PATIENT NAME: Consuela Gordon

AGE: 36

SEX: Female

DOB: December 11, 19XX

DATE OF VISIT: October 9, 20XX

CHIEF COMPLAINT: "My usual doctor moved out of state, so I'm changing to this clinic."

HISTORY OF PRESENT ILLNESS: The patient does not have any complaints at this time.

PAST MEDICAL HISTORY:

Medical: Usual childhood illnesses. She has occasional migraine headaches but has not had one in about 6 months. No current or chronic illnesses. She specifically denies any HTN, lipid disorders, diabetes, or cancer. Denies hospitalizations other than for childbirth.

Surgical: Appendectomy at age 14, done as an out-patient with uneventful recovery. She does not recall the name of her surgeon. She lived in Ohio at the time of the operation. Denies major trauma requiring surgery.

Gynecological: G3, P2, AB1. Menarche age 12. Regular 28-day cycles. Took oral contraceptives for approximately 8 years; has not taken for 2 years since her husband had a vasectomy. She had a Pap smear approx. 15 months ago and was told it was normal. Has not had mammography. Patient states that she does breast self-examination "sporadically"; estimates that she does 4 to 5 self-exams per year.

Medications: She takes OTC Aleve 1 or 2 tablets as needed for minor headache or muscle aches. She takes Imitrex injections as needed for migraines.

Allergies: Allergic to codeine; states she gets severe nausea if she takes but denies associated rash or respiratory problems. She is allergic to shellfish and experiences hives and swelling of the lips if consumed.

Health Maintenance: Last complete physical approximately 15 months ago. Pt states "everything was normal." Patient denies ever having a blood transfusion. She is unsure of the date of her last tetanus immunization. States that she doesn't recall having any immunizations "as an adult." She has never had TB skin testing that she recalls; has not had an ECG. Remembers having a chest x-ray after the birth of one of her children but does not remember when that was. She is not sure why she had the chest x-ray but states she developed a fever after delivery.

FAMILY HISTORY: Father is living, age 68, and is in fair health. Mother is living, age 63 and in good health. One brother, age 39, who had stomach ulcers but is otherwise in good health. There is no history of familial diseases.

PSYCHOSOCIAL HISTORY: The patient is married and has 2 children, ages 8 and 5. They live in a two-story home. She has a master's degree in economics. She teaches part-time at a community college. All family members are insured through her husband's employer. She is fluent in English and Spanish, speaks English at home because her husband does not speak Spanish. Her only sexual partner is her husband. She previously smoked 1/2 pack of cigarettes per day for approx. 9 years; quit when she wanted to get pregnant with her first child and has not smoked since. She drinks 1 or 2 glasses of wine most days of the week and more on "special occasions." She denies any recreational or illicit drug use. She does not have any religious preference or special practices. She sometimes practices meditation when she does yoga. She says it is important for her to be involved in decision making regarding her health, and she would seek advice from a close friend who is a nurse. She prefers to try self-treatment with OTC and herbal products for minor illnesses but is not averse to conventional medical treatment. She does not have any food intolerances, only the shellfish allergy. She eats at least 2 servings of fruits daily and 1 to 2 servings of vegetables daily. She limits red meat to one serving per week. She avoids fried foods and tries to keep cholesterol and fat intake low. She does not follow any specific dietary guidelines. She does not have more than two caffeinated beverages a day. She is willing to accept blood transfusion or organ transplantation if needed; she is a registered donor. She does not have a living will or medical power of attorney. She states her husband would make medical decisions for her if she was unable. She exercises 4 to 5 times a week for 45 to 60 minutes, either jogging or yoga.

REVIEW OF SYMPTOMS:

Constitutional: Denies fever, chills, night sweats, fatigue.

Eyes: Photophobia at times, only in association with migraine headaches. Resolves with treatment of HA. Denies any change in vision, double vision, eye pain. Unsure of date of last eye exam. Has never worn glasses or contact lenses.

ENT: Denies any change in hearing or loss of hearing. Denies ear pain, tinnitus. Denies loss of smell or change in sense of smell. No history of nasal polyps. Denies rhinorrhea, sneezing, sinus infections, epistaxis. Last dental exam about 4 months ago for general cleaning. Wisdom teeth extracted at age 19 without complications. Denies odontalgia, bleeding of gums.

CV: States "rings feel tight for a few days, then after my period everything goes back to normal." Denies chest pain, palpitations, exercise intolerance. States that her parents were told she had a heart murmur as a child; does not recall any surgery or other intervention. Has never been told that she has a murmur as an adult.

Respirations: Denies dyspnea, cough, shortness of breath. No history of asthma.

GI: Occasional nausea associated with migraines, usually without vomiting if HA is treated early enough. She has noticed weight loss of approx. 5 lb in the past 4 to 6 weeks without any change in diet or exercise. She states that she feels like she is eating the same amount or more, saying that occasionally she will feel hungry sooner after a regular meal. Denies abdominal pain, bloating, vomiting. Bowel habits have not changed significantly, although patient states she might have 2 or 3 bowel movements some days but generally has only one. Denies diarrhea; no hemorrhoids.

(Continued)

GU: Denies urinary urgency, frequency, hematuria, incontinence.

Gynecological: per PMH. Denies vaginal discharge, dyspareunia. No history of sexually transmitted infections. Last breast self-exam 2 months ago, no masses felt. Last clinical exam about 15 months ago; Pap smear at that time was "normal" per pt.

MSK: Denies joint pains, loss of movement in any joints. Had fracture of the right radius and ulna at age 13, wore cast; no problems since.

Integumentary: Has noticed increased dryness of skin in the past few months. Denies associated pruritus. Has been using a moisturizing lotion with some improvement. Denies lesions or moles. Denies changes in texture of hair or nails.

Neurological: Has had migraine headaches since early 20s. Used to occur almost monthly, but after having her children says they have occurred much less frequently. She goes 6 months or longer without any HAs. When they occur, she generally wakes up early morning with the headache. If she uses the Imitrex right away, HA will resolve within an hour or 2. If she delays using Imitrex, she will usually experience nausea and photophobia. Cannot identify any specific HA triggers. Has never needed more than one dose of Imitrex to resolve HA. Denies head trauma, seizure activity.

Psychiatric: States that she sometimes feels "anxious or jumpy for no reason." She has had 2 or 3 episodes of feeling this way in the past 2 weeks. Cannot identify any precipitating factor. States, "I just go about my business and wait for it to go away. This isn't like me; I'm not usually a worry-wart." She denies sleep disturbances, hallucinations, depression.

Endocrine: Denies polydipsia, polyuria. Denies heat or cold intolerance.

Hematological/Lymphatic: Denies easy bruising or episodes of easy or prolonged bleeding. Has not noticed any enlarged lymph nodes.

Allergic/Immune: Denies allergic rhinitis, atopy.

PHYSICAL EXAMINATION:
General: This is a 36-year old Hispanic woman who appears her stated age. She is articulate and a good historian. She is alert and oriented and does not appear anxious at the present time. Grooming and affect are appropriate.

Vital Signs: T 99.1 P 84 R 20 BP 122/74. Ht 5'7" Wt 138 BMI 21.6

Skin: Good turgor, no lesions. No excessive dryness noted; no dryness or flaking of scalp or hair.

HEENT: Head normocephalic, atraumatic. PEARL bilaterally. TMs intact bilaterally without erythema or effusion. Bony landmarks well visualized. Nares patent bilaterally. No polyps. Nasal mucosa pink and moist, no rhinorrhea. Oropharnyx without tonsillar enlargement, erythema, or exudates. Buccal mucosa moist without lesions. Natural dentition, teeth stable. No gingivitis.

Neck: Supple with full ROM. No adenopathy. No thyromegaly, no masses.

CV: Heart RRR, no murmurs or gallops. PMI nondisplaced. No peripheral edema.

Respirations: Breath sounds clear all fields. Diaphragmatic excursion is symmetrical.

Abdomen: Soft, nondistended. No organomegaly or masses. Bowel sounds are present and physiological in all four quadrants.

Rectal exam: Soft brown stool in vault. Hemoccult negative. Good sphincter tone.

Back: Spine straight without scoliosis or kyphosis. No tenderness. Full ROM of spine. No CVA tenderness.

EXT: Full ROM all extremities. No joint swelling or erythema.

Neurological: Cranial nerves II to XII intact. Sensory intact. Motor is 5/5. Patellar reflexes 3/4, all others 2/4; no clonus. Negative Romberg. Gait is balanced and coordinated without ataxia.

ASSESSMENT:
1. Unintentional 5 lb weight loss. R/O thyroid disorder; with anxiety and hyperreflexia, Graves' disease is likely.
2. Migraine headaches, stable.

PLAN:
1. CBC, CMP, TSH, T3, T4, UA. Consider endocrinology referral depending on lab results.
2. Continue Imitrex injectable, 0.6 mg Subcutaneous PRN migraine HA. Rx given.
3. Return in 1 week to review lab results.
4. Schedule well-woman exam within next month.

Suzette Barnes, NP

Abbreviations

These abbreviations were introduced in Chapter 2. Beside each, write the meaning as indicated by the content of this chapter.

AV _____

BMI _____

BP _____

CAD _____

CBC _____

CC _____

CMP _____

CN _____

COPD _____

CV _____

CVA _____

DOB _____

DOE _____

DTR _____

ECG, EKG _____

ENT _____

EOM _____

G3, P2, AB1 _____

GI _____

GU _____

GYN _____

H&P _____

HA _____

Hct _____

HEENT _____

Hgb _____

HIV _____

HPI _____

Ht _____

HTN _____

LDL _____

MSK _____

OLD CHARTS _____

OTC _____

P _____

PEARL _____

PMH _____

PQRST _____

PRN _____

PSA _____

Pt _____

R, RR _____

R/O _____

ROM _____

ROS _____

RRR _____

SH _____

S/P _____

SOAP _____

SOB _____

T _____

TB _____

TMs _____

TSH _____

T_3 _____

T_4 _____

UA _____

UTD _____

WBC _____

WNL _____

Wt _____

Chapter 3

Adult Preventive Care Visits

OBJECTIVES

- Describe the major components of an adult preventive care visit.
- Discuss the importance of documenting a patient's personal and family medical history.
- Identify several screening questionnaires used to identify tobacco, alcohol, and substance abuse.
- State the five Ps of the sexual history.
- Identify specific information that should be documented for the patient who is a victim of intimate partner violence.
- Explain the Occupational Safety and Health Administration's mission and describe occupational hazards that should be identified.
- List conditions that are screened for in the family history.
- Identify the "red flags" in a family history.
- Identify age- and gender-specific screening guidelines that are commonly used in preventive care visits.
- Discuss the goals of patient education and counseling related to preventive care.
- Identify areas of concern that should be addressed during geriatric prevention visits.

According to the most recent National Ambulatory Medical Care Survey (2008), ambulatory medical care in physician offices is the largest and most widely used segment of the American health-care system. During 2006, an estimated 902 million visits were made to physician offices. New patients accounted for 12.2% of visits, whereas established patients accounted for 87.8%. Approximately 19.2% of all visits were for preventive care.

Preventive care is defined as medical care that focuses on disease prevention. This takes place at primary, secondary, and tertiary prevention levels. *Primary prevention* avoids the development of a disease. Most population-based health promotion activities, such as vaccines, immunization, and hand washing, are primary preventive measures. *Secondary prevention* activities are aimed at early disease detection, thereby increasing opportunities for interventions to prevent progression of the disease and emergence of symptoms. These activities include screening measures to detect a specific condition, such as using mammography to screen for breast cancer. *Tertiary prevention* aims to eliminate, or at least delay, the onset of complications and disability due to the disease. Most medical interventions fall into this category. One example of tertiary prevention is striving for euglycemic control in a patient with diabetes.

Health maintenance is a term that is often used interchangeably with preventive care. Health maintenance is a guiding principle that emphasizes health promotion and disease prevention rather than the management of symptoms and illness. It includes the full array of counseling, screening, and other preventive services designed to minimize the risk for premature illness and death and to ensure optimal physical, mental, and emotional health throughout the natural life cycle.

It is far better to try to prevent a condition than to have to treat it. The cost of disease management creates a tremendous economic burden for government payers and private insurance carriers as well as society in general. In addition to the economic cost of disease, there is the physical and psychological impact on the quality of life of patients and their families. For these reasons, screening guidelines for

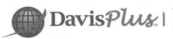 **DavisPlus** | Visit **http://davisplus.fadavis.com** for complete learning activities on actual EMR software at, Keyword: Sullivan

certain conditions have been developed. The term *screening* refers to tests and examinations used to detect a disease, like cancer, in people who do not have any symptoms. Current U.S. screening recommendations are focused on diseases that occur most frequently and that have the highest morbidity and mortality rates. The Agency for Healthcare Research and Quality (AHRQ) has developed an Adult Preventive Care Timeline, which has screening recommendations related to heart disease, cancer, health risks, sexual health, bone health, and immunizations. The timeline is shown in Appendix A. Many federal and state agencies and specialty organizations, such as the American Heart Association and the American Cancer Society, also publish guidelines for screening. Although many of the recommendations are the same, there are variations in frequency of screening. It is beyond the scope of this book to include all the recommendations that have been published; instead, the most generally accepted guidelines are summarized. The focus of this chapter is documenting preventive care visits for adult patients; pediatric patient visits are discussed in Chapter 4.

Documenting Preventive Care

The adult preventive care visit generally follows the format of the comprehensive history and physical examination (see Chapter 2) but is often more narrow in scope. Preprinted forms, such as the adult medical history form shown in Figure 3-1, may be used to collect much of the patient's history, including personal and family medical history. If using such a form, it is important to review it thoroughly with the patient and obtain more information about any positive responses. Specifically document that the form was reviewed with the patient. Throughout the remainder of this chapter, several screening tools or questionnaires are referenced. Such tools are an excellent aid for obtaining and documenting important information during the preventive care visit.

When using printed forms or providing written material, health-care providers should assess their patients' level of health literacy. The U.S. Department of Health and Human Services (HHS) defines *health literacy* as the degree to which individuals have the capacity to obtain, process, and understand basic health information needed to make appropriate health decisions and services needed to prevent or treat illness. It is beyond the scope of this book to address this subject; however, information is widely available.

Components of a preventive care visit include the following:

- Risk factor identification based on personal and family health history
- Age- and gender-specific screening
- Appropriate laboratory and diagnostic screening tests
- Patient education and counseling
- Assessment of immunization status and administering immunizations as appropriate

Risk Factor Identification Based on Personal History

Indications for screening are often based on the patient's age. For example, the American Cancer Society recommends that women 40 years and older have an annual screening mammogram. However, screening recommendations may be different depending on certain personal risk factors. Therefore, a key purpose of obtaining the patient's personal medical history is to identify what conditions the patient is at risk for and the screening measures appropriate for those conditions. Some risk factors are associated with personal habits, such as alcohol or tobacco use or dietary intake. It is important to determine whether these risk factors are present; recognize, however, that inquiring about risk factors could appear judgmental. Inform your patient that you need to ask some questions that could be sensitive in nature, and let the patient know that you ask these questions of all your patients. Approaching these matters in a nonjudgmental, professional, matter-of-fact manner should enhance patient disclosure of sensitive information. Following are some of the risk factors that you should inquire about, and you should specifically document their presence or absence as part of the personal medical history.

Exercise

Document the type of activity (e.g., walking, weight lifting, aerobics), frequency, and duration (e.g., 30 minutes every other day). The current recommendation is for moderate activity five or more days of the week for at least 30 minutes that encompasses a combination of cardiovascular and weight training. Lack of exercise or a sedentary lifestyle is a risk factor for certain conditions, such as cardiovascular disease and stroke.

If the patient exercises, inquire about any history of exercise-induced symptoms such as syncope, chest pain, difficulty breathing, or anaphylaxis or urticaria. Exercise-related syncope is more ominous if it occurs during exercise than during the postexertional state and always requires investigation because it may be the only symptom to precede sudden cardiac death. It is important to recognize excessive exercise syndromes. In women, this may manifest as a triad of symptoms: disordered eating, amenorrhea, and osteoporosis. Excessive exercise syndromes may result in premature osteoporotic fractures due to permanent loss of bone mineral density (BMD). Also document whether there is any use of performance-enhancing drugs or supplements.

To be completed by patient

Date: __/__/__
Name: _____ Age: _____ Date of birth: __/__/__ ☐ Male ☐ Female
Mailing address: _____
Home phone: _____ Work phone: _____ Other phone: _____
Emergency contact name and phone number: _____
Employer's name & address: _____

Please list all the people living in your household and their relationship to you.

Name	Age	Relationship

Personal Health History: Do you have, or have you ever had, any of the following?
(Check all boxes that apply.)

☐ Allergies   ☐ Bowel problems   ☐ Heart problems   ☐ Nerve problems
☐ Anemia   ☐ Breathing problems   ☐ High blood pressure   ☐ Seizures

☐ Alcohol/Drug addiction ☐ Cancer (type _____) ☐ High cholesterol   ☐ Skin problems
☐ Arthritis   ☐ Depression   ☐ Kidney problems   ☐ Stroke
☐ Asthma   ☐ Diabetes   ☐ Liver problems   ☐ Thyroid problems

☐ Back pain   ☐ Eye problems   ☐ Migraine headaches   ☐ Ulcers

☐ Blood transfusion ☐ Serious injury (type _____)

Current Medications (please include prescription and over-the-counter medications):

Name of Medication	Dose (mg)	Taken how many times a day?

Please indicate if you have allergies to any of the following:

___ penicillin ___ sulfa ___ codeine ___ latex ___ vaccines ___ nuts ___ shellfish ___ nickel ___ contrast dye
Other: _____
If any food allergies, please list: _____

Family History: (check all that apply)

	Alcoholism	Asthma or allergies	Cancer (type)	Depression	Diabetes	Heart Disease	High blood pressure	Stroke	Cause of death	Age at death
Father										
Mother										
Siblings										
Grandparents										

(Continued)

Social History:
Marital status: ☐ married ☐ single
Tobacco use: ☐ none ☐ chew tobacco ☐ cigar/pipe ☐ cigarettes _____ packs/day for _____ years quit date ____
Alcohol use: ☐ none drinks/week _____ Type of drink _____
☐ other drug use (type) _____
Exercise: ☐ daily _____ times/week Intensity: ☐ low ☐ medium ☐ high
☐ aerobic ☐ weight training
Seat Belt use: ☐ yes ☐ no Helmet or other safety measures: ☐ yes ☐ no

Immunizations/Screening Exams (date of most recent):
☐ hepatitis B _____ ☐ Pneumovax _____ ☐ tetanus _____ ☐ flu shot _____
☐ stool for blood _____ ☐ chest x-ray _____ ☐ TB test _____ ☐ colonoscopy _____

Women only:
Pap Smear _____ Any abnormal Pap smears? ☐ yes ☐ no
Mammogram _____ Any abnormal mammogram? ☐ yes ☐ no
Do you perform breast self-exams? ☐ yes ☐ no If yes, how often? _____
Age you started your periods: _____ Are they regular? ☐ yes ☐ no
Number of days: _____
Do you still have periods? ☐ yes ☐ no
Have you ever taken hormone replacement therapy? ☐ yes ☐ no
Have you had bone density testing? ☐ yes ☐ no
If yes, when and where was most recent? _____
How many times have you been pregnant? _____
How many children do you have? _____
Number of vaginal deliveries: _____ Number of C-sections: _____

Men only:
Prostate exam: _____ Any abnormal prostate exams ☐ yes ☐ no
Testicular exam: _____ Do you perform testicular self-exams? ☐ yes ☐ no

Figure 3-1 Adult medical history form.

Diet and Nutrition

The goal of obtaining a nutritional history is to aid the health-care provider in identifying dietary deficiencies or excesses and educating the patient about how to improve their nutritional status. Assess dietary habits by asking about a typical day's food intake. Include number of meals per day; frequency of eating out and types of eating establishments frequented (such as fast food, restaurant, cafeteria); number of fruit and vegetable servings per day; portion size, frequency, and type of protein (such as meat, poultry, seafood, dairy or soy products); and fiber intake. Determine how much fat (especially saturated), sugar, and processed foods are consumed each day. Instead of gathering this information by interviewing the patient, you may ask the patient to record all food intake for a predetermined amount of time. A copy of the food diary should then be placed in the patient's chart. If the patient follows a vegetarian diet, document which type (e.g., vegan, lacto-ovo vegetarian) and assess for nutritional inadequacies. Vegetarians who consume eggs or dairy products may not have any nutritional deficiencies; however, strict vegans may have deficiencies in amino acids, zinc, calcium, iron, and vitamins D and B_{12}. Document the use of vitamins and supplements taken, if any.

Document the amount of water and other beverages consumed. The quantity of caffeine consumed per day should be documented in standard units of measure, such as how many cups of coffee or tea, number of soft drinks, energy drinks, and amount of caffeine-containing foods.

Body Mass Index

Obesity is a serious, chronic disease that is known to reduce life span, increase disability, and lead to many serious illnesses. Studies have confirmed a direct correlation between increases in body mass index (BMI) and increases in the prevalence of type 2 diabetes, hypertension, heart disease, stroke, and arthritis. The BMI is calculated based on the patient's height and weight. Although these measurements are obtained as part of the physical examination rather than the history, it is important to determine the BMI for every patient because being overweight or obese is a major risk factor for many health problems. BMI is calculated by using the following formula:

Weight (kg) ÷ Stature (cm) ÷ Stature (cm) × 10,000 *or,*
Weight (lb) ÷ Stature (in) ÷ Stature (in) × 703

BMI calculators are readily available at many Internet sites. BMI tables, such as the adult table shown in Figure 3-2, are available from many sources.

Body Mass Index Table

	Normal						Overweight					Obese										Extreme Obesity															
BMI	19	20	21	22	23	24	25	26	27	28	29	30	31	32	33	34	35	36	37	38	39	40	41	42	43	44	45	46	47	48	49	50	51	52	53	54
Height (inches)																	Body Weight (pounds)																			
58	91	96	100	105	110	115	119	124	129	134	138	143	148	153	158	162	167	172	177	181	186	191	196	201	205	210	215	220	224	229	234	239	244	248	253	258
59	94	99	104	109	114	119	124	128	133	138	143	148	153	158	163	168	173	178	183	188	193	198	203	208	212	217	222	227	232	237	242	247	252	257	262	267
60	97	102	107	112	118	123	128	133	138	143	148	153	158	163	168	174	179	184	189	194	199	204	209	215	220	225	230	235	240	245	250	255	261	266	271	276
61	100	106	111	116	122	127	132	137	143	148	153	158	164	169	174	180	185	190	195	201	206	211	217	222	227	232	238	243	248	254	259	264	269	275	280	285
62	104	109	115	120	126	131	136	142	147	153	158	164	169	175	180	186	191	196	202	207	213	218	224	229	235	240	246	251	256	262	267	273	278	284	289	295
63	107	113	118	124	130	135	141	146	152	158	163	169	175	180	186	191	197	203	208	214	220	225	231	237	242	248	254	259	265	270	278	282	287	293	299	304
64	110	116	122	128	134	140	145	151	157	163	169	174	180	186	192	197	204	209	215	221	227	232	238	244	250	256	262	267	273	279	285	291	296	302	308	314
65	114	120	126	132	138	144	150	156	162	168	174	180	186	192	198	204	210	216	222	228	234	240	246	252	258	264	270	276	282	288	294	300	306	312	318	324
66	118	124	130	136	142	148	155	161	167	173	179	186	192	198	204	210	216	223	229	235	241	247	253	260	266	272	278	284	291	297	303	309	315	322	328	334
67	121	127	134	140	146	153	159	166	172	178	185	191	198	204	211	217	223	230	236	242	249	255	261	268	274	280	287	293	299	306	312	319	325	331	338	344
68	125	131	138	144	151	158	164	171	177	184	190	197	203	210	216	223	230	236	243	249	256	262	269	276	282	289	295	302	308	315	322	328	335	341	348	354
69	128	135	142	149	155	162	169	176	182	189	196	203	209	216	223	230	236	243	250	257	263	270	277	284	291	297	304	311	318	324	331	338	345	351	358	365
70	132	139	146	153	160	167	174	181	188	195	202	209	216	222	229	236	243	250	257	264	271	278	285	292	299	306	313	320	327	334	341	348	355	362	369	376
71	136	143	150	157	165	172	179	186	193	200	208	215	222	229	236	243	250	257	265	272	279	286	293	301	308	315	322	329	338	343	351	358	365	372	379	386
72	140	147	154	162	169	177	184	191	199	206	213	221	228	235	242	250	258	265	272	279	287	294	302	309	316	324	331	338	346	353	361	368	375	383	390	397
73	144	151	159	166	174	182	189	197	204	212	219	227	235	242	250	257	265	272	280	288	295	302	310	318	325	333	340	348	355	363	371	378	386	393	401	408
74	148	155	163	171	179	186	194	202	210	218	225	233	241	249	256	264	272	280	287	295	303	311	319	326	334	342	350	358	365	373	381	389	396	404	412	420
75	152	160	168	176	184	192	200	208	216	224	232	240	248	256	264	272	279	287	295	303	311	319	327	335	343	351	359	367	375	383	391	399	407	415	423	431
76	156	164	172	180	189	197	205	213	221	230	238	246	254	263	271	279	287	295	304	312	320	328	336	344	353	361	369	377	385	394	402	410	418	426	435	443

Figure 3-2 Adult body mass index table.

Different tables are used for children and teens. Four different BMI categories have been identified:

- Underweight = less than 18.5
- Normal weight = 18.5 to 24.9
- Overweight = 25 to 29.9
- Obesity = 30 or greater

At the prevention visit, it is important to explore why the patient is obese, teach the patient that this is a reversible risk factor, and encourage weight management, nutrition, and exercise. Recognition of weight loss, accountability, and health-care provider support remain key elements of patient success.

Tobacco Use

Tobacco use is the leading preventable cause of premature death in the United States. It is estimated that directly or indirectly, tobacco causes more than 400,000 deaths annually, a figure that represents nearly 20% of all deaths. These deaths have been attributed to a number of conditions defined as tobacco-related, including heart disease (115,000 deaths), cancer (136,000), chronic pulmonary disease (60,000), and cerebrovascular accidents (27,000). Health-care providers should screen all patients for tobacco use. Document whether the tobacco use is smoked (cigarettes, pipe, cigar) or smokeless (snuff and chewing tobacco). Documentation should include the amount used per day and how long the patient has been using tobacco. Cigarette use is usually reported as a pack-year history. This figure is determined by multiplying the number of packs per day (PPD) by the total number of years smoked. Pipe and cigar smoking is indicated by frequency per day. Smokeless tobacco use is documented as the number of cans or pouches used per day, or sometimes per week. It is important to educate a patient currently using any form of tobacco on the health risks associated with tobacco use and to document specifically the education provided. You should ask whether the patient is interested in quitting. Here is one example of how tobacco use and education could be documented:

The patient chews tobacco, approximately one pouch every 2 days for the past 12 years. I discussed specific health risks associated with smokeless tobacco, including oral cancers (cancer of the throat, tongue, and larynx), leukoplakia, gum disease, cardiovascular disease, hypertension, and early mortality. Patient stated that he is not ready to quit. I advised patient that cessation aids are available should he desire to quit.

If the patient formerly smoked but has quit, document the year quit and the pack-year history. Take every opportunity to provide positive reinforcement to any patient who has quit smoking. Unfortunately, some patients who quit using tobacco products will start again, so ask about tobacco use at every visit.

Application Exercise 3.1

Calculate the pack-year history for a patient who has smoked two PPD for 20 years: _____

Calculate the pack-year history for a patient who has smoked one-half PPD for 15 years: _____

Alcohol Use

Alcohol consumption is associated with a number of physical and social problems, including reduced physical coordination, reduced mental alertness, poor decision making, double vision, and mood swings. Long-term chronic consumption of high levels of alcohol leads to higher risk for heart disease, liver disease, circulatory problems, peptic ulcers, various forms of cancer, and irreversible brain damage. Screening for alcohol use should be a part of every preventive care visit. Document the type of alcohol, amount, and frequency of consumption. If the amount or frequency of alcohol use is a concern, screen for alcohol abuse or dependence. This can be accomplished through administration of the CAGE questionnaire, which was developed by Dr. John Ewing, founding director of the Bowles Center for Alcohol Studies, University of North Carolina at Chapel Hill. CAGE is an internationally used assessment instrument for identifying problems with alcohol and takes less than 1 minute to administer. *CAGE* is an acronym formed from the italicized letters in the questionnaire:

C Have you ever felt the need to **C**ut down on drinking?

A Have people **A**nnoyed you by criticizing your drinking?

G Have you ever felt **G**uilty about drinking?

E Have you ever taken a drink first thing in the morning (**E**ye-opener) to steady your nerves or get rid of a hangover?

Patients who answer affirmatively to two questions are seven times more likely to be alcohol dependent than the general population. Those who answer negatively to all four questions are one-seventh as likely to have alcoholism as the general population.

The sensitivity of the CAGE questionnaire was thought to be 75%. More recent studies, however, show that the sensitivity is lower, particularly in populations with a lower prevalence of alcohol use, such as women and elderly people. The CAGE questionnaire also may fail to identify binge drinkers.

Because of the risk for fetal harm, it is particularly important to screen for alcohol use in women who are pregnant or who may become pregnant. Studies have shown that the T-ACE questionnaire, a four-item screening questionnaire based on the CAGE screening tool, is considered accurate in detecting drinking problems in pregnant women.

The T-ACE questions are:

T–Tolerance: How many drinks does it take to make you feel high?

A–Have people **annoyed** you by criticizing your drinking?

C–Have you ever felt you ought to **cut down** on your drinking?

E–Eye-opener: Have you ever had a drink first thing in the morning to steady your nerves or get rid of a hangover?

Affirmative answers to questions A, C, and E are each scored one point. A reply of more than two drinks to the T question is scored two points. The T-ACE is considered to be positive with a score of two or more. Women who screen positive should receive further assessment and brief intervention to help reduce the risk to the developing fetus and to maximize pregnancy outcome.

One of the most accurate tests available to screen for problem drinking is the Alcohol Use Disorders Identification Test (AUDIT), which was developed by the World Health Organization. It is accurate 94% of the time and is also accurate across ethnic and gender groups. Furthermore, it has a greater sensitivity in populations with a lower prevalence of alcoholism than does the CAGE screening tool. The test comprises 10 multiple-choice questions that are scored on a point system. AUDIT can be administered as a paper-and-pencil test. The disadvantage of the AUDIT test is that it takes longer to administer and is more difficult to score than the shorter tests. The questions and scoring guide are shown in Figure 3-3. A score of eight or more indicates an alcohol problem.

Documentation is as simple as stating the screening tool used and the score, such as "CAGE score = 4" or "AUDIT score of 9."

Other Substance Abuse

Hazardous substance use, abuse, and dependence are more prevalent in the United States than some of the conditions that are routinely screened for, yet healthcare providers sometimes fail to identify patients with substance abuse issues. One tool that screens for substance abuse is the Drug Abuse Screening Test (DAST-10) developed by Harvey Skinner, PhD. It is a 10-item, yes/no, self-report instrument that asks questions about involvement with drugs in the past 12 months and should take less than 8 minutes to complete. The DAST-10 is intended for use with patients 18 years and older. In this screening tool, "drug abuse" refers to the use of prescribed or over-the-counter drugs in excess of the directions and any nonmedical use of drugs. The tool and scoring guidelines are shown in Figure 3-4.

Another tool used for substance abuse screening is the National Institute of Drug Abuse Modified Alcohol, Smoking, and Substance Involvement Screening Test (NIDA Modified ASSIST). The screening may be administered in a written version or even accessed online. If using a written version, provide a blank cover page to protect patient confidentiality and place the completed questionnaire in the patient's medical record. The NIDA Modified ASSIST may be used to screen for tobacco, alcohol, and substance use and dependence. The first question asks, "Which of the following substances have you used in your lifetime?" (a) tobacco products, (b) alcoholic beverages, (c) cannabis, (d) cocaine, (e) prescription stimulants, (f) methamphetamine, (g) inhalants, (h) sedatives or sleeping pills, (i) hallucinogens, (j) street opioids, (k) prescription opioids, (l) other. If the answer is "none," the screening is complete. If any of the substances have been used, the next question asks if they have been used in the past 3 months. Other questions ask how often the patient has a strong desire or urge to use; how often use of the substance has led to health, social, legal, or financial problems; and how often use of the substance has caused the patient to fail to do what was normally expected of them. Answers include never, once or twice, monthly, weekly, or daily or almost daily. Three yes/no questions complete the screening: (1) Has a friend or relative ever expressed concern about your use of the drug? (2) Have you ever tried and failed to control, cut down, or stop using the drug? (3) Have you ever used the drug by injection? If the answer to the last question is yes, ask about the pattern of injecting and recommend HIV and hepatitis B and C testing. For complete information on administering and scoring the NIDA Modified ASSIST screen, please visit the National Institute of Drug Abuse website at www.drugabuse.gov.

Sexual History

Patients and providers alike may not be comfortable talking about the sexual history, sex partners, or sexual practices. It is important to emphasize to patients that taking a sexual history is a necessary part of a regular medical history. A sexual history allows the provider to identify individuals at risk for sexually transmitted diseases (STDs; also sexually transmitted infections, or STIs), such as syphilis, human papillomavirus (HPV), HIV, pelvic inflammatory disease (PID), and hepatitis, and helps to identify appropriate anatomical sites for certain STD tests. As with all parts of the history, the sexual history may need to be modified to be culturally appropriate for some patients based on culture or gender dynamics.

The contents of a sexual history that should be documented can be remembered by the five Ps: Partners,

Questions	0 Points	1 Point	2 Points	3 Points	4 Points
How often do you have a drink containing alcohol?	Never	Monthly or less	2–4 times a month	2–3 times per week	4 or more times a week
How many drinks containing alcohol do you have on a typical day when you are drinking?	1 or 2	3 or 4	5 or 6	7–9	10 or more
How often do you have 6 or more drinks on one occasion?	Never	Less than monthly	Monthly	2–3 times per week	4 or more times a week
How often during the past year have you found that you were not able to stop drinking once you started?	Never	Less than monthly	Monthly	2–3 times per week	4 or more times a week
How often during the past year have you failed to do what was normally expected of you because of drinking?	Never	Less than monthly	Monthly	2–3 times per week	4 or more times a week
How often during the past year have you needed a first drink in the morning to get yourself going after a heavy drinking session?	Never	Less than monthly	Monthly	2–3 times per week	4 or more times a week
How often during the past year have you had feelings of guilt or remorse after drinking?	Never	Less than monthly	Monthly	2–3 times per week	4 or more times a week
How often during the past year have you been unable to remember what happened the night before because you had been drinking?	Never	Less than monthly	Monthly	2–3 times per week	4 or more times a week
Have you or has someone else been injured as a result of your drinking?	No		Yes, but not in the past year		Yes, during the past year
Has a relative, friend, doctor, or health-care worker been concerned about your drinking or suggested you cut down?	No		Yes, but not in the past year		Yes, during the past year

Figure 3-3 Alcohol Use Disorders Identification Test (AUDIT). A score of 8 or more on the AUDIT generally indicates harmful or hazardous drinking. Questions 1 to 8 are scored 0, 1, 2, 3, or 4 points. Questions 9 and 10 are scored 0, 2, or 4 only. (From Babor TF, et al. *The Alcohol Use Disorders Identification Test: Guidelines for Use in Primary Care,* 2nd ed. Geneva, Switzerland: World Health Organization, Department of Mental Health and Substance Dependence, 2001.)

Practices, Protection from STDs, Past history of STDs, and Prevention of pregnancy. Specific questions that can be asked to obtain the history in each of the five areas are shown in Appendix B. Appropriate screening measures can then be tailored to the patient based on risk factors identified by the sexual history.

Intimate Partner Violence

Sometimes referred to as domestic violence, family violence, or relationship violence, *intimate partner violence* (IPV) refers to violence occurring between people who are, or were formerly, in an intimate relationship. IPV can occur on a continuum of economic,
psychological, and emotional abuse, to physical and sexual violence. Although men are among the victims of IPV, evidence suggests that most victims are women and that women are more vulnerable to its health impacts. IPV screening can be conducted by asking three simple questions:

1. Within the past year, have you been hit, slapped, kicked, or otherwise physically hurt by someone?
2. Are you in a relationship with a person who threatens or physically hurts you?
3. Has anyone forced you to participate in sexual activities that made you feel uncomfortable?

The following questions concern information about your possible involvement with drugs (not including alcoholic beverages) during the past 12 months. Carefully read each statement and decide if your answer is "Yes" or "No." Then check the appropriate response beside the question.

In the following statements "drug abuse" refers to:
        1. The use of prescribed or over-the-counter drugs in excess of the directions, and
        2. Any nonmedical use of drugs.

The various classes of drugs may include cannabis (marijuana, hashish), solvents (e.g., paint thinner), tranquilizers (e.g., Valium), barbiturates, cocaine, stimulants (e.g., speed), hallucinogens (e.g., LSD), or narcotics (e.g., heroin).

1. Have you used drugs other than those required for medical reasons?	Yes	No
2. Do you abuse more than one drug at a time?	Yes	No
3. Are you unable to stop using drugs when you want to?	Yes	No
4. Have you ever had blackouts or flashbacks as a result of drug use?	Yes	No
5. Do you ever feel bad or guilty about your drug use?	Yes	No
6. Does your spouse (or parents or friends) ever complain about your involvement with drugs?	Yes	No
7. Have you neglected your family because of your use of drugs?	Yes	No
8. Have you engaged in illegal activities in order to obtain drugs?	Yes	No
9. Have you ever experienced withdrawal symptoms (felt sick) when you stopped using drugs?	Yes	No
10. Have you had medical problems as a result of your drug use (e.g., memory loss, hepatitis, convulsions, bleeding)?	Yes	No

One point is given for each "Yes" answer.

Score	Degree of Probability Related to Drug Abuse	Suggested Action
0	No problems	None at this time
1–2	Low level	Monitor; reassess at later date
3–5	Moderate level	Further investigation required
6–8	Substantial level	Assessment required
9–10	Severe level	Assessment required

Figure 3-4 Drug Abuse Screening Test (DAST-10). (Courtesy of Dr. Harvey A. Skinner, Dean, Faculty of Health, York University, Toronto, Canada.)

With disclosure of IPV, the provider's responsibilities include acknowledging the abuse, making a safety assessment, assisting with a safety plan, providing appropriate referrals, and documenting. Documentation should specifically include the victim's description of current and past abuse, the name of the alleged perpetrator and relationship to the victim, and any information or referrals provided to the victim. A detailed description of all physical injuries should be documented, including the type of injury, location (in relation to fixed landmarks or standard anatomical regions), length, width, shape, color, depth, degree of healing, and other relevant details, such as swelling. Include a detailed description of the patient's psychological demeanor, noting gestures, facial expressions, and other relevant aspects. Use a body diagram to establish the location of all visible injuries and scars. Photographs may be included in the documentation and should be identified by the patient's name, date the photograph was taken, identity of person taking the photograph, and setting in which the photograph was taken.

Safety Measures

Adults are at risk for injury resulting from motor vehicle crashes; therefore, safety screening should include documentation of seat belt use and risky behavior while driving, such as drinking alcohol and use of cell phones or text messaging. If the patient rides a motorcycle or bicycle, inquire about helmet use. Consider safety in the home as well, and document whether there are weapons or firearms in the home, presence of smoke detectors, and any safety equipment in the home, such as grab bars in a tub or shower area. If the patient has a pool, document the presence of a fence around the pool and a pool alarm. In instances of water recreation or sports, document the use of sunscreen, personal flotation devices, and eye protection.

Occupational History

The U.S. Congress created the Occupational Safety and Health Administration (OSHA) in 1970. Its mission is to prevent work-related injuries, illnesses, and occupational fatalities by issuing and enforcing standards for workplace safety and health. OSHA's role is to ensure safe and healthful working conditions. Some of the specific exposures that OSHA monitors can be grouped as follows:

- Mechanical: equipment-related injury, puncture wounds, falls/slips/trips, impact force, compressed air, high-pressure fluid injection
- Physical: noise, ionizing radiation, heat or cold stress, electricity, dehydration
- Biological: bacteria, fungi (mold), virus, tuberculosis, blood-borne pathogens (e.g., hepatitis, HIV)
- Chemical: acids, bases, heavy metals (e.g., lead), solvents (e.g., petroleum), particulates (e.g., asbestos), fumes (e.g., noxious gases, vapors), fire
- Psychosocial: work-related stress (e.g., too much overtime), harassment (e.g., sexual, verbal, emotional), burnout
- Musculoskeletal: carpal tunnel syndrome (CTS) and back pain, which account for one third of all serious injuries suffered by American workers

Determine the patient's specific job duties and assess for risk for work-related injury or any possible exposures. If an individual is exposed to potential hazards, ask whether the employer provides screening. Document the type of screening and how often the screening is done. Document the use of personal protective devices, such as goggles, and hearing protection.

Oral Health

According to the Centers for Disease Control and Prevention (CDC), nearly one third of all adults in the United States have untreated tooth decay. One in seven adults aged 35 to 44 years has gum disease; this increases to one in every four adults aged 65 years and older. In addition, nearly one fourth of all adults have experienced some facial pain in the past 6 months. Oral cancers are most common in older adults, particularly those older than 55 years who smoke and are heavy drinkers. Unfortunately, many adults do not get regular dental care. Documentation related to oral health should include the number of dental caries, identification of missing or broken teeth, condition of the patient's gums, and the patient's personal oral hygiene habits, such as the frequency of brushing and flossing and use of fluoride toothpaste.

Blood or Blood Product Transfusions

A number of infectious diseases can be passed from the donor to the recipient through transfusion of blood or blood products. Among these are HIV, human T-lymphotropic virus types 1 and 2 (HTLV-1, HTLV-2), hepatitis B and C, *Treponema palladum*, malaria, Chagas' disease, and Creutzfeldt-Jakob (or "mad cow") disease. According to the American Society of Anesthesiologists, the risk for contracting HIV, hepatitis C, hepatitis B, or HTLV-1 from a blood transfusion is about 1 in 34,000 transfused units, with hepatitis B and hepatitis C accounting for 88% of this risk.

Noninfectious complications of blood transfusions include hemolytic transfusion reaction, allergic reaction, anaphylaxis, febrile nonhemolytic transfusion reaction, iron overload from repeated transfusions causing an acquired hemochromatosis, and bacterial infection from contamination, especially from platelets because they are stored at room temperature. The risk for contracting diseases through blood transfusion are higher in less developed countries where screening may not occur and the process of collecting, storing, and using blood and blood products may not be regulated.

If a patient has had a blood or blood product transfusion, document the date and type of product transfused (e.g., whole blood, packed cells, fresh-frozen plasma) and the reason. Document whether there were any complications from the transfusion. When a person's need for a transfusion can be anticipated, as in the case of scheduled surgery, autologous donation can be used to protect against disease transmission and eliminate the problem of blood type in compatibility.

Risk-Factor Identification Based on Family History

Obtaining a detailed family history enables health-care providers to assess risk due to the complex interactions of genes, lifestyle, and exposures experienced by family members, as well as susceptibility due to single genes. Conditions known to have a genetic familial tendency include diabetes, cardiovascular disease, hypertension, hyperlipidemia, cancer, asthma, and osteoporosis. Establishing genetic risk factors may enable an earlier or more accurate diagnosis and allows the provider and patient to determine the degree of intervention needed, such as preventive measures, surveillance, or management. Common diseases and the recommended screening test for each are shown in Table 3-1.

It is common practice to inquire about the medical history of parents, siblings, and grandparents; however, there are several hereditary conditions that

Table 3-1 Common Diseases and Recommended Screenings

Family History	Recommended Screening Test
Cancer	
Breast	Clinical breast examination Mammogram
Ovarian	Bimanual pelvic examination, no recommended screening test, ultrasound and carcinoembryonic antigen (CEA) if there is clinical suspicion
Prostate	Digital rectal examination Prostate-specific antigen (PSA)
Colon	Fecal occult blood test (FOBT) Sigmoidoscopy or colonoscopy[1]
Heart Disease	
Hypertension	Blood pressure evaluation
Hyperlipidemia	Diet evaluation Cholesterol panel
Psychiatric Disease	
Depression	Psychiatric history Depression screening evaluation
Schizophrenia	Psychiatric history
Suicide	Psychiatric history Depression screening evaluation
Alcoholism	CAGE questions
Autoimmune Disease	
Rheumatoid arthritis	History and physical examination Rheumatoid factor (RF) Sedimentation rate
Systemic lupus erythematosus	Antinuclear antibody (ANA) Sedimentation rate
Endocrine Disease	
Diabetes	Fasting blood sugar (FBS) Glucose challenge test[2] Hemoglobin A_{1c} (HgbA$_{1c}$)[2]
Thyroid disease	Thyroid-stimulating hormone (TSH) T_3[2] Free T_4[2]

[1]Patients who have a family history of colon cancer should have a colonoscopy rather than a sigmoidoscopy.
[2]If clinically indicated.

require information about multiple generations to understand various inheritance patterns, such as with certain cancers. At a minimum, the family history should include the age, health status, and presence of diseases of first-degree relatives, defined as parents, grandparents, and siblings. Document the age of the relative, presence of any conditions that have a genetic or familial tendency, and current health status of the individual. Age and cause of death should be documented for deceased relatives. It may be necessary to remind the patient that a family history is only pertinent for blood relatives, not spouses, in-laws, or adopted persons. When an

adopted person is unaware of his or her family history, this should be documented to alert the health-care team that the patient may be at risk for any genetic conditions.

There are certain findings from the family history that are particularly important. These include early age at onset, two or more first-degree relatives with the same disorder or related conditions, a family member with two or more related conditions, disease occurring in the less often affected sex, and conditions that are refractory to usual treatment or prevention strategies. These are considered "red flags" in the family history and indicate a higher level of risk for family members. Algorithms have been created for certain diseases, such as coronary artery disease (CAD) and cerebrovascular accident (CVA), which consider these characteristics and stratify family history into three risk categories (weak, moderate, and strong). Recent literature is filled with studies evaluating statistical models that predict risk for disease or some other adverse event. The purpose of a risk prediction model is to stratify individuals accurately into clinically relevant risk categories. This risk information can be used to guide clinical decision making about preventive interventions for persons or disease screening for populations identified as high risk.

Assessing family history as part of risk stratification is a key initiative of the CDC and HHS. The CDC tool is Family Healthware, an interactive, Web-based tool that assesses familial risk for six diseases (coronary heart disease, stroke, diabetes, and colorectal, breast, and ovarian cancer) and provides a "prevention plan" with personalized recommendations for lifestyle changes and screening. The tool collects data on health behaviors, screening tests, and disease history of a person's first- and second-degree relatives. Algorithms in the software analyze the family history data and assess familial risk based on the number of relatives affected, their age at disease onset, gender, how closely related the relatives are to each other and to the user, and the combinations of diseases in the family. A second set of algorithms uses the data on familial risk level, health behaviors, and screening to generate personalized prevention messages. This tool can be accessed at www.cdc.gov/genomics/famhistory/famhx.htm.

"My Family Health Portrait" was developed by HHS through the Office of the Surgeon General. Part of this initiative is to encourage discussion among family members about their health history. The tool helps patients assemble and organize family history information and makes a pedigree, which can then be printed and presented to their health-care provider. It does not offer medical advice or screening recommendations. The tool is accessible at https://familyhistory.hhs.gov.

Appropriate Laboratory and Diagnostic Screening Tests

Various governmental agencies and specialty societies, such as the American Cancer Society and the American Heart Association, publish recommendations for periodic screening tests. Insurance companies may have their own schedules for screening tests. It is beyond the scope of this book to discuss all the screening tests that could be performed, but general screening recommendations are presented. Many of the recommended screening tests that are appropriate for the general adult population are shown in Table 3-2. Other tests are gender specific and are discussed in the next section. Determining which screening tests to order is based on conditions and diseases that the patient is at risk for as revealed by the medical, family, and social history. Consult the HHS AHRQ website for the most current U. S. Preventive Services Task Force (USPSTF) evidence-based recommendations.

Table 3-2 Screening Recommendations

Screening Test	Recommended Ages (yr)	
	Male	Female
Total cholesterol	35–65[1]	45–65[1]
Venereal disease research laboratory (VDRL)	≥20[2]	≥20[2]
Flexible sigmoidoscopy	≥50[3]	≥50[3]
Colonoscopy	≥50[3,4]	≥50[3,4]
Digital rectal examination	≥40[5]	≥40[5]
FOBT	≥40[6]	≥40[6]
ECG	≥40[2]	≥40[2]
CXR	≥20[2]	≥20[2]
TSH	≥20[2]	≥20[2]
CBC	≥20[2]	≥20[2]
CMP	≥20[2]	≥20[2]
Fasting blood sugar	≥20[2]	≥20[2]
Urinalysis (UA)	≥20[2]	≥20[2]
Hearing assessment	≥20[2]	≥20[2]
PPD	≥20[2]	≥20[2]
Glaucoma screening	Refer high-risk patients to eye specialist for screening	Refer high-risk patients to eye specialist for screening

[1]Unless clinically indicated earlier by history.
[2]If clinically indicated.
[3]Fecal occult blood testing should precede the decision to perform a flexible sigmoidoscopy or colonoscopy. Positive fecal occult blood testing would indicate a colonoscopy instead of a flexible sigmoidoscopy. Recommended every 5 years.
[4]Colonoscopy for high-risk individuals as indicated by history, every 10 years.
[5]At the time of the flexible sigmoidoscopy or colonoscopy.
[6]Annually.

Gender-Specific Screening

Screening for Women

In addition to the history and physical examination that you will perform for all adult well visits and the screening recommendations outlined in Table 3-2, the female preventive care visit typically includes additional diagnostic studies. Often referred to as a well-woman examination (WWE), the visit includes focus on the gynecologic history (including sexual history and IPV screening, as discussed earlier) for women of childbearing age, and education about menopause and postmenopausal health concerns when appropriate. In addition to a standard physical examination, a clinical breast examination and pelvic examination should be performed. Other screening examinations, such as those shown in Table 3-3, may be clinically indicated.

When performing a clinical breast examination, it is appropriate to educate the patient about how to perform breast self-examination. Patient education about normal findings at the time of the examination helps the patient become familiar with her body and monitor any changes that might occur. Document any patient education in the plan, even if you perform this at the same time you are doing a physical examination. The plan may also include an order for a mammogram if clinically indicated.

Screening for STDs and gynecologic cancers is part of the pelvic examination. Obtain a Papanicolaou (Pap) test to screen for cervical cancer. Bimanual pelvic examination should be performed to assess the uterus and search for any adnexal masses. It is important to document whether there is any difficulty performing any part of the pelvic examination. Certain patient characteristics may lead to a clinically unsatisfactory examination. The patient may be anxious and unable to relax, or the patient may be very obese, making it difficult or even impossible to palpate some anatomic structures. Rather than simply omitting the part of the examination that was difficult or unsatisfactory, you should document the difficulties encountered and describe why the examination was unsatisfactory. If a patient refuses any part of the examination or refuses to have a screening test that is indicated, you should document the patient's refusal in the appropriate system (i.e., if the patient refuses the rectal examination, document in the genitourinary system) or in the plan if a recommended test is refused.

Screening for Men

The male preventive health visit, also called the well-man examination, should include a genital examination and inguinal hernia check as well as the general

Table 3-3	Screening Recommendations for Women

Screening Test	Frequency
Pelvic examination	Performed in conjunction with a Pap test in patients who have a cervix, after age 40 annually
Papanicolaou (Pap) test	Pap testing recommended every 3 years after two normal annual tests for all women who have been or are sexually active and who have a cervix. If the patient is taking contraceptive medication or hormone replacement therapy, annual Pap tests are performed. No evidence has proved the upper age limit to discontinue Pap testing.
Clinical breast examination	Every 3 years from age 20 to 40 unless clinically indicated
Mammogram	Annually after age 40 years; sooner if clinically indicated
Rubella serology or vaccination	Women of childbearing age
Bone density scan	65 years and older; sooner if clinically indicated

physical examination. In patients 18 to 30 years of age, perform a testicular examination to screen for testicular cancers. A prostate and rectal examination should be performed, as indicated in Table 3-4. Test the stool for occult blood as part of screening for colorectal cancer. Guidelines for prostate-specific antigen (PSA) as a screening for prostate cancer are controversial. For many years, the guideline was to begin at age 50 years. In 2009, the American Urological Association recommended that screening begin at age 40 years. The American Cancer Society no longer recommends routine PSA screening for all men. Instead, its guidelines call for health-care providers and patients to weigh the benefits and the risks of screening before deciding on a course of action. If the patient refuses to allow any part of the examination, document the refusal as well as any education provided to the patient on the importance of the examination component that was refused.

MEDICOLEGAL ALERT !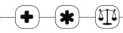

If any part of the examination is deferred, document the reason, so that readers of the medical records will not have to speculate. Deferral implies that the examination is not done at this time for a specific reason. "Deferral" should not be documented if the patient is actually refusing a recommended examination or test. If the patient refuses, educate the patient on the importance of performing the examination or test; if the patient persists in refusing, you should respect his or her right to refuse but document any education provided and the risks associated with refusing the examination or test.

Assessing Immunization Status
Review of immunization status is an important component of the adult health maintenance visit. Immunizations are used to prevent disease, and there are several that should be maintained through adulthood.

Many patients are not aware of the need for immunizations unless they are required for certain activities, occupations, or college entrance. If the patient was fully immunized during childhood, immunizations that they are likely to need as adults include diphtheria-tetanus, hepatitis B, herpes zoster, HPV, varicella, influenza, and pneumonia. If the patient was not fully immunized during childhood, a catch-up schedule is available. The CDC is the best source for up-to-date information on adult immunizations, schedules, and the medical indications for specific immunizations, and may be accessed at www.cdc.gov.

Health Education and Counseling
According to the latest National Ambulatory Medical Care Survey (2008), health education and counseling were documented as being ordered or provided at 36.5% of office visits. The most frequent education or counseling provided related to diet or nutrition and exercise. The preventive health visit is a convenient time to educate and counsel patients. Any patient education or counseling provided should be specifically documented. It is important to reinforce and praise patients for positive health behaviors and equally important to educate patients about the risks associated with negative health behaviors, such as tobacco use or sedentary lifestyle. Studies have shown that the health-care provider's advice can have a strong influence on patient behavior. Patients may not be ready to

Table 3-4	Screening Recommendations for Men

Screening Test	Frequency
Prostate-specific antigen screening	Annually after age 50 years
Prostate examination	Annually after age 50 years
Testicular examination	18 years and older
Hernia examination	18 years and older

change their behavior at any particular visit, but they may move closer to making a change when the information is reinforced over multiple visits.

MEDICOLEGAL ALERT !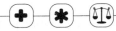

Documenting that you have counseled the patient on the risks of negative health habits and the management of chronic disease is an important part of medicolegal risk management. Providers have been sued for not providing patient education and counseling. One such case involved a 33-year-old woman who was obese and hypertensive and smoked. She had frequent visits to the clinic for various complaints. Routine screening tests revealed marked hypercholesterolemia and an abnormal ratio of high-density lipoprotein (HDL) to low-density lipoprotein (LDL). The health-care provider never counseled the patient regarding her risk for coronary artery disease. Several years later, the patient presented to an emergency room with crushing chest pain that radiated to her arms and neck. The diagnosis of myocardial infarction was confirmed, but by the time the diagnosis was made, the window of opportunity for thrombolytic therapy had closed. The patient sued the clinic and the health-care provider for malpractice. The health-care provider was found negligent for not educating and counseling the patient about her risk factors for developing heart disease.

It is highly recommended that you provide educational information in writing when possible. This not only serves to reinforce information that was given verbally but also gives patients information that they can read at their own pace and at a time convenient for them. Many professional organizations offer patient handouts on common conditions. Resources are available in print and electronically, and many can be customized to a particular practice setting or specialty. When handouts are given, ask follow-up questions about the content at the next visit and determine whether the patient has any related questions.

Assessing Geriatric Risk Factors

Patients older than 65 years are frequent consumers of health-care services. The preventive care visit provides an opportunity to address the unique issues associated with aging. Baseline and periodic geriatric assessments should be used to identify the medical, psychosocial, and environmental factors that affect a patient's health and level of functioning. Numerous screening instruments have been developed to detect common geriatric problems in order to improve functional outcomes and quality of life. Figure 3-5, the Geriatric Health Questionnaire (developed by Gerald Jogerst, MD), is a combination of several screening instruments and may be used as a brief yet comprehensive functional assessment. Abnormal responses to screening questionnaires should be followed with further testing or interventions or more in-depth instruments as indicated.

Common Geriatric Problems

Because quality-of-life issues are largely determined by functional status, periodic assessment of older patients should cover the following fundamental areas of concern:

• Activities of daily living (ADLs)
• Instrumental activities of daily living (IADLs)
• Sensory deficits
• Cognition
• Mood
• Gait and mobility, including recent falls
• Nutritional status

Functional Impairment

Functional impairment is defined as difficulty performing or requiring the assistance of another person to perform ADLs and IADLs. The ability to perform these tasks should be evaluated as a baseline at about 65 years of age but may be done earlier if indicated by the presence of chronic disease or significant morbidities. This provides a benchmark against which to measure future levels of function and to determine the need for support services or placement (e.g., in an assisted living facility or nursing home), for medical or surgical interventions (e.g., total hip or knee replacement), or for rehabilitative services (e.g., occupational or physical therapy).

Two commonly used tools to screen patients and document their functional ability are the Katz Index of ADLs and Lawton IADL Scale. The Katz Index ranks adequacy of performance in the six functions of bathing, dressing, toileting, transferring, continence, and feeding. Clients are scored yes/no for independence in each of these six functions. A score of six indicates full function; four indicates moderate impairment; and two or less indicates severe functional impairment. The Lawton IADL Scale is an appropriate instrument to assess independent living skills, such as the ability to use the telephone, shopping, food preparation, doing laundry, housekeeping, ability to handle finances, responsibility for one's own medication, and transportation. These skills are considered more complex than the basic ADLs measured by the Katz Index. The Lawton IADL instrument is most useful for identifying how a person is functioning at the present time and for identifying improvement or deterioration over time. It measures eight domains of function. Women are scored

Geriatric Health Questionnaire

Patient's Name: _____ Date: _____

Instructions: Please circle answers.

1. General Health:

In general, would you say your health is:
- ☐ Excellent
- ☐ Very Good
- ☐ Good
- ☐ Fair
- ☐ Poor

How much bodily pain have you had during the past 4 weeks?
- ☐ None
- ☐ Very Mild
- ☐ Mild
- ☐ Moderate
- ☐ Severe
- ☐ Very Severe

2. Activities of Daily Living

Are you fully independent (can do the activity yourself), need assistance from another person, or are dependent and unable to do the task at all? Check the correct box.

Activity	Independent	Need Assistance	Dependent
Walking	☐	☐	☐
Dressing	☐	☐	☐
Bathing	☐	☐	☐
Eating	☐	☐	☐
Toileting	☐	☐	☐
Driving	☐	☐	☐
Using telephone	☐	☐	☐
Shopping	☐	☐	☐
Preparing meals	☐	☐	☐
Housework	☐	☐	☐
Taking medications	☐	☐	☐
Managing finances	☐	☐	☐

3. Geriatric Review of Systems:

a. Do you have difficulty driving, watching TV, or reading because of poor eyesight? Yes No

b. Can you hear normal conversation voice? Yes No
   Do you use hearing aids? Yes No

c. Do you have problems with your memory? Yes No

d. Do you often feel sad or depressed? Yes No

e. Have you unintentionally lost weight in the last 6 months? Yes No

f. Do you have trouble with control of your bladder? Yes No
   Do you have trouble with control of your bowels? Yes No

g. How many falls have you had in the past year? _____

h. Do you drink alcohol? Yes No
   If yes, how many drinks per week? _____

4. Do you live with anyone? Yes No

If yes, who?
- ☐ Spouse
- ☐ Child
- ☐ Other
- ☐ Relative
- ☐ Friend

Who would help you in an emergency? _____

Who would help you with health-care decisions if you were not able to communicate your wishes? _____

(Continued)

5. How many medicines do you take, including prescribed, over the counter, and vitamins? _____
    What is your system for taking your medications?
        ☐ Pill box
        ☐ Family help
        ☐ List or chart
        ☐ None

6. Are you sexually active?   Yes   No

7. Has anyone intentionally tried to harm you?   Yes   No

8. Have you had a shot to prevent pneumonia?   Yes   No

9. Please draw the face of a clock with all the numbers and the hands set to indicate 10 minutes after 11 o'clock.

Memory: 3 item recall after 1 minute   (pen, dog, watch)   # recalled _____

Patient Signature: _____   Date: _____

Reviewing Physician: _____   Date: _____

Figure 3-5 Geriatric Health Questionnaire. (From Rakel D. *Textbook of Family Medicine,* 7th ed. Philadelphia: Saunders, 2007.)

on all eight areas of function; historically, for men, the areas of food preparation, housekeeping, and laundering are excluded. Patients are scored according to their highest level of functioning in each category. A summary score ranges from 0 to 8 for women, and 0 through 5 for men; the higher the score, the greater the person's level of independence.

Sensory Deficits

The prevalence of visual and auditory impairment is high in elderly people and may contribute to an individual's inability to function independently and in a safe manner. Vision should be checked using the Snellen chart and the patient referred for further evaluation if corrected vision is greater than 20/40. Regular screening for glaucoma, the second highest cause of blindness in the United States, should be recommended for all patients who are 60 years and older. Patients at higher risk (African Americans and those with a family history of glaucoma) should start regular screening at 40 years of age.

Hearing loss is the third most prevalent chronic condition in older adults and has important effects on their physical and mental health. Hearing loss inhibits the ability to interpret speech. This in turn may reduce a patient's ability to communicate, which can result in social isolation, depression, and anxiety, and pose environmental safety issues, such as the inability to hear warning alarms or someone knocking on the door. The USPSTF currently recommends screening of older adults for hearing impairment by periodically questioning them about their hearing, counseling them about the availability of hearing aid devices, and making referrals for abnormalities when appropriate. The optimal frequency of such screening has not been determined and is left to clinical discretion.

The Hearing-Dependent Daily Activities (HDDA) Scale is shown in Figure 3-6. It is a rapid and easy method of assessing the impact of hearing loss on daily life. This scale has been shown to correlate well with pure tone audiometry, which is the standard test for assessment of hearing loss. Patients are asked

The table below presents the Hearing-Dependent Daily Activities (HDDA) questionnaire used to evaluate the affect of hearing loss in older persons. Providers should score "Always" and "No, I Can't" as 0 points, "Occasionally" and "With Some Difficulty" as 1 point, and "Never" and "Yes, Without Difficulty" as 2 points.

No.	Questions	Always	Occasionally	Never
1.	Have you noticed that you don't hear as well as you used to?			
2.	Has anybody told you that you don't hear well?			
3.	Does your family tell you that you turn up the volume of the television or radio very loudly?			
4.	When you're talking to someone, do you have to ask the person to speak louder?			
5.	When you're talking to someone, do you have to ask the person to repeat what they're saying various times?			
		No, I Can't	With Some Difficulty	Yes, Without Difficulty
6.	Can you understand when someone is speaking to you in a low voice?			
7.	Can you understand when someone is speaking to you on the telephone?			
8.	Can you hear the sound of a coin dropping on the floor?			
9.	Can you hear the sound of a door closing?			
10.	Can you hear when someone approaches you from behind?			
11.	Can you hear when someone is speaking to you in a noisy setting such as a pub or restaurant?			
12.	Can you hold a conversation in a group setting when several people are speaking at the same time?			

Figure 3-6 Hearing-Dependent Daily Activities (HDDA) Scale. (From American Academy of Family Physicians. Hidalgo JL-T, et al. The hearing-dependent daily activities scale to evaluate impact of hearing loss in older people. *Ann Fam Med*. 2008;6:441-447.)

12 questions about their level of hearing and understanding. Each question has a range of three possible answers. The lower the score, the greater the impact of hearing loss on the patient's daily activities.

Cognition

Dementia is a chronic, progressive loss of cognitive and intellectual functions. Early screening for dementia becomes more important with the advent of newer treatment regimens. The Mini-Cog test is a 3-minute instrument to screen for cognitive impairment in older adults in the primary care setting. The Mini-Cog uses a three-item recall test for memory and a simply scored clock-drawing test (CDT). The latter serves as an "informative distractor," helping to clarify scores when the memory recall score is intermediate. The Mini-Cog was as effective as or better than established screening tests in both an epidemiologic survey in a mainstream sample and a multiethnic, multilingual population comprising many individuals of low socioeconomic status and education level. In comparative tests, the Mini-Cog was at least twice as fast as the mini-mental state examination. The Mini-Cog is less affected by subject ethnicity, language, and education and can detect a variety of different dementias. Moreover, the Mini-Cog detects many people with mild cognitive impairment (cognitive impairment too mild to meet diagnostic criteria for dementia). For scoring, one point is given for each recalled word. The CDT is scored as either "normal" (patient places the correct time and the clock appears grossly normal) or "abnormal" (incorrect time or abnormal clock). A score of zero is positive for cognitive impairment. An abnormal CDT with a score of 1 or 2 on the three-word recall test is positive for cognitive impairment. A normal CDT and a score of 1 or 2 on the word recall test is negative for cognitive impairment.

Mood

Depression is common in elderly people and may go undetected unless specifically screened for. If the patient gives a positive response to either of the two questions below, further inquiry is needed.

- Over the past month, have you often been bothered by feeling sad, depressed, or hopeless?
- During the past month, have you often been bothered by little interest or pleasure in doing things?

The Geriatric Depression Scale (GDS) is designed specifically to screen for depression in older adults. The GDS questions are answered yes or no. This simplicity enables the scale to be used with ill or moderately cognitively impaired individuals. Two different scales are available: a long form that contains 30 questions, and a short form that contains 15 questions. Either form may be used as part of a comprehensive geriatric assessment. The scoring for the long form, shown in Figure 3-7, sets a range of 0 to 9 as "normal," 10 to 19 as "mildly depressed," and 20 to 30 as "severely depressed." The short form has a similar scale, with 0 to 4 being "normal," 5 to 7 "mildly depressed," 8 to 11 "moderately depressed," and 12 to 15 "severely depressed."

Gait and Mobility

Falls are a significant cause of morbidity and mortality in elderly people; therefore, the focus should be on preventing falls. Environmental factors that can help prevent falls include adequate lighting, use of grab bars or assistive devices such as canes or walkers, a clutter-free environment, and removing throw rugs or having nonskid backs on all rugs. If there are pets in the house, patients should be alert to their location to avoid tripping over them. Nonenvironmental factors that may cause falls include decrease in vision; lack of flexibility; loss of muscle strength, especially in the legs; and changes in sleep patterns. Other important risk factors for falls in elderly people are medication use and chronic health conditions. High-risk medications include calcium channel blockers, analgesics, sedatives, and hypnotics. Conditions such as heart disease, peripheral vascular disease, neuropathies, and bladder incontinence can also increase the risk for falling.

Several tools exist to help determine a person's risk for falling. One very simple test is the Timed Up and Go test. The score is recorded as the number of seconds it took to complete the test and gives an assessment of the patient's mobility. Another tool is the Berg Balance Test, which is a performance-based assessment tool that is used to evaluate standing balance during functional activities. The patient is scored on 14 different tasks, such as reaching, bending, transferring, and standing. Elements of the test are representative of daily activities that require balance, such as sitting, standing, leaning over, and stepping. Some tasks are rated according to the quality of the performance of the task, whereas others are evaluated by the time required to complete the task. Scores for each item range from 0 (cannot perform) to 4 (normal performance). Overall scores range from 0 (severely impaired balance) to 56 (excellent balance). The Tinetti Performance Oriented Mobility Assessment tool is a test that evaluates both balance and gait. It starts with a component to measure balance, very similar to the Timed Up and Go test described earlier. In addition, the gait is evaluated for step length and height, symmetry, and continuity. Other factors such as trunk motion and walking stance are included in the scoring. The score indicates the patient's risk of falling as low, medium, or high; the lower the score, the greater the risk of falling.

Nutrition

Aging is accompanied by physiologic changes that can negatively affect nutritional status. Sensory impairments that occur with aging, such as decreased sense of taste and smell, may result in decreased appetite. Poor oral health and dental problems can lead to difficulty chewing, inflammation, and a monotonous diet that is poor in quality, all of which increase the risk for malnutrition. Progressive loss of vision and hearing, as well as osteoarthritis, may limit mobility and affect an elderly person's ability to shop for food and prepare meals. Energy needs decrease with age, yet the need for most nutrients remains relatively unchanged, resulting in an increased risk for malnutrition.

The Mini Nutritional Assessment—Short Form (MNA-SF) provides an easy way to screen elderly patients for malnutrition in less than 5 minutes. The form consists of six questions and has been validated as an efficient screening tool. The score for screening is derived from six components—reduced food intake in the preceding 3 months; weight loss during the preceding 3 months; mobility; psychological stress or acute disease in the preceding 3 months; neuropsychological problems; and BMI. The MNA-SF has predictive validity for adverse health outcome, social functioning, and rate of visits to the general practitioner as well as length of hospital stay, likelihood

Geriatric Depression Scale, Long Form

1. Are you basically satisfied with your life?
2. Have you dropped many of your activities and interests?
3. Do you feel that your life is empty?
4. Do you often get bored?
5. Are you hopeful about the future?
6. Are you bothered by thoughts you can't get out of your head?
7. Are you in good spirits most of the time?
8. Are you afraid that something bad is going to happen to you?
9. Do you feel happy most of the time?
10. Do you often feel helpless?
11. Do you often get restless and fidgety?
12. Do you prefer to stay at home, rather than going out and doing new things?
13. Do you frequently worry about the future?
14. Do you feel you have more problems with memory than most?
15. Do you think it is wonderful to be alive now?
16. Do you often feel downhearted and blue?
17. Do you feel pretty worthless the way you are now?
18. Do you worry a lot about the past?
19. Do you find life very exciting?
20. Is it hard for you to get started on new projects?
21. Do you feel full of energy?
22. Do you feel that your situation is hopeless?
23. Do you think that most people are better off than you are?
24. Do you frequently get upset over little things?
25. Do you frequently feel like crying?
26. Do you have trouble concentrating?
27. Do you enjoy getting up in the morning?
28. Do you prefer to avoid social gatherings?
29. Is it easy for you to make decisions?
30. Is your mind as clear as it used to be?

Original scoring for the scale; one point for each of these answers.

1. no	11. yes	21. no
2. yes	12. yes	22. yes
3. yes	13. yes	23. yes
4. yes	14. yes	24. yes
5. no	15. no	25. yes
6. yes	16. yes	26. yes
7. no	17. yes	27. no
8. yes	18. yes	28. yes
9. no	19. no	29. no
10. yes	20. yes	30. no

Scale

0–9	Normal range
10–19	Mild depression
20–30	Severe depression

Figure 3-7 Geriatric Depression Scale, long form. (From Brink TL, Yesavage JA, Lum O, Heersema P, Adey MB, Rose TL. Screening tests for geriatric depression. *Clinical Gerontologist 1:* 37-44, 1982.

of discharge to a nursing home, and mortality. The complete tool and scoring criteria may be accessed at www.mna-elderly.com.

Another screening tool for use with elderly patients is the Malnutrition Universal Screening Tool (MUST). This tool derives a score classifying malnutrition risk as low, medium, or high on the basis of three components—BMI, history of unexplained weight loss, and acute illness effect. MUST was developed primarily for use in the community (where it predicts admission rates and need for general practitioner visits) but has also been shown to have high predictive validity in the hospital environment (length of hospital stay, mortality in elderly wards, discharge destination in orthopedic patients). Complete information on using this screening tool and scoring criteria can be found at www.bapen.org.uk.

To reinforce the content of this chapter, please complete the worksheets that follow.

1. List the five components of the adult preventive care examination.

_____
_____
_____
_____
_____

2. List at least five risk factors that should be screened for in the personal history.

_____
_____
_____
_____
_____

3. List at least three diseases that are related to tobacco use.

_____
_____
_____

4. List the four questions that make up the CAGE questionnaire.

_____
_____
_____
_____

5. List one advantage of the AUDIT screening tool compared with the CAGE questionnaire.

_____
_____

6. List at least five substances that are screened for with the NIDA Modified ASSIST.

_____
_____
_____
_____
_____

7. List the five Ps of the sexual history.

_____

_____

_____

_____

_____

8. List three questions that are used to screen for IPV.

_____

_____

_____

9. List at least four facts that should be documented when a patient discloses IPV.

_____

_____

_____

_____

10. List at least three potential complications associated with blood transfusion.

_____

_____

_____

11. List at least four conditions that have a genetic predisposition that should be screened for when taking a patient's family medical history.

_____

_____

_____

_____

12. List at least five activities of daily living.

_____

_____

_____

_____

_____

13. List at least five independent activities of daily living.

_____

_____

_____

_____

_____

14. List at least five factors that may contribute to falls in elderly patients.

_____

_____

_____

_____

_____

15. Inez Lewis is a 68-year-old woman who presents for her annual WWE. She has a personal history of hypertension and a family history of glaucoma. List at least five screening examinations that could be ordered for Ms. Lewis.

_____

_____

_____

_____

_____

_____

16. Gene Ankar is a 52-year-old man who presents for his annual well-man examination. List two specific physical examination components and at least three screening tests that could be ordered for this patient, based on USPSTF recommendations.

_____

_____

_____

_____

_____

_____

Sexual History

Jennifer Erwin, a 23-year-old woman, comes in for her annual WWE. The sexual history documented for this visit is shown below. Read it and then answer the questions that follow.

In the past 2 months, Ms. Erwin has had 3 partners. In the past year, she has had approximately 9 or 10 partners. She denies anal intercourse. Does engage in oral sex. She had been treated for an STD once in the past. She is on Seasonique oral contraceptive.

1. What additional information should have been included in Ms. Erwin's sexual history?

_____

_____

_____

_____

2. What counseling or education would you provide to Ms. Erwin during this visit?

_____

_____

_____

_____

3. What physical examination should be done during this visit?

_____

_____

4. List at least three screening examinations or tests (including those recommended by the USPSTF) that should be done during this visit.

_____

_____

Geriatric Screening

Mr. Jonas Hammel is an 84-year-old man who comes in for his annual examination. He lives alone but is accompanied by his daughter-in-law Linda, who is concerned that Mr. Hammel seems to have trouble remembering things lately. Mr. Hammel has had an unintentional weight loss of 14 pounds since his last examination 1 year ago. During the examination, you administer the Mini-Cog test. You name three items (ball, tree, chair) and have Mr. Hammel repeat them, which he is able to do without difficulty. You instruct him to draw a clock and to indicate 10 minutes after 8:00. His attempt at the clock-drawing test is shown below. Later, you ask him to recall the three items; he is able to recall only "tree."

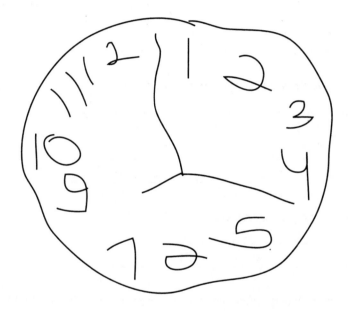

1. Based on the information above, how would you interpret Mr. Hammel's Mini-Cog results?

_____

2. What additional screening examinations could be conducted as part of the evaluation of Mr. Hammel's weight loss?

_____

_____

3. Based on the USPSTF Adult Preventive Care Timeline, what other screening tests could be done at this visit?

_____

_____

_____

4. Based on his age, Mr. Hammel could be screened for other risk factors; name at least four.

_____

_____

_____

_____

Worksheet 3.4

Family History Screening

Mr. Keith Shipley is a 42-year-old man who is new to your practice. He has a personal history of hypertension and dyslipidemia. Results of his family history screening are shown below. After reading the history, answer the questions that follow.

Father: 77 years old, alive, fairly good health. Has rheumatoid arthritis, HTN, high cholesterol, and BPH.

Mother: 72 years old. Treated for colon cancer at age 56. Fair health at present.

Brother: 45 years old. Diagnosed with colon cancer 4 years ago. Had surgery.

Sister: 39 years old, alive and well. No known health problems.

PGF: health history is unknown.

PGM: died of stroke at age 81.

MGF: died of complications of pneumonia at age 72.

MGM: died at age 64; unsure of cause of death.

1. Identify the red flags from this patient's family history.

_____

_____

_____

2. What conditions with a known genetic familial tendency should Mr. Shipley be screened for at this time?

_____

_____

_____

3. Based on USPSTF recommendations, what additional screening should Mr. Shipley have at this time?

_____

_____

_____

4. What patient counseling or education should be provided to Mr. Shipley and documented in his medical record?

_____

_____

_____

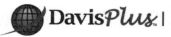 **DavisPlus** | Visit **http://davisplus.fadavis.com** for complete learning activities on actual EMR software at, Keyword: Sullivan

Adult Immunizations

Consult the current adult immunization recommendations available at the CDC website (www.cdc.gov/VACCINES/RECS/schedules/adult-schedule.htm#print). Answer the questions below.

1. What vaccines are indicated for a 40-year-old man who has sex with men and who had his last tetanus immunization 6 years ago?

_____

_____

2. Which three vaccines are contraindicated in pregnant women?

_____

_____

3. What vaccines are recommended for a 21-year-old woman who plans to start nursing school in 6 months who received one HPV vaccine at age 12?

_____

_____

4. What vaccines are recommended for a 63-year-old woman who volunteers at a public library and has diabetes?

_____

_____

5. A 34-year-old man undergoes splenectomy following an accident in which he sustained blunt abdominal trauma. Which vaccines are indicated for this patient?

_____

_____

Worksheet 3.6

Abbreviations

These abbreviations were introduced in Chapter 3. Beside each, write the meaning as indicated by the context of this chapter.

ADL _____

AHRQ _____

AUDIT _____

BMD _____

BPH _____

CAD _____

CDC _____

CDT _____

CTS _____

DAST-10 _____

FBS _____

FOBT _____

GDS _____

HDDA _____

HDL _____

HHS _____

HPV _____

HTLV-1 _____

HTLV-2 _____

IADL _____

IPV _____

MNA-SF _____

MUST _____

NIDA Modified ASSIST _____

OSHA _____

PID _____

PPD _____

STD _____

STI _____

USPSTF _____

VDRL _____

WWE _____

Chapter 4

Pediatric Preventive Care Visits

OBJECTIVES

- Discuss the goals of the Medicaid Early and Periodic Screening, Diagnosis, and Treatment (EPSDT) program.
- Identify measurements that are used as part of growth screening.
- Discuss developmental milestones and screening tools used to evaluate attainment of these milestones.
- Identify laboratory tests that are part of newborn screening and preventive care visits.
- Identify resources for pediatric immunization schedules.
- Discuss the importance of providing and documenting anticipatory guidance for parents and guardians of pediatric patients.
- Discuss risk factor identification in the pediatric and adolescent populations.
- Discuss the importance of obtaining an adolescent psychosocial history and tools that may be used to gather and document it.
- Identify components of a sports preparticipation history and physical examination.

Pediatric preventive care visits, or well-child visits, are often enjoyable for the provider and may provide an opportunity for you to interact with a patient who is not "ill." In obtaining the subjective information, you will often have to rely on parents or caregivers of the patient to provide the medical history. Because children at certain ages are unable to voice their problems or concerns, you may have to rely more heavily on the objective data you obtain during a visit. Observing interactions between the child and parents or caregiver becomes an important part of the pediatric preventive care visit.

Age is an important consideration when conducting and documenting well-child visits. Age is documented in months when the child is 24 months or younger and in years and months for children older than 24 months (e.g., "17 months," and "3 years, 8 months"). Patients younger than 18 years are generally considered to be pediatric patients, although some guidelines include patients up to 21 years of age. Most screening and immunization guidelines are age specific; therefore, it is important to document the date of birth accurately and calculate the child's age at each visit.

Documenting preventive care visits for pediatric and adolescent children is often facilitated by the use of standardized forms. Many providers use forms that have been specifically developed for the Early and Periodic Screening, Diagnosis, and Treatment (EPSDT) program. This federally mandated program is the child health component of Medicaid and is the most comprehensive child health program in either the public or private sector. EPSDT requires states to assess a child's health needs through initial and periodic examinations and evaluations to ensure that health problems are diagnosed and treated early, before they become more complex and their treatment becomes more costly. States must perform medical, vision, hearing, and dental checkups according to standardized schedules.

Most states have adopted their own EPSDT forms to ensure compliance with federal requirements and

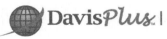 Visit **http://davisplus.fadavis.com** for complete learning activities on actual EMR software at, Keyword: Sullivan

to serve as a guideline for conducting periodic screening examinations. These forms are readily available on the Internet by using the state name and EPSDT as the search term. The American Academy of Pediatrics (AAP) has developed a set of Pediatric Visit Documentation Forms for well-child visits from the initial visit at 2 weeks of age up to the 2-year well-child visit. The forms may be viewed and ordered from the organization's website at www.aap.org. Health history forms such as the one shown in Figure 4-1 may also be used and can be tailored to a specific practice setting.

Components of Pediatric Preventive Care Visits

The components of well-child visits generally follow the format of the comprehensive history and physical

---

To be completed by parent or guardian   **Today's Date:** __/__/__

Child's Name: _____ Date of Birth: __/__/__ ☐ Male ☐ Female
Mother's Name: _____ Father's Name: _____
Address: _____
Home Phone: _____ Mother's Work Phone: _____ Father's Work phone: _____
Sibling's names and ages: _____
Person completing form/relationship: _____

Birth and Development History:
Mother's age at time of delivery: _____   Type of delivery: ☐ vaginal ☐ cesarean
Birth weight: _____
Problems during pregnancy: _____ Obstetrician: _____
Feeding: ☐ breast ☐ bottle   Type of formula: _____ Vitamins: ☐ yes ☐ no

Medical History: (Check if the child has ever had any of the following)

☐ Allergies   ☐ Bladder infection   ☐ Eye problems   ☐ Feeding problems
☐ Anemia   ☐ Breathing problems   ☐ Hearing problems   ☐ Skin problems
☐ Asthma   ☐ Bowel problems   ☐ Kidney problems   ☐ Sleep problems
☐ Bedwetting   ☐ Easy bruising/   ☐ Liver problems   ☐ Seizures
                        bleeding

☐ Serious injury (type _____)

Current Medications (please include prescription and over-the-counter medications):

Name of Medication	Dose (mg)	Taken how many times a day?

Medication allergies: ☐ None _____

Please list any hospitalizations (other than delivery) or surgeries.

Year	Procedure or Reason for Hospitalization	Doctor	Which hospital?

Social History:
Parents' marital status: ☐ married ☐ single ☐ separated ☐ divorced
Any smokers in the house? ☐ yes ☐ no
If divorced or separated, who has legal custody? _____
Car Seat/Seat Belt use: ☐ yes ☐ no   Helmet or other safety measures: ☐ yes ☐ no
Smoke detector in the house? ☐ yes ☐ no   Do you have a pool? ☐ yes ☐ no   If yes, is it fenced? ☐ yes ☐ no

Immunizations (list dates and any severe reactions):
DTP/Td _____   Oral polio _____
MMR _____   HIB-c _____   varicella _____
Cocci (skin test) _____   TB skin test _____

Figure 4-1 Pediatric medical history form.

examination (see Table 2.1), with minor variations related to age. EPSDT-mandated components of pediatric preventive care (or screening) visits include the following:

- Growth screening
- Developmental screening
- Laboratory screening tests
- Assessment of immunization status and administration as appropriate
- Anticipatory guidance, counseling, and education
- Risk factor identification

Growth Screening

Growth and development are important parameters that should be assessed routinely during well-child visits. Growth generally refers to the increase in size of the body as a whole or its separate parts. Growth charts are used to assess and compare a child's growth with a nationally representative reference population and are available for boys, birth to 36 months; girls, birth to 36 months; boys 2 to 20 years; and girls, 2 to 20 years. Growth charts provide an overview of the normal growth trajectory of children, thus alerting the provider to what is atypical or disturbed. Standardized growth charts are available from the Centers for Disease Control and Prevention (CDC) and can be viewed at and downloaded from the organization's website at www.cdc.gov/growthcharts. The measurements typically recorded during the first 2 years of life are length (or height), weight, and head circumference. After the age of 2 years, head circumference may not be measured at every visit if the child's development has been consistent. Body mass index (BMI) should be calculated and documented beginning at 2 years of age, when an accurate stature can be obtained, to screen for childhood obesity.

A sample growth chart for plotting length and weight for age is shown in Figure 4-2. To plot the length, find the age across the top of the length graph and then find the length in inches along the left axis. Follow each line to the intersecting point and mark. To plot the weight, find the child's age across the bottom of the weight graph and the weight in pounds along the right axis. Follow each line to the intersecting point and mark. You will notice lines curving across the chart with small numbers corresponding to each line at the right side of the chart. These numbers refer to percentiles. Percentile is the most commonly used clinical indicator to assess the size and growth patterns of individual children in the United States. Percentiles rank the position of an individual by indicating what percentage of the reference population the individual would equal or exceed. For example, on the weight-for-age growth charts, a 5-year-old girl whose weight is at the 25th percentile weighs the same or more than 25% of the reference population of 5-year-old girls and weighs less than 75% of 5-year-old girls.

Application Exercise 4.1

On the sample growth chart shown in Figure 4-2, plot the length and weight for Kevin, a 21-month-old boy. His length is 33 inches, and his weight is 29 pounds. Determine Kevin's percentile for length and weight.

Application Exercise 4.1 Answer
Compare your marks on the graph with those shown in Figure 4-3.

Excess weight and obesity in children are significant public health problems in the United States. The number of adolescents who are overweight has tripled since 1980, and the prevalence among younger children has more than doubled. The CDC recognizes four categories of weight status: underweight (less than 5th percentile), healthy weight (5th percentile to less than 85th percentile), overweight (85th to 95th percentile), and obese (equal to or greater than 95th percentile). Obesity disproportionately affects certain minority youth populations. The National Health and Nutrition Examination Survey (2008), or NHANES, found that African American and Mexican American adolescents ages 12 to 19 years were more likely to be overweight, at 21% and 23%, respectively, than non-Hispanic white adolescents (14%). Being overweight during childhood and adolescence increases the risk for developing high cholesterol, hypertension, respiratory ailments, orthopedic problems, depression, and type 2 diabetes. The incidence of type 2 diabetes has increased dramatically in children and adolescents, particularly in American Indian, African American, and Hispanic/Latino populations. The CDC, together with the National Center for Health Statistics, developed a graph for plotting BMI percentiles. It is shown in Figure 4-4 and is available at www.cdc.gov/growthcharts. BMI calculators are readily available online at various Internet sites.

Developmental Screening

Developmental milestones are physical or behavioral signs of development or maturation of infants and children. Rolling over, crawling, walking, and talking are considered developmental milestones and provide important information regarding the child's development. The milestones are different for each age range. The milestones are identifiable skills that can serve as

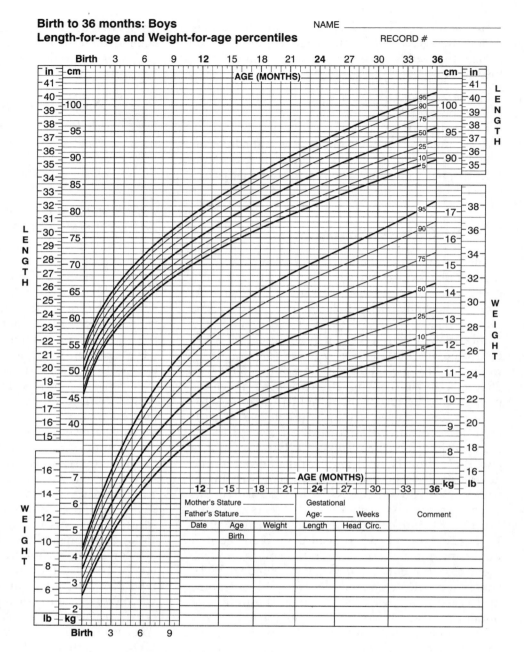

Figure 4-2 A sample growth chart. (Developed by the National Center for Health Statistics in collaboration with the National Center for Chronic Disease Prevention and Health Promotion [2000] and modified 4/20/01.)

a guide to normal development. Typically, simple skills need to be reached before the more complex skills can be learned. There is a general age and time when most children pass through these periods of development.

There are also specific speech and language milestones. Children vary in their development of speech and language; however, there is a natural progression or "timetable" for mastery of speech and language skills.

Developmental screening includes subjective information from parents and caregivers and objective information observed by the clinician. If a child fails to meet developmental milestones at the appropriate age, or if there is any suspicion of developmental delay,

formal developmental testing is usually warranted. There are numerous developmental tests that can be used to screen for developmental delay. Some are aimed at parents, whereas health-care providers complete others. The Denver Developmental Screening Test II (DDST-II) is a 125-item standardized measure that is designed to determine whether a child's development is within the normal range. It includes a set of questions for parents and tests for the child on 20 simple tasks and items that fall into four sectors: personal-social (25 items), fine motor adaptive (29 items), language (39 items), and gross motor (32 items). The number of items administered during an assessment will vary with the child's age and ability. The DDST-II scoring

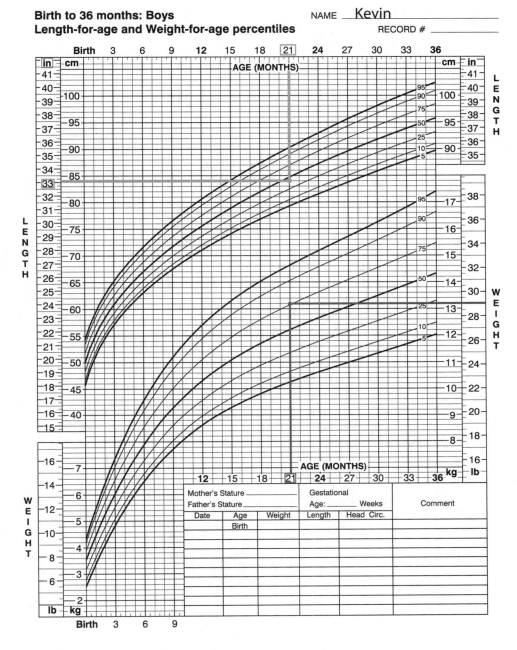

Birth to 36 months: Boys
Length-for-age and Weight-for-age percentiles

NAME _Kevin_____

RECORD # _____

Figure 4-3 A sample growth chart showing Kevin's weight and length. Kevin's weight is in the 75th percentile, and his length is in the 50th percentile. (Developed by the National Center for Health Statistics in collaboration with the National Center for Chronic Disease Prevention and Health Promotion [2000] and modified 4/20/01.)

process, which is described in the screening manual, requires that the individual test items be interpreted before the entire test is interpreted. Screeners must be properly trained and pass a proficiency test before using the DDST-II for clinical purposes.

The Bayley Scales of Infant Development, 3rd edition (2009), also known as Bayley-III, are recognized as one of the most comprehensive tools to assess children from as young as 1 month old. With Bayley-III, it is possible to obtain detailed information even from nonverbal children as to their functioning. Children are assessed in the five key developmental domains of cognition, language, social-emotional, motor, and adaptive behavior. Bayley-III identifies infant and toddler strengths and competencies as well as weaknesses. It also provides a valid and reliable measure of a child's abilities, in addition to giving comparison data for children with high-incidence clinical diagnoses. It takes between 45 and 60 minutes to administer. A specific kit must be purchased to administer the Bayley-III.

One tool that parents can complete is the Parents' Evaluation of Developmental Status (2007), or PEDS. PEDS contains 10 open-ended questions that elicit parents' concerns about their child. It is both an evidence-based surveillance tool and a screening test. PEDS can be used from birth to 8 years of age.

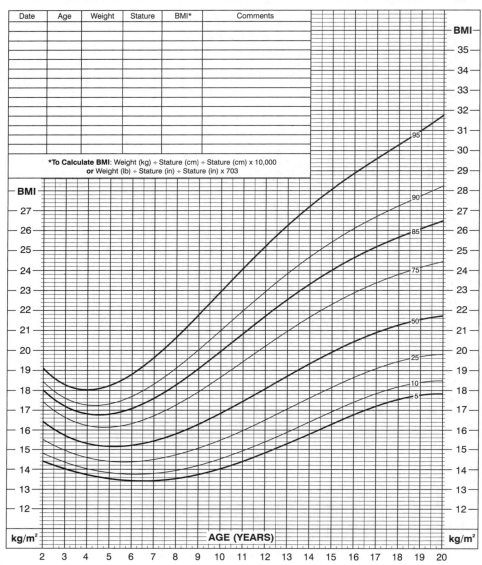

2 to 20 years: Girls
Body mass index-for-age percentiles

NAME _____

RECORD # _____

Figure 4-4 Body mass index graph. (Developed by the National Center for Health Statistics in collaboration with the National Center for Chronic Disease Prevention and Health Promotion [2000] and modified 10/16/00.)

It takes just a few minutes to administer and score if conducted as an interview. Less time is required if parents complete the questionnaire while waiting or at home before the visit. There is also a version that is used to assess attainment of developmental milestones, known as PEDS-DM. These tools are available in English, Spanish, and Vietnamese. Information is readily available from Ellsworth and Vandermeer Press or at www.pedstest.com.

Another screening tool that uses parent reporting is the Ages and Stages Questionnaires, 3rd edition (ASQ-3). It contains 21 age-specific questionnaires, which allow for accurate screening anytime between 1 month and 5½ years of age. Questions are asked to which parents answer "yes," "sometimes," or "not yet."

It takes approximately 10 to 15 minutes for parents to complete the questionnaire and 2 to 3 minutes for scoring. There is an initial cost for the kit, which provides a user guide, scoring sheets, and a master set of all 21 questionnaires for printing and photocopying. The third edition is available in English and Spanish; the second edition is available in French. Contact Paul H. Brooks Publishing Co., Inc. for more information.

Laboratory Screening Tests

The federal Maternal and Child Health Bureau (MCHB) of the Health Resources and Services Administration (HRSA) has been involved with newborn screening and genetic testing and services since the early 1960s. The goal of screening is to decrease or to eliminate the catastrophic effects of preventable mental retardation. Genetic disease gained recognition with the introduction of the newborn screening program for phenylketonuria (PKU). In the United States, the early screening of children for special health-care needs and congenital disorders begins in the newborn period. Under the direction of state public health agencies, all infants are tested for certain genetic conditions, such as hemoglobinopathies, metabolic disorders, hearing loss, and other congenital conditions.

Although there are no national newborn screening standards at this time, agencies such as the MCHB, CDC, and AAP are working toward establishing a standardized screening panel. The panel of newborn disorders screened for varies from state to state. States routinely test blood collected from newborns for up to 30 metabolic and genetic diseases; the 6 most commonly included are medium-chain acyl-CoA dehydrogenase (MCAD) deficiency, congenital hypothyroidism, PKU, neonatal hyperbilirubinemia, biotinidase deficiency, and sickle cell anemia. Many of these tests are administered at the hospital before the infant's discharge. States may require certain screenings to be performed more than once. The National Newborn Screening and Genetics Resource Center has a U.S. map on its website, where you can select a state and then view a table of the required screenings (http://genes-r-us. uthscsa.edu/resources/consumer/statemap.htm).

The CDC recommends routine screening for lead exposure between the ages of 9 and 12 months and again at 24 months, but public health authorities in each state are responsible for setting state and local policy. A screening questionnaire of three questions may also be used to determine whether lead screening is needed. Children whose parents respond "yes" or "not sure" to any of these three risk assessment questions should be considered for screening:

1. Does your child live in or regularly visit a house or child care facility built before 1950?
2. Does your child live in or regularly visit a house or child care facility built before 1978 that is being or has recently been renovated or remodeled?
3. Does your child have a sibling or playmate who has or had lead poisoning?

Assessing Immunization Status

Vaccine-preventable disease levels are at or near record lows. Even though most infants and toddlers have received all recommended vaccines by 2 years of age, many underimmunized children remain, leaving

the potential for outbreaks of disease. Many adolescents are underimmunized as well, missing opportunities to protect themselves against diseases such as hepatitis B, influenza, and pneumococcal disease. Every pediatric visit, whether for preventive care or evaluation of an illness or injury, is an opportunity to assess the child's immunization history and determine whether immunizations need to be administered. The CDC and the National Immunization Program publish recommendations for childhood (birth to 6 years of age) and adolescent (7 to 18 years of age) immunizations. They also publish a catch-up schedule for children who were not immunized at the recommended ages. The recommendations are updated annually; visit the CDC website at www.cdc.gov to obtain the most current schedule.

MEDICOLEGAL ALERT !

Some parents or guardians may not want their child to receive immunizations. If the parents or guardians refuse immunizations, you should ask why they are refusing. The parents may have misinformation about the risks of immunizations, they may not understand the reason for immunizations, or they may refuse immunizations because of cultural or religious beliefs. It is important to provide education to the parents about the benefits and risks of immunizations, but ultimately, the parents have the right to refuse. Any attempts you make at educating the parents on the benefits and risks of immunizations should be documented, along with any written material or other resources you may have given them.

Anticipatory Guidance

Anticipatory guidance refers to specific topics that should be discussed with parents and caregivers of pediatric patients at age-appropriate levels. As children grow and develop, we anticipate that they will be involved in certain activities. For instance, many children learn to ride bicycles at about 4 to 5 years of age. Anticipating that this may occur should prompt you to educate parents and caregivers that they should talk to the child about bicycle safety, wearing a helmet, wearing reflective clothing, and so forth. Table 4-1 presents topics that should be addressed with parents and caregivers based on the age of the child. Many EPSDT forms list the specific anticipatory guidance that should be discussed at each age-specific visit. Be sure to document which topics are discussed with the parent or caregiver.

Table 4-1	Age-Specific Anticipatory Guidance

Age at Visit	Topics to Discuss
Birth to 2 weeks	Good parenting practices; postpartum adjustment; infant care/sleep positioning; injury prevention; closeness with the baby; individuality of infants; breastfeeding or bottle feeding; signs of illness
1 month	Injury prevention; sleep practices; sleep positioning; bladder and bowel habits; nutrition; infant development; when to call the doctor; infant care; plans for next visit
2 months	Injury prevention; nutrition; sleep positioning/practices; fever education; family relationships; other child care providers; talk to baby; pacifiers, bottle tooth decay
4 months	Injury prevention; choking, aspiration; teething; solid foods; sleep positioning; thumb sucking; baby-proof home; appropriate child care providers
6 months	Injury prevention; cup, finger foods; no bottle in bed; pool and tub safety; teething; poisons—ipecac; nutrition; sleep positioning
9–12 months	Baby-proof home and pool; shoes—protection, not support; talk to child; self-feeding; sleep; discipline; praise; dental hygiene
15–18 months	Safety; tantrums; eating; discipline/limits; sleeping; snacks; dental hygiene; no bottles; sibling interaction; read to child; toilet training; aspiration
2–3 years	Decreased appetite, brushing teeth; toilet training; read to child; independence/dependence; car, home, and swimming pool safety; preschool; control of TV viewing
4–5 years	Preschool and school readiness (attention span, easy separation from parents); seat belts; street safety; should know full name, address, and phone number; household chores; no playing with matches; sexual curiosity
6–9 years	Water, seat belts, skateboard, and bicycle safety; dental hygiene; peer relations; nutrition; limit setting; regular physical activity; parental role model; communication
10–14 years	Safety issues; nutrition; dental hygiene; peer pressure; smoking, alcohol, and drugs; puberty; safe sex/contraception/STD prevention; communication
15–18 years	Safety issues; dental hygiene; smoking, alcohol, and drugs; safe sex/contraception/STD prevention; communication, dating, peer pressure, motor vehicle safety; sports safety; staying in school

Adapted from Early Periodic Screening Diagnosis and Treatment (EPSDT) program guidelines. The EPSDT is a national Medicaid program. More information is available at http://www.hcfa.gov/medicaid/epsdthm.htm.

Risk Factor Identification

For infants and younger children, risk factors for developing diseases or conditions are often related to the mother's health during pregnancy. Therefore, a maternal history should be documented for all children 2 years of age or younger and may be indicated in older children if there is concern for developmental delay or if the child has physical abnormalities. The maternal history can be divided into two main components: genetic and teratology history and infection history.

In addition to assessing risk factors related to maternal health, exploration of the genetic and teratology history should include questions regarding the father and families of both parents. The disorders that should be screened for are shown in Figure 4-5. Specific questions for maternal history include metabolic disorders (such as type 1 diabetes), prior pregnancy loss or stillbirth, medications (including supplements, vitamins, herbs, and over-the-counter medications), street drugs, alcohol use during pregnancy, and occupational or environmental hazards.

Risk factor screening for prenatal exposure to mumps, rubella, rubeola, varicella-zoster, or other viral illnesses is part of the infection history. Determine whether there is maternal hepatitis B, HIV, human papillomavirus, syphilis, gonorrhea, chlamydia, or other sexually transmitted infections. Inquire about a history of toxoplasmosis, cytomegalovirus, or group B streptococcus. Exposure to any of these infections poses a risk for fetal malformation or birth defects.

Data show that health risks in adolescents are more social in origin than medical. The American Medical Association's Department of Adolescent Health developed the Guidelines for Adolescent Preventive Services (GAPS) with the goal of improving health-care delivery to adolescents using primary and secondary interventions to prevent and reduce adolescent morbidity and mortality. The use of GAPS enables the health-care provider to restructure the visit from a focus on traditional assessment of wellness to identification and treatment of at-risk behaviors such as drinking, unprotected sex, nicotine use, or thoughtless or careless approaches to life. GAPS consists of 24 recommendations that encompass health-care delivery, health guidance, screening, and immunizations.

Specific screening tools have been developed for gathering the psychosocial history of adolescents.

Screening for Genetic and Teratology Risk Factors

Thalassemia	Huntington chorea
Neural tube defect (spina bifida, meningomyelocele)	Mental retardation
Congenital heart disease	Autism
Tay-Sachs, Canavan, Neimann-Pick disease	Hemophilia
Sickle cell disease or trait	Rh sensitized
Muscular dystrophy	Down syndrome
Cystic fibrosis	Other inherited genetic or chromosomal disorder

Figure 4-5 Screening for genetic and teratology risk factors.

One commonly used tool can be remembered by the mnemonic HEEADSSS, which stands for home, education/employment, eating, activities, drugs, sexuality, suicide/depression, and safety. Henry Berman, MD, developed the original HEADS questionnaire in 1972. In 1985, it was expanded by Drs. Cohen and Goldering to HEADSS (adding suicide/depression screening), and this version was used for nearly 20 years. In 2004, it was updated again to address morbidity and mortality factors. The second "E" (eating) was added to encourage exploration of eating habits and screen for obesity and the third "S" (safety) to screen for unintentional injury and violence. The questions that comprise the HEEADSSS assessment are shown in Figure 4-6; notice that questions are identified as "essential," "as time permits," and "optional when a situation requires further questioning." Whenever possible, the interview should be conducted without the presence of parents, family members, or other involved adults.

Three out of four adolescent deaths are caused by unintentional injury (e.g., motor vehicle crashes, drownings, poisonings, burns) and violence (e.g., homicide, suicide). Risk factor screening should include questioning about violence—either as an observer, a victim, or an offender. The FISTS mnemonic is helpful to remember screening questions related to fights, injuries, sexual violence, threats, and self-defense strategies. Specific questions for each of these categories are shown in Figure 4-7.

Unfortunately, children and adolescents may also be the targets of intentional violence. Child abuse is one of the leading causes of injury-related infant and child mortality. The Child Abuse Prevention and Treatment Act (CAPTA) defines abuse as a recent act or failure to act that results in death, serious physical or emotional harm, sexual abuse or exploitation, or imminent risk for serious harm; involves a child; and is carried out by a parent or caregiver who is responsible for the child's welfare. Four types of abuse are generally recognized: neglect, physical abuse, sexual abuse, and emotional abuse. These types of abuse are more typically found in combination than alone. Each state is responsible for defining child abuse and maltreatment within its own civil and criminal codes.

The most common type of abuse is neglect. Neglect is the failure of a parent, guardian, or other caregiver to provide for a child's basic needs. Physical abuse is nonaccidental physical injury that is inflicted by a parent, caregiver, or other person who has responsibility for the child. Such injury is considered abuse regardless of whether the caregiver intended to hurt the child. Sexual abuse includes any sexually explicit conduct or simulation thereof for the purpose of producing a visual depiction of such conduct, or the rape, molestation, prostitution, or other form of sexual exploitation of children or incest with children. Emotional abuse is a pattern of behavior that impairs a child's emotional development or sense of self-worth. This may include constant criticism, threats, or rejection, as well as withholding love, support, or guidance. Emotional abuse is often difficult to prove and, therefore, child protective services may not be able to intervene without evidence of harm or mental injury to the child. Emotional abuse is almost always present when other forms are identified. Table 4-2, adapted from the Child Welfare Information Gateway, summarizes the signs that suggest abuse based on characteristics of the child or the parent or adult caregiver.

If any type of abuse is suspected, standardized tools are available to assist the health-care provider with additional screening and documentation. The Childhood Trauma Questionnaire (CTQ) is a 28-item self-report inventory intended to measure childhood or adolescent abuse and neglect. The central constructs underlying the questionnaire are

Home
Who lives with you?
Where do you live?
Do you have your own room?
What are relationships like at home?
To whom are you closest at home?
To whom can you talk at home?
Is there anyone new at home? Has someone left recently?
Have you moved recently?
Have you ever had to live away from home? If yes, why?
 • Have you ever run away? If yes, why?
 • Is there any physical violence at home?

Education and Employment
What are your favorite subjects at school? Your least favorite subjects?
How are your grades? Any recent changes? Any dramatic changes in the past?
Have you changed schools in the past few years?
What are your future education/employment plans/goals?
Are you working? Where? How much?
 • Tell me about your friends at school.
 • Is your school a safe place? Why or why not?
 • Have you ever had to repeat a class? Have you ever had to repeat a grade?
 • Have you ever been suspended? Expelled? Have you ever considered dropping out?
 • How well do you get along with the people at school? At work?
 • Have your responsibilities at work increased?
Do you feel connected to your school? Do you feel as if you belong?
Are there adults at your school you feel you could talk to about something important? Who?

Eating
What do you like and not like about your body?
Have there been any recent changes in your weight?
Have you dieted in the last year? How? How often?
Have you done anything else to try to manage your weight?
How much exercise do you get in an average day? Week?
What do you think would be a healthy diet? How does that compare to your current eating patterns?
 • Do you worry about your weight? How often?
 • Do you eat at home in front of the TV? Computer?
 • Does it ever seem as though your eating is out of control?
 • Have you ever made yourself throw up on purpose to control your weight?
 • Have you ever taken diet pills?
What would it be like if you gained (lost) 10 pounds?

Activities
What do you and your friends do for fun? (with whom, where, and when?)
What do you and your family do for fun? (with whom, where, and when?)
Do you participate in any sports or other activities?
 • Do you have any hobbies?
 • Do you read for fun? What?
 • How much TV do you watch in a week? How about video or computer games?
 • What music do you like to listen to?

Drugs
Do any of your friends use tobacco? Alcohol? Other drugs?
Does anyone in your family use tobacco? Alcohol? Other drugs?
Do you use tobacco? Alcohol? Other drugs?
Is there any history of alcohol or drug problems in your family?
Does anyone at home use tobacco?
 • Do you ever drink or use drugs when you're alone? (Assess frequency, intensity, patterns of use or abuse, and how
    youth obtains or pays for drugs, alcohol, or tobacco)

Sexuality
Have you ever been in a romantic relationship?
Tell me about the people that you've dated. OR Tell me about your sex life.
Have any of your relationships ever been sexual relationships?
What does the term "safe sex" mean to you?
 • Are you interested in boys? Girls? Both?
 • Have you ever been forced or pressured into doing something sexual that you didn't want to do?
 • Have you ever been touched sexually in a way that you didn't want?
 • Have you ever been raped, on a date or any other time?
 • How many sexual partners have you had altogether?

(continued)

- Have you ever been pregnant or worried that you might be pregnant? (females)
- Have you ever gotten someone pregnant or worried that that might have happened? (males)
- What are you using for birth control? Are you satisfied with your method?
- Do you use condoms every time you have intercourse?
- Does anything ever get in the way of always using a condom?
- Have you ever had a sexually transmitted disease or worried that you had an STD?

Suicide and Depression
Do you feel sad or down more than usual? Do you find yourself crying more than usual?
Are you "bored" all the time?
Are you having trouble getting to sleep?
Have you thought a lot about hurting yourself or someone else?
- Does it seem that you've lost interest in things that you used to really enjoy?
- Do you find yourself spending less and less time with friends?
- Would you rather just be by yourself most of the time?
- Have you ever tried to kill yourself?
- Have you ever had to hurt yourself (by cutting yourself, for example) to calm down or feel better?
- Have you started using alcohol or drugs to help you relax, calm down, or feel better?

Safety
Have you ever been seriously injured? (How?) How about anyone else you know?
Do you always wear a seat belt in the car?
Have you ever ridden with a driver who was drunk or high? When? How often?
Do you use safety equipment for sports and/or other physical activities (for example, helmets for bicycling or skateboarding)?
Is there any violence in your home? Does the violence ever get physical?
Is there a lot of violence at your school? In your neighborhood? Among your friends?
Have you ever been physically or sexually abused?
- Have you ever been in a car or motorcycle accident? (What happened?)
- Have you ever been picked on or bullied? Is that still a problem?
- Have you gotten into physical fights in school or your neighborhood? Are you still getting into fights?
- Have you ever felt that you had to carry a knife, gun, or other weapon to protect yourself? Do you still feel that way?

Italics = essential questions
- Bulleted items = as time permits
Bold italics = optional or when situation requires

Figure 4-6 The HEEADSSS psychosocial interview for adolescents.

Fighting:
- How many fights have you been in during the past year?
- When was your last fight?

Injuries:
- Have you ever been injured in a fight?
- Have you ever injured someone else in a fight?

Sexual Violence:
- Has your partner ever hit you?
- Have you ever hit (hurt) your partner?
- Have you ever been forced to have sex against your will?
- Do you think that couples can stay in love when one partner makes the other one afraid?

Threats:
- Has someone carrying a weapon ever threatened you?
- What happened?
- Has anything changed since then to make you feel safer?

Self-Defense
- What do you do if someone tries to pick a fight with you?
- Have you ever carried a weapon in self-defense?

Figure 4-7 FISTS screening questions.

Table 4-2 Signs of Child Abuse

Type of Abuse	Child Characteristics	Parent/Adult Characteristics
Neglect	Frequently absent from school; begs or steals food or money; lacks needed medical or dental care, immunizations, or glasses; is consistently dirty or has severe body odor; lacks sufficient clothing for the weather; states that there is no one at home to provide care	Appears indifferent to the child; seems apathetic or depressed; behaves irrationally or in a bizarre manner; is abusing alcohol or drugs
Physical	Has unexplained burns, bites, bruises, broken bones, or black eyes; has fading bruising or other marks noticeable after an absence from school; seems frightened of the parents and protests or cries when it is time to go home; shrinks at the approach of adults; reports injury by a parent or another adult caregiver	Offers conflicting, unconvincing, or no explanations for the child's injury; describes the child as "evil" or in some other very negative way; uses harsh physical discipline with the child; has a history of abuse as a child
Sexual	Has difficulty walking or sitting; suddenly refuses to change for gym or to participate in physical activities; reports nightmares or bedwetting; experiences a sudden change in appetite; demonstrates bizarre, sophisticated, or unusual sexual knowledge or behavior; runs away; becomes pregnant or contracts a sexually transmitted disease, particularly if younger than 14 years; reports sexual abuse by a parent or another adult caregiver	Is unduly protective of the child or severely limits the child's contact with other children, especially of the opposite sex; is secretive and isolated; is jealous or controlling with family members
Emotional	Shows extremes in behavior, such as overly compliant or demanding, extreme passivity or aggression; is either inappropriately adult or infantile; is delayed in physical or emotional development; has attempted suicide; reports a lack of attachment to the parent	Constantly blames, belittles, or berates the child; is unconcerned about the child and refuses to consider offers of help for the child's problems; overtly rejects the child

Adapted from Child Welfare Information Gateway.

emotional abuse, physical neglect and abuse, and sexual abuse. The items are written at a sixth grade reading level, and the CTQ is suitable for ages 12 years and older. The examinee responds to 28 questions on a five-point Likert scale, with answer choices ranging from "never true" to "very often true." It takes approximately 5 minutes to complete the questionnaire. The results are reported as severity classifications of none or minimal; low to moderate; moderate to severe; and severe to extreme.

The Youth at Risk Screening Questionnaire is directed at parents or adult caregivers. A list of 51 behaviors is given, and parents are asked to indicate if the item describes a youth they are concerned about. Each item is assigned a point value of 1, 5, 10, 15, or 20. The total score reflects the level of risk that the youth's behavior will escalate without intervention. A score of 5 to 16 indicates low risk; 17 to 32, moderate risk; 33 to 84, high risk; and 85 or more, extremely high risk. The questionnaire may be completed online; once submitted, a results page appears along with a brief list of resources, helpful interpretation material, and additional screening resources.

The online version is available at www.crisiscounseling. org/Riskassessment.htm.

Another screening tool is the Childhood Maltreatment Interview Schedule—Short Form (CMIS-SF). The short form was adapted from the full CMIS, published by John Briere, PhD, in 1992. The form is intended to be completed by interviewing the patient rather than by self-report. Questions typically start with the phrase, "Before age 17..." and go on to ask about specific events that may have occurred, such as a parent having problems with drugs or alcohol or an adult yelling at, insulting, ridiculing, or humiliating the child. If the response is positive, follow-up questions are asked about how often, who was involved, and so forth. The questions explore psychological, emotional, and physical abuse.

Health-care providers are required by law to make a report of child maltreatment. For more information, see the Child Welfare Information Gateway publication, *Mandatory Reporters of Child Abuse and Neglect*: www.childwelfare.gov/systemwide/laws_policies/ statutes/manda.cfm. An additional resource for information and referral is the Childhelp® National Child Abuse Hotline (800.4.A.CHILD).

Age-Specific Physical Examinations

The content of the physical examination of pediatric patients includes each of the systems shown in Table 2-1. You are encouraged to follow the "head-to-toe" order when conducting a physical examination, but exceptions are made for pediatric patients. If possible, you should auscultate the lungs, heart, and abdomen when the child is quiet and not crying. Some components of the examination are likely to elicit crying, such as examining the ears and the oropharynx and conducting parts of the musculoskeletal examination. Regardless of the order in which the examination is performed, you should always document in the order shown in Table 2-5.

There are many excellent references available that teach physical examination techniques. It is beyond the scope of this book to present the entire physical examination for all the age-specific well-child visits. Once a child reaches school age, the physical examination is essentially the same as the adult physical examination. Table 4-3 presents a summary of physical examination components that should be documented specifically when performing infant and toddler examinations. Table 4-4 shows neurological reflexes that should be tested and documented during infancy. If you detect any abnormalities on physical examination, be sure that your assessment and plan address what additional testing, if any, is indicated and what follow-up will be needed.

Table 4-3 Documentation of Important Components of Age-Specific Physical Examinations

System Examination Component	Age	Comments
Skin		
Color for jaundice, cyanosis, other discoloration	All ages; most critical in neonate	Jaundice that appears within the first 24 hours after birth is likely to be pathologic jaundice due to hemolytic disease of newborn; jaundice that persists beyond 2–3 weeks should raise suspicions of biliary obstruction or liver disease; important to document presence or absence of Mongolian spot because it may be misdiagnosed as ecchymosis, raising concern of intentional injury
Rash or lesions	All ages	Many benign skin lesions and rashes common in childhood
HEENT		
Head	Birth until sutures and fontanelles closed	Anterior fontanelle at birth measures 4–6 cm in diameter, closes between 4 and 26 months of age; posterior measures 1–2 cm at birth, usually closes by 2 months
Eyes	Birth to 24 months	
Red reflex		Absence may indicate congenital glaucoma, cataract, retinal detachment, or retinoblastoma
Strabismus		If present after 10 days of age, may indicate poor vision or central nervous system disease
Mouth		
Teeth	First eruption, then throughout life	First eruption at about 6 months, then usually a tooth each month until 2 years, 2 months
Tonsils	All ages	May be enlarged in healthy child; peak growth of tonsillar tissue between 8 and 16 years
Palate	Most critical in infancy	Document whether any cleft or bifid uvula
Neck		
Lymph nodes	All ages	May not be palpable until toddler
Nuchal rigidity	All ages	Not a reliable sign of meningeal irritation until after age of 2 years
Respiratory		
Lung sounds	Every visit	Look for a cause of any abnormal breath sounds
Cardiovascular		
Heart rate, rhythm, and sounds	Every visit	Document character of any murmur present and include in assessment and plan; Still's murmur common in preschool- and school-age children, usually benign

Continued

Table 4-3	Documentation of Important Components of Age-Specific Physical Examinations—cont'd

System Examination Component	Age	Comments
Gastrointestinal		
Umbilical cord	Birth until healed	Document that parent/caregiver was educated on cord care
Bowel sounds	Every visit	Absence of bowel sounds is always abnormal; look for cause
Rectum	Birth	Assess and document patency
Male Genitourinary		
Testes	Most critical at birth	Both testes should be descended; if cannot palpate both, consultation is warranted
Scrotum	Most critical at birth	Inspect for masses; if present, document whether transparent on transillumination; hydroceles common in newborns
Penis, including foreskin	All ages	Nonretractable at birth, but must visualize the urinary meatus and document presence or absence of hypospadias; document sexual maturity using Tanner's stages[1]
Female Genitourinary		
Breasts	All ages	In newborn, may express white liquid for up to 2 weeks; document breast development
External genitalia	All ages	Often a milky-white or blood-tinged vaginal discharge in first few weeks; inspect hymen; document external genital development using Tanner's stages[1]
Musculoskeletal		
Clavicle	Birth	Fracture may occur during delivery
Spine	Birth through adolescence	Assess for spina bifida at birth; screen for scoliosis until adolescence
Hips	Birth through 6 months	Document findings of Barlow and Ortolani tests; if there is congenital hip dysplasia, the best outcome is when treatment is initiated in the first 6 weeks of life
Neurological		
Cranial nerves	Birth to 24 months, then annually if normal	Consult physical examination reference for strategies to assess cranial nerves in newborns, infants, and young children
Reflexes	Many reflexes present at birth will disappear in infancy; see Table 4.4 for reflexes that should be tested in infancy	

[1]Refer to a physical diagnosis reference for explanation and more information.

Pediatric Sports Preparticipation Physical Examination

Many pediatric patients will want to participate in sports activities and usually will need medical clearance to do so. The preparticipation physical examination may be the only time a healthy adolescent will see a health-care provider, so it is important to include some age-appropriate screening questions and anticipatory guidance. A comprehensive medical history that includes questions about a personal and family history of cardiovascular disease is an important component of the preparticipation evaluation. A personal history of congenital or acquired heart disease, as well as a history of hypertension or murmurs, should be documented. Symptoms of chest discomfort, shortness of breath, palpitations, syncope, or near-syncope with exercise are important. A known family history of hypertrophic cardiomyopathy, Marfan syndrome, or atherosclerosis, as well as a history of unexplained sudden death in family members younger than 50 years, are all of concern. Asking about the use of cocaine or anabolic steroids is particularly appropriate. All components of an age-specific physical examination should be completed, with particular emphasis on the respiratory, cardiac, and musculoskeletal systems.

Table 4-4   Neurological Reflexes That Should Be Tested During Infancy*

Reflex	Ages	Comments
Palmar grasp	Birth to 3–4 months	Persistence beyond 4 months suggests cerebral dysfunction
Plantar grasp	Birth to 6–8 months	Persistence beyond 8 months suggests cerebral dysfunction
Moro (startle reflex)	Birth to 4–6 months	Persistence beyond 4 months suggests neurological disease; persistence beyond 6 months is strongly suggestive of disease; asymmetrical response suggests fracture of clavicle, humerus, or brachial plexus injury
Asymmetrical tonic neck	Birth to 2 months	Persistence beyond 2 months suggests neurological disease
Rooting	Birth to 3–4 months	Absence of rooting indicates severe generalized or central nervous system disease
Placing and stepping	4 days after birth, variable age to disappear	Absence of placing may indicate paralysis; babies born by breech delivery may not have placing reflex
Parachute	Develops around 4–6 months and does not disappear	Delay in appearance may predict future delays in voluntary motor development
Trunk incurvation (Galant's reflex)	Birth to 2 months	Absence suggests a transverse spinal cord lesion or injury

*Refer to a physical examination reference for a full description of each reflex and maneuver to elicit.

The cardiac examination should include auscultation with provocative maneuvers to screen for hypertrophic cardiomyopathy because this is the most common cause of sudden death in young male athletes. The recommended musculoskeletal examination is provided in Table 4-5.

Young women are less likely to experience sudden death on the athletic field than young men. In female athletes, however, several predispositions should be considered. Anorexia nervosa and other eating disorders are more common among female athletes than among male athletes. Screening questions about desires to change weight or displeasure with body habitus identify many of these women. Female runners are more likely to develop stress fractures than are male runners. Osteoporosis occurs in amenorrheic female athletes, and this finding should prompt further consideration of the possibility of an eating disorder.

To reinforce the content of this chapter, please complete the worksheets that follow.

Table 4-5   Musculoskeletal Portion of Sports Preparticipation Physical Examination

Examination Component and Maneuver	Assessment
Neck—move neck in all directions	Range of motion
Shoulders—shrug against resistance	Test strength of shoulder, neck, and trapezius muscles
Arms—hold out to side and apply pressure	Strength of deltoid muscle
Arms—hold out to side, bend 90 degrees at elbows, raise and lower arms	External rotation and stability of glenohumeral joint
Arms—hold out straight, then bend and straighten elbow	Range of motion of elbow
Arms—hold down, bend 90 degrees at elbows, pronate and supinate forearm	Range of motion of elbows and wrists, muscle strength of forearms and wrists
Hand—make a fist, clench and then spread fingers	Range of motion of fingers, strength and stability of joints and muscles
Squat and duck walk	Hip, knee, and ankle range of motion; joint strength and stability
Stand straight with arms to side, back to examiner	Symmetry, leg-length discrepancy
Bend forward from waist with knees straight	Scoliosis of spine
Stand and raise up on toes and walk on heels	Ankle joint strength and stability and calf muscle strength

Worksheet 4.1

1. List five components of pediatric health maintenance visits.

_____

_____

_____

_____

2. List three growth parameters that should be measured and documented from birth to 24 months of age.

_____

_____

_____

3. At what age is BMI screening introduced?

_____

4. Name three widely used resources available from the CDC.

_____

_____

_____

5. List at least three tools that are used to screen children for achievement of developmental milestones.

_____

_____

_____

6. List at least four of the six most commonly included laboratory tests that are part of mandatory newborn screening.

_____

_____

7. For each of the ages listed, list at least three topics that should be discussed with parents/caregivers as part of anticipatory guidance.

6 months:

_____

_____

2–3 years:

_____

_____

10–14 years:

_____

_____

8. List at least four conditions (maternal or paternal) that should be explored as part of the genetic and teratology history.

_____

_____

_____

9. List at least four infections that could cause fetal malformation or birth defects that should be explored as part of the maternal infections.

_____

_____

10. What does the FISTS mnemonic stand for?

_____

_____

_____

_____

11. List the four recognized types of child abuse.

_____

_____

12. List at least two screening tools that can be used to assess for child abuse or maltreatment.

_____

_____

13. List at least four topics that should be explored when taking the history of a child who presents for a preparticipation sports examination.

_____

_____

14. What three systems should be emphasized when examining a child who presents for a preparticipation sports examination?

_____

_____

_____

Worksheet 4.2

Plotting Growth Measurements

Madison Greer is brought in by her parents for a 24-month-old well-child visit. Shown below are measurements obtained at today's visits, along with measurements from her 6-month and 12-month well-child visits. Plot each of these measurements on the growth chart provided.

	6-month-old	**12-month-old**	**24-month-old**
Weight:	15 pounds	20 pounds	26 pounds
Length:	25 inches	28½ inches	33½ inches
Head circumference:	16½ inches	17½ inches	18½ inches

Source: Developed by the National Center for Health Statistics in collaboration with the National Center for Chronic Disease Prevention and Health Promotion, 2000.

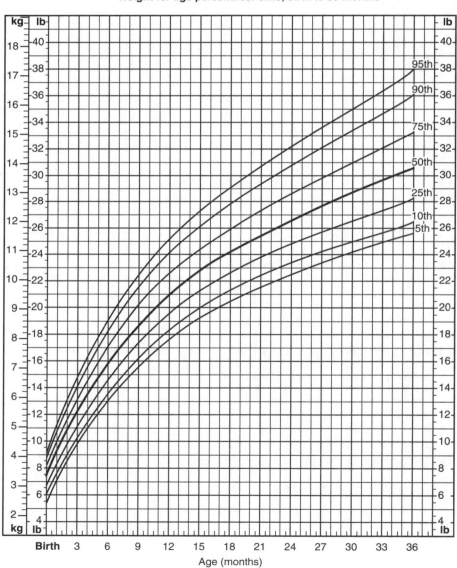

Weight-for-age percentiles: Girls, birth to 36 months

Length-for-age percentiles: Girls, birth to 36 months

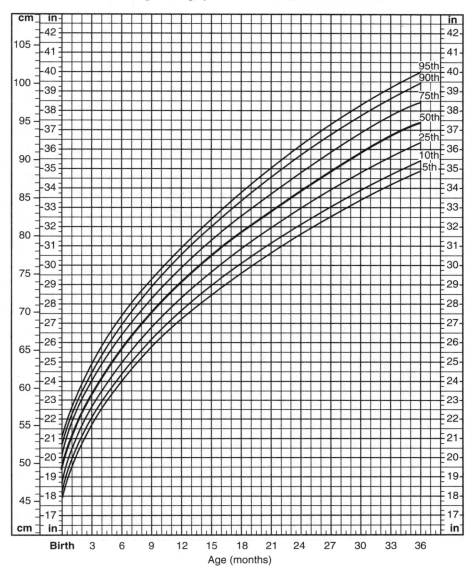

Age (months)

Source: Developed by the National Center for Health Statistics in collaboration with the National Center for Chronic Disease Prevention and Health Promotion, 2000.

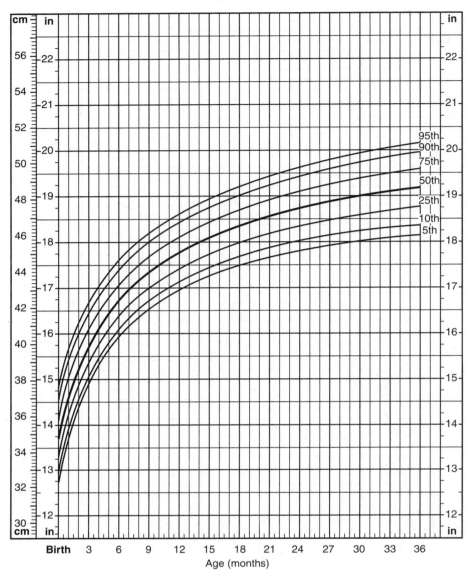

Head circumference-for-age percentiles: Girls, birth to 36 months

95th
90th
75th
50th
25th
10th
5th

Age (months)

Birth 3 6 9 12 15 18 21 24 27 30 33 36

Source: Developed by the National Center for Health Statistics in collaboration with the National Center for Chronic Disease Prevention and Health Promotion, 2000.

Indicate the percentile for each of the measurements above.

	6-month-old	**12-month-old**	**24-month-old**
Weight:	_____	_____	_____
Length:	_____	_____	_____
Head circumference:	_____	_____	_____

Consult a pediatric textbook or history and physical examination textbook and determine whether or not these measurements are within normal limits.

Connor Atchinson is a 24-month-old boy who is brought in for a well-child visit. Shown below are measurements obtained at today's visits, along with measurements from his 6-month and 12-month well-child visits. Plot each of these measurements on the growth chart provided.

	6-month-old	**12-month-old**	**24-month-old**
Weight:	8.5 kg	10.4 kg	12 kg
Length:	68.5 cm	76 cm	86 cm
Head circumference:	44.4 cm	46.2 cm	47.6 cm

Weight-for-age percentiles: Boys, birth to 36 months

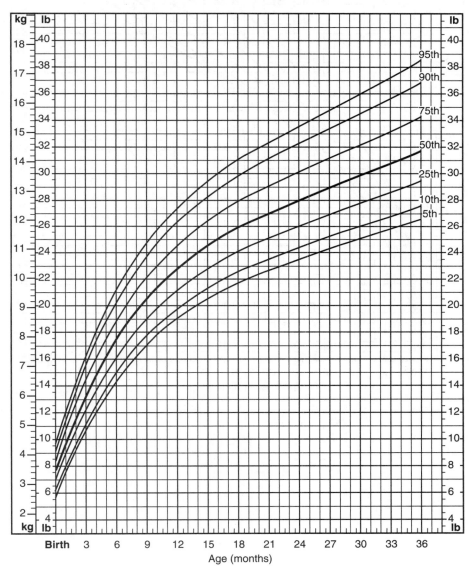

Source: Developed by the National Center for Health Statistics in collaboration with the National Center for Chronic Disease Prevention and Health Promotion, 2000.

Length-for-age percentiles: Boys, birth to 36 months

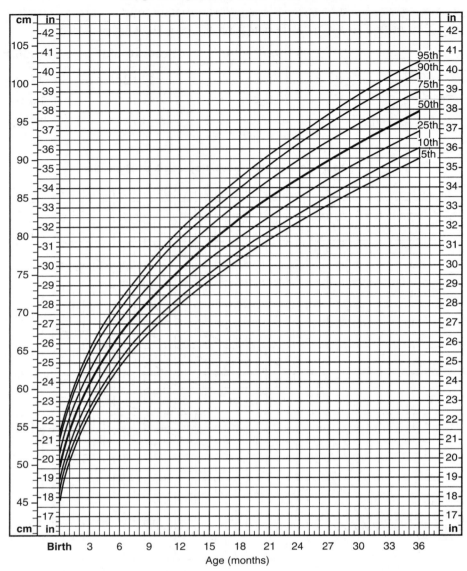

Source: Developed by the National Center for Health Statistics in collaboration with the National Center for Chronic Disease Prevention and Health Promotion, 2000.

Head circumference-for-age percentiles: Boys, birth to 36 months

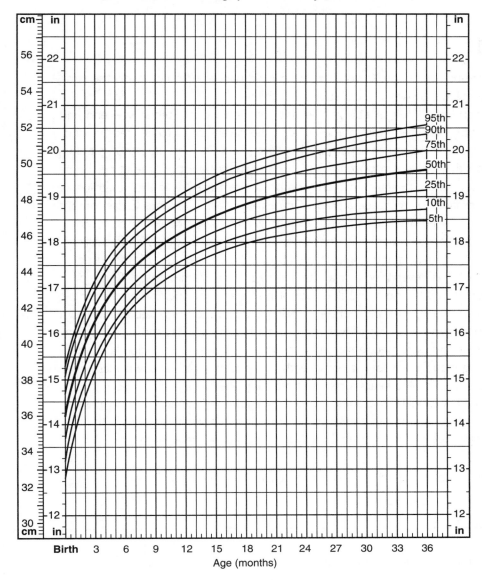

Source: Developed by the National Center for Health Statistics in collaboration with the National Center for Chronic Disease Prevention and Health Promotion, 2000.

Indicate the percentile for each of the measurements above.

	6-month-old	**12-month-old**	**24-month-old**
Weight:	_____	_____	_____
Length:	_____	_____	_____
Head circumference:	_____	_____	_____

Consult a pediatric textbook or history and physical examination textbook and determine whether or not these measurements are within normal limits.

Sample HEEADSSS Write-Up

Below is a sample HEEADSSS write-up for Allison Kawolski, a 15-year-old patient who comes to the family practice office. After reading the write-up, answer the questions that follow.

AK lives at home with her mother and two younger siblings. She visits her father every other weekend, and the father, stepmother, and one stepbrother live in that home. AK says she is very close to her mother and has a good relationship with her. Not as close to her father, but they "get along OK." She does not get along well with her stepmother or stepbrother. AK is also close to her aunt and spends a lot of time at her home. AK feels that she has a good support system in her mom, aunt, and band director. AK is in the 9th grade at Ridgeline High School. She has never failed or repeated a grade. Grades are mostly Bs, some Cs last report card. She is in band and in several clubs. She worked this past summer as a lifeguard at a water park, but does not work during the school year. AK volunteers as a dog-walker at the humane society and usually goes two Saturdays a month. Her father smokes and drinks alcohol but "isn't a drunk." Her mother used to smoke but quit a few years ago. AK has never tried a cigarette and says, "they are disgusting." Some of her friends smoke, but she is not pressured by them and does not plan to start smoking. She has never experimented with drugs. AK has had three sexual partners—all male partners. She has talked to her mom about taking OCPs. AK says she understands that the pill will not protect her from STDs and says she hopes her partner will use a condom. She knows of someone from her school who committed suicide last year, but says she can't imagine ever doing that. Denies feeling consistently or frequently sad or down. Has never contemplated suicide and thinks it is "stupid." AK wears a seat belt regularly. She has a learner's permit but no driver's license yet. Rides her bike occasionally and doesn't wear a helmet when riding. No guns in either of her parents' homes. Knows of one boy who brings a knife to school, but she doesn't hang out with him. Witnesses fights at school occasionally but has never been directly involved. Feels safe at home.

1. Based on the information in this write-up, list any risk factors that you identified for Allison.

_____

_____

2. Critically analyze the content of this write-up. Identify other topics or additional information that should have been included in this write-up.

_____

_____

_____

_____

3. Do you feel additional screening is needed at this time? Why or why not? If yes, what screening should be done?

_____

_____

_____

4. What anticipatory guidance should be provided to Allison's mother at this visit?

_____

_____

_____

Worksheet 4.4

Abbreviations

These abbreviations were introduced in Chapter 4. Beside each, write the meaning as indicated by the content of this chapter.

AAP _____

ASQ-3 _____

CAPTA _____

CMIS-SF _____

CTQ _____

DDST-II _____

DTP _____

EPSDT _____

FISTS _____

GAPS _____

HEEADSSS _____

HIB-c _____

HRSA _____

MCAD _____

MCHB _____

MMR _____

NHANES _____

OCP _____

PEDS _____

PEDS-DM _____

PKU _____

Td _____

Chapter 5

SOAP Notes

OBJECTIVES

- Define the Subjective, Objective, Assessment, and Plan components of a SOAP note.
- Organize pertinent positive and negative aspects of the history in the Subjective portion of the note.
- Organize pertinent positive and negative findings of the physical examination in the Objective portion of the note.
- Generate Assessments by analyzing information from the Subjective and Objective portions of the note.
- Document Assessments using terminology consistent with *International Classification of Diseases, 9th Revision* (ICD-9) codes.
- Identify components of patient management that should be documented in the Plan section of the note.
- Evaluate sample SOAP notes and complete worksheets.

After a comprehensive history and physical examination (H&P) has been documented, it is usually not necessary to include that level of detail at subsequent visits to the same provider. One variation of the comprehensive H&P is the SOAP note. SOAP stands for Subjective, Objective, Assessment, and Plan. The SOAP note represents one format to document a patient encounter systematically and logically. The SOAP format is used in many different practice settings. It is important to understand that sections of the SOAP note are interrelated. The completeness and accuracy of the history (subjective information) will help guide what you look for when performing a problem-specific physical examination (objective information) and formulating differential diagnoses. Together, the subjective and objective information should lead you to, and should support, the assessment. Once you have made an assessment, you can establish a plan of care.

It is beyond the scope of this book to address interviewing techniques and interpersonal skills; you should employ your best communication techniques when interviewing the patient and obtaining the history that will make up the subjective portion of the SOAP note. (Several reference texts that deal with medical interviewing are listed in the bibliography.) Although all parts of a SOAP note are important, the ability to take and record an accurate medical history from a patient is one of the most important tasks to be mastered in medicine. In 1947, Platt claimed that in most cases the diagnosis can be made with the history alone. In 1975, Hampton and colleagues attempted to evaluate the relative contributions of history taking, the physical examination, and laboratory tests in making medical diagnoses. Nearly 20 years later, Peterson and colleagues undertook a study to quantitate the relative contributions of the history, physical examination, and laboratory investigation in making medical diagnoses. They found that history taking led to the final diagnosis in 61 of 80 patients, or 76% of encounters.

The author's experience over the years substantiates the findings of Platt, Hampton, and Peterson. Obtaining an adequate history will often take the most time during a patient encounter; the time spent documenting the subjective portion of a SOAP note will often correlate.

Subjective

The elements of the comprehensive H&P that are typically included as Subjective information in a SOAP note are as follows:

- Chief complaint (CC)
- History of present illness (HPI)

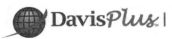

DavisPlus | Visit **http://davisplus.fadavis.com** for complete learning activities on actual EMR software at, Keyword: Sullivan

- Pertinent past medical history (PMH)
- Pertinent family history (FH)
- Pertinent psychosocial history (SH)
- Any specialized history related to the chief complaint (for instance, obstetrical and gynecological history for a female patient who presents with irregular menses)
- Pertinent review of systems (ROS)

The subjective portion of the note is information that the "subject" or patient tells you. Sometimes, subjective information is obtained from someone other than the patient. A spouse or family member, a caregiver, and members of the health-care team could all offer subjective information. If someone other than the patient provides the history, document who provided the history and their relationship to the patient.

On occasion, you might want to use quotation marks to identify information as a direct quote from the patient and to indicate that you have recorded the patient's exact words. This is particularly useful if the patient describes something important (such as pain) or if the patient does not answer a question to your satisfaction. For instance, when asked if she takes any medication, a patient responds "Yes, I take a little red pill for my blood pressure." You could guess what that little red pill may be, but for the sake of accuracy, it would be better to document this information using the patient's words (patient takes "a little red pill" for hypertension). The use of quotation marks lets other readers know the information within the marks is not your paraphrase or restatement of something the patient told you but the words of the patient. Notice that the word "hypertension" was substituted for "blood pressure." It is acceptable to do this because the patient is stating a fact and you are translating the lay term into an accepted and more specific medical term that will have consistent meaning to others who will read the note.

One of the most challenging aspects of documenting the subjective information is determining what elements of the history are pertinent. It takes years of practicing medicine to understand the importance of certain associated signs and symptoms and how they relate to the chief complaint. Many conditions have a certain pattern of presentation. A man having a myocardial infarction is likely to present with chest pain or pressure, sometimes radiating to the neck, jaw, or arm; nausea, dyspnea, and diaphoresis are often part of the symptom complex of infarction. Not only should you ask about all these signs and symptoms as you gather the medical history, but you should also document the absence or presence of each of these signs and symptoms. Some findings from the history will support or suggest one diagnosis more than another. These findings are "pertinent positives" because their presence is pertinent to the overall history. The absence of other findings, called "pertinent negatives," likewise may suggest a certain diagnosis and help rule out other diagnoses because of their absence. Consider the history of a 22-year-old man who presents with low-grade fever and right lower quadrant abdominal pain. The differential diagnosis of acute appendicitis should come to mind. Patients with this condition typically present with anorexia, or loss of appetite. If this man is anorexic, that is a pertinent positive finding and would support the differential of appendicitis. If he states that he is hungry and wants to know how soon he can eat, the absence of anorexia is a pertinent negative, and although it does not rule out appendicitis, it makes it less likely. When documenting certain areas of the history, such as associated signs and symptoms, it is helpful to list all pertinent positives together, and then to list the pertinent negatives. Pattern recognition is one way a diagnosis is made. Documenting the pertinent positives and negatives in the patient's history will often help readers recognize the pattern of the condition the patient is exhibiting.

The documentation of pertinent positives and negatives should be detailed enough to narrow the differential diagnoses and eventually lead to the most likely diagnosis. Try to anticipate what information other readers want to know, such as the presence or absence of certain findings, and be sure that information is included in your documentation. For example, if an 18-month-old child presents with a history of fever and a rash, and the parent states the child is inconsolable, the differential diagnosis of meningitis should come to mind. Your documentation should reflect that you considered the diagnosis of meningitis; therefore, it should include the presence or absence of symptoms that are associated with meningitis. Lethargy is one such symptom; therefore, if the child is attentive and looking around the room and interactive with his environment, these are negatives in the child's history that lead you away from the diagnosis of meningitis or make it less likely.

Application Exercises

There are at least two ways to develop documentation skills: (1) practice, practice, and practice, and (2) critically analyze documentation. We give you the opportunity to do both throughout this text. Read the subjective information documented in the following two examples, and answer the questions.

Application Exercise 5.1

This 42-year-old man presents with left knee pain. He injured his knee while playing softball. His pain has gradually worsened over the past week. He has not noticed any swelling. He denies any numbness below the knee. He has not had any prior knee surgery. He is allergic to penicillin. He denies tobacco use. He works full-time in computer sales.

Based on this example, answer the following questions:

1. How long has the patient had left knee pain?
2. Has he tried anything to relieve the pain?
3. What pertinent positives and negatives are documented? Should any other pertinent elements have been documented?
4. Does the patient have any chronic medical conditions?
5. Has the patient had any surgery?
6. Does the patient take any medications?

As you can see, this entry did not allow you to answer these questions. However, the information should be part of the history related to the patient's chief complaint of knee pain and should be documented as subjective information. This information is important to anyone who may be involved in the patient's care. Read Application Exercise 5.2, and then answer these same questions.

Application Exercise 5.2

This 42-year-old man presents with complaints of left knee pain. He originally injured his left knee about a month ago while playing softball. He states that he slid into a base and his foot caught against the bag, which twisted his knee. In the past week, the pain has gradually worsened. He describes the pain as "a deep ache." He has not noted any swelling of the knee. The pain is worse when he has to stand for more than half an hour at a time and when he walks and goes upstairs. The patient has taken ibuprofen 400 mg occasionally for the pain, with some relief. He denies any numbness or tingling of the extremity or previous injury to the knee. He does not have any chronic medical problems and specifically denies having a history of hypertension or ulcers. He has never had surgery. He does not take any medications on a regular basis. He is allergic to penicillin, which causes a rash. He is married, has two children, and is employed full-time in computer sales. He denies any tobacco use; drinks "a few beers a week," and denies recreational drug use.

Application Exercise 5.2 is longer than Application Exercise 5.1. It is also more thorough and helps answer the questions a reader was not able to answer after reading Application Exercise 5.1. Application Exercise 5.2 does a better job of documenting aggravating and alleviating factors and pertinent positives and negatives. Notice also the use of quotation marks ("a few beers a week") to indicate a verbatim response from the patient. There will be times when you want to include the patient's exact words in your documentation; ideally, you should ask follow-up questions in order to determine exactly how often the patient consumes alcohol and how much he consumes. This would give you a better idea of whether the patient has any health risks associated with alcohol use.

MEDICOLEGAL ALERT !

When a condition or symptom involves anything that is symmetrical, specify the area of concern and do so consistently. In Application Exercise 5.2, the patient complained of left knee pain. Always check that you document left knee when you are referring to history and report left knee findings from the physical examination. Most conditions involving the left extremity warrant examination of and comparison to the right extremity. Even one discrepancy in use of left or right could raise doubts as to which area is being examined or treated. Malpractice lawyers will look for such discrepancies and will be sure to point them out, which might damage your credibility.

Objective

The elements of the comprehensive H&P that are typically included as Objective information in a SOAP note are as follows:

- Vital signs
- A general assessment of the patient
- Physical examination findings
- Results from laboratory or diagnostic studies

The objective information is what you or others can observe. It is typically documented in the order listed above. Vital signs may be documented on a flow sheet or some other place in the chart, especially if the patient is hospitalized. If the vital signs are recorded elsewhere, it is a good idea to record them again in the objective section. Recording the specific readings of the vital signs is preferred over "vital signs stable" or "vital signs within normal limits." It is easier and more convenient for others who will read the note to see the actual numbers, and this allows them to make their own interpretation of the vital signs.

A general assessment is not always included in a note in an office-based encounter but is very helpful in certain settings or with certain more serious or urgent chief complaints. General assessments are written to help identify a patient and paint a picture of the patient's overall presentation and status. Identifying information typically documented includes the patient's age and gender and sometimes the patient's race. Consider two patients who present to an urgent care center with shortness of breath. The general assessment for the first patient is documented as "a 28-year-old man who is cyanotic, using accessory muscles and gasping for breath." General assessment of the second patient is documented as "a 28-year-old man sitting comfortably who is acyanotic and has no tachypnea or increased respiratory effort and is able to speak in complete sentences." The approach to these two patients will be different based on the observations made about each patient. Although most providers automatically make this assessment mentally, it is good practice to document it specifically, especially in settings where patients are seen based on severity of their condition and not the order in which they arrive.

Just as it is challenging to know how much history to obtain and document in the subjective portion, it may also be a challenge to obtain and document the physical examination and other objective information. The objective information should flow logically from the subjective and should reflect your differential diagnoses just as the subjective does. Physical examination is usually taught in a system-based manner, and this may help you to know how much examination to do, which systems to examine, and how much examination to document. Some chief complaints will be associated with a specific system; back pain, for instance, is associated with the musculoskeletal system, so the physical examination would focus on the musculoskeletal system. Because the musculoskeletal and the neurological systems are interrelated, you would also perform and document a neurological examination of a patient presenting with back pain. The differential diagnosis of a complaint will help determine which systems are examined. A 34-year-old woman presenting with abdominal pain has a differential diagnosis of appendicitis, cholecystitis, ovarian cyst, sexually transmitted disease, ectopic pregnancy, and so on. The documentation should indicate that both the gastrointestinal and the genitourinary systems were examined.

The physical examination is typically done in a head-to-toe format. This approach can be modified as needed, omitting systems that do not need to be examined, or saving the examination of a system for last because of discomfort for the patient. Regardless of the order in which the examination is performed, it should be documented in head-to-toe order. The suggested order of documenting a physical examination is shown in Table 2-5. You should be aware that there are variations of this format. Some providers will document the respiratory and cardiac examinations under the heading CHEST. Some will document pulses under a heading of EXTREMITIES rather than in the cardiovascular system. These are acceptable variations. The content of the documentation is usually far more important than the format.

Just as there are pertinent positive and negative findings from the history, there will typically be pertinent positive and negative findings from the physical examination. The history of a patient who presents with a sore throat includes the pertinent positives of sudden onset, fever, pain with swallowing, and a muffled voice, prompting the differential diagnosis of streptococcal pharyngitis. On physical examination, you would expect to see tonsillar enlargement, erythema of the tonsils and pharynx, and possibly exudates. Presence of any of these findings is considered a pertinent positive and makes the diagnosis of streptococcal pharyngitis more likely than if the findings were not there. The absence of any of these findings would be a pertinent negative.

Formats for Documenting Objective Information

Two formats are commonly used for documenting the objective information portion of a SOAP note. Example 5.1 shows the narrative format, and Example 5.2 shows the system-heading format. Either format is acceptable. Some health-care providers prefer the system-heading format because the use of headings makes it easier to find specific information. Instead of reading the entire objective section, a reader can go quickly and easily to the system related to the chief complaint. If using the system-heading format, omit the heading for any system not examined. It is not necessary to include the heading and then document "not examined" or "not pertinent."

EXAMPLE 5.1

Narrative Format

The patient is a 6-year-old Hispanic female who is alert and cooperative. Her temperature is 99.2, respirations 20, pulse is 88, and BP is 96/60. Her skin is dry and intact without any rashes or lesions. The turgor is good. The head is normocephalic and atraumatic. The pupils are equal, round, and reactive to light. The tympanic membranes are intact bilaterally without erythema or effusion. Cone of light and bony landmarks are visible bilaterally. The ear canals are without swelling or discharge. The nose is patent without any rhinorrhea. Oropharynx is without erythema or exudates, and the mucous membranes are moist and intact. The neck is supple without any lymphadenopathy. The breath sounds are clear to auscultation without any adventitious sounds. There are no sternal retractions. Heart is regular rate and rhythm without murmur. The abdomen is soft and nondistended. The bowel sounds are physiological in all four quadrants. There is no organomegaly, and no masses are palpated. The extremities show full range of motion of all joints, and there is no clubbing, cyanosis, or edema. Cranial nerves II to XII are grossly intact, and there are no focal neurological deficits.

EXAMPLE 5.2

Systems Headings Format

General: The patient is a 6-year-old Hispanic female who is alert and cooperative. Her temperature is 99.2, respirations 20, pulse is 88, and BP is 96/60.

Skin: Dry and intact without any rashes or lesions. The turgor is good.

HEENT: The head is normocephalic and atraumatic. The pupils are equal, round, and reactive to light. The tympanic membranes are intact bilaterally without erythema or effusion. Cone of light and bony landmarks are visible bilaterally. The ear canals are without swelling or discharge. The nose is patent without any rhinorrhea. Oropharynx is without erythema or exudates, and the mucous membranes are moist and intact.

Neck: The neck is supple without any lymphadenopathy.

Respiratory: The breath sounds are clear to auscultation without any adventitious sounds. There are no sternal retractions.

Cardiovascular: Heart is regular rate and rhythm without murmur.

Abdomen: Soft and nondistended. The bowel sounds are physiological in all four quadrants. There is no organomegaly and no masses are palpated.

Extremities: Full range of motion of all joints, and there is no clubbing, cyanosis, or edema.

Neurological: Cranial nerves II to XII are grossly intact, and there are no focal neurological deficits.

Documenting Diagnostic Test Results

Results of laboratory or other diagnostic tests are commonly documented in the objective portion of a SOAP note. Tests that may be ordered for a 34-year-old woman who presents with abdominal pain include a complete blood count, chemistry profile, urinalysis (UA), urine pregnancy test, and abdominal ultrasound. The results of these studies would generally follow the documentation of the physical examination.

Give the name of the test first, then the result (e.g., CBC shows a WBC of 5.8, Hgb of 11, and Hct of 34). If all the results are within normal limits, you may document as "the CBC is WNL." If one component of a panel of tests is abnormal, but the rest are normal, you could document "CMP shows a potassium of 5.2; otherwise, the results are WNL." Other readers will appreciate having the test result specifically documented because this will give them the opportunity to make their own interpretation of the results and save the time of having to look up results that may be documented elsewhere in the medical record.

MEDICOLEGAL ALERT !

Failure to follow-up on abnormal laboratory tests or studies can be a component of alleged malpractice. Every office should have a protocol for tracking laboratory results as they come into the office. You must notify the patient of any abnormal test results and have a follow-up plan to determine why the results are abnormal. Failure to recognize that there is an abnormal test result, or failure to follow-up on an abnormal test result, could have disastrous results.

If you plan to order diagnostic tests but do not have the results at the time you are documenting, this is usually documented as part of the plan instead of an objective finding. This is because there are no results to observe or document yet. Consider the scenario of a 17-year-old patient who presents with right ankle pain. After gathering all the history, or subjective information, you perform the physical examination (objective information). You decide to order an x-ray of the ankle. If you cannot perform the x-ray on site, the patient will have to go to an outpatient facility. Dr. Jones, the radiologist at the facility, typically phones you immediately with the results of the x-ray, so you ask the patient to return to your office after the x-ray is taken. When you get the results, you document "x-ray of the right ankle is negative for any fracture or other acute findings per Dr. Jones." If you can perform the x-ray on site, or if the patient returns with the radiographs taken at another facility, you would view the films and document the interpretation as your own (e.g., "I did not see any fracture or other acute findings on the x-ray of the right ankle.").

Interventions Done During the Visit

Interventions done during the visit are often documented as part of the objective section. Suppose the patient described earlier with the ankle pain is seen at 5:30 p.m. You cannot take x-rays on site, and the outpatient facility where he would have an x-ray done is closed for the day. In the meantime, you apply a posterior splint and instruct the patient on crutch walking. These interventions are documented in the objective section of the note. Obtaining an x-ray is part of your plan, which will be discussed later in this chapter. If the patient were instructed to return tomorrow after x-rays are taken, that would also be part of the plan.

Application Exercise 5.3

Look at the following information and indicate which is subjective (S) or objective (O).

_____ The right hand is swollen.

_____ There is no tenderness to palpation of the right knee.

_____ My left arm feels numb and has a tingling sensation.

_____ Patient is hard of hearing.

_____ No respiratory distress is noted.

_____ Patient denies allergies to any medication.

Application Exercise 5.4

Read the following subjective documentation:

The patient complains of experiencing shortness of breath over the past 3 days. It started gradually and is progressively worsening. The shortness of breath is worse with any activity. He has also noted swelling of his feet and ankles. The patient has had an occasional nonproductive cough. He specifically denies any chest pain or hemoptysis. He has not had any fever or chills, congestion, or sore throat. His past medical history is significant for myocardial infarction 5 years ago. He takes carvedilol daily. He denies smoking or other tobacco use.

Based on the subjective information documented above, examination of which two systems should be documented in the objective portion of the SOAP note?

_____

_____

List at least three specific components that should be examined in each of these two systems.

_____

_____

_____

Application Exercise 5.5

Adhering to the recommended head-to-toe order of documenting the physical examination in the objective portion of a SOAP note, indicate the order in which the following should be documented.

_____ The neck is supple without adenopathy or masses.

_____ BP 120/72, P 80, R 16, T 97.8.

_____ Faint crackles are noted at the base of the lungs bilaterally.

_____ The patient is a 72-year-old man who appears his stated age and is in no acute distress.

_____ No hemorrhages or AV nicking seen on funduscopic examination.

_____ The abdomen is soft and nondistended. Bowel sounds are present in all four quadrants.

_____ The heart rhythm is irregularly irregular.

Assessment

Careful analysis and interpretation of the subjective and objective data should lead to a logical assessment. Impression, diagnosis, and assessment are terms used interchangeably. Upon reading the chief complaint, a list of possible causes, also known as a differential diagnosis, is formulated. Table 5-1 shows examples of differential diagnoses for four common complaints.

As subjective and objective data are assimilated, the list of differential diagnoses becomes more refined. Laboratory and other diagnostic studies may help confirm a suspected diagnosis, although such studies are not always necessary to reach a final diagnosis, as in the

Table 5-1	Examples of Differential Diagnoses Based on Chief Complaint
Chief Complaint	**Differential Diagnoses**
Headache	Tension headache, migraine headache, cervical myofasciitis, sinusitis, cerebrovascular accident, space-occupying lesion
Eye pain	Trauma, conjunctivitis, corneal abrasion, sinusitis, orbital cellulitis, glaucoma, keratitis, ocular migraine, hordeolum
Vaginal discharge	Candidiasis, bacterial vaginosis, trichomonas, chlamydia, gonorrhea
Diarrhea	Infection, irritable bowel syndrome, food intolerance/allergy, ulcerative colitis, antibiotic induced

case of sinusitis. A definitive (or final) diagnosis is based on diagnostic evidence. For example, a patient may present to the clinic complaining of dysuria, and the differential diagnosis of urinary tract infection (UTI) is considered. A pertinent positive finding from the physical examination is mild tenderness across the lower abdomen. The UA shows 2+ leukocytes, trace protein, and blood, but is otherwise negative. The UA is suggestive of a UTI but does not confirm the diagnosis. Other conditions considered in the differential diagnosis could be causing her symptoms and the UA findings. If the result of a urine culture is positive. the diagnosis of a UTI can be made definitively. There are times when you will not be able to make a definitive diagnosis at a single visit, such as when additional testing is indicated but not readily available and must be scheduled for a later time. If a definitive diagnosis has not been reached, a symptom is listed as the assessment. Example 5.3 compares symptoms and definitive diagnoses and shows ICD-9 codes for each.

EXAMPLE 5.3

Symptom		Definitive Diagnosis	
Dysuria	788.1	Urinary tract infection	599.0
Knee pain	719.46	Osteoarthritis	715.9
Ear pain	388.70	Otitis media	382.9
Right lower quadrant pain	789.03	Appendicitis	540.9
Fatigue	780.79	Anemia	285.9

The first assessment listed should usually correlate with the presenting complaint. As you uncover other diagnoses, list them in order of importance or impact on the chief complaint. Comorbidities that may influence the patient's medical course should also be listed. Refer to Example 5.4.

EXAMPLE 5.4

S: This patient complains of experiencing an aching, occasionally sharp pain in right lower leg over the past 2 days. He noticed an open sore on the leg this morning. He has felt feverish and slightly nauseated since last night. He rates the pain severity as 5/10 at rest; standing worsens the pain to 8/10. He has not had any relief with Tylenol or elevation of leg. Measurement of the fasting blood sugars range from 200 to 275, and 2-hour postprandial blood sugars range from 250 to 325. Last HgbA1C done 3 months ago and was 8.3.

PMH: Significant for type 2 diabetes and HTN.

Medications: Metformin 1000 mg BID; Glyburide 5 mg BID; Lisinopril 20 mg daily.

Allergies: NKDA

Social: 30-pack-year history of cigarette smoking; quit 2 years ago. Denies alcohol or drug use.

O: General assessment: 68-year-old man who is alert and oriented but looks mildly distressed.

VS: BP 156/94; P 94; R 20; and T 97.0. Wt 235, Ht 70"

Heart: RRR without murmur.

Lungs: Adventitious breath sounds throughout all lung fields.

Extremities: There is a 2-cm superficial ulceration on the right lower leg proximal to the lateral malleolus with 4-cm area of surrounding erythema and increased warmth. Dorsalis pedis pulses are 1+ and equal. There is decreased sensation from the mid-calf to the toes bilaterally.

A: Ulcer right lower leg	707.10
Cellulitis right lower leg	682.6
Type 2 DM, poorly controlled	250.02
Diabetic Neuropathy	250.6
Hypertension	401.1

The ulcer and cellulitis of the right lower extremity represent the presenting complaint, whereas the poorly controlled type 2 diabetes, neuropathy, and hypertension are comorbid conditions that may affect his overall medical course and outcome.

MEDICOLEGAL ALERT !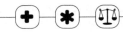

It is inappropriate to label a patient with an unproven diagnosis. This can adversely affect the patient's present and future health care, would be inappropriate coding, could become a medicolegal issue, and may tarnish your reputation.

Differential Diagnosis

When a definitive diagnosis cannot be determined, a list of potential diagnoses—or the differential diagnosis (DDX)—should be documented, reflecting conditions that are being considered and that may require further workup. It is beyond the scope of this text to address the process of developing and refining differential diagnoses. Although generating a list of differential diagnoses is a basic skill that can be learned with practice, it takes extensive clinical training and a wealth of clinical experience to develop the higher-order critical thinking skills needed to synthesize and analyze data in order to refine and continually narrow the differential diagnoses and arrive at a logical most likely or definitive diagnosis. There is certainly truth in the axiom, "if it is never considered, it will never be diagnosed"; therefore, a health-care provider must be able to generate differential diagnoses for every problem with which a patient presents. It is one thing to know that a patient has a herniated disk with radicular symptoms and then to consult a medical textbook about the particulars of that condition. It is another thing altogether to have a patient in front of you who presents with back pain or numbness in the leg and to have to go through the process of investigating a symptom and arriving at a certain diagnosis. We recognize that the process is a complex and multifaceted one, and we make no attempt to teach clinical reasoning or medical decision making. We aim to present only a brief discussion of the importance of documentation that reflects the subjective and objective data gathered about a symptom, documenting an assessment or assessments that reflect analysis of such data and support a plan of care. It may be helpful for the novice health-care provider to consult symptom-based books as a starting point to developing differential diagnoses (see Bibliography for specific references).

When documenting the DDX, list in order of most likely to least likely. The list does not need to be all-inclusive but should demonstrate thoughtful analysis of the available data. This allows other readers to follow your reasoning and should demonstrate when additional workup is warranted. In some practice settings, laboratory and imaging services are readily available; having the results of diagnostic studies at the time of the encounter may establish a definitive diagnosis. When these services are not available, documentation of the plan should reflect which studies are needed and how the results will guide the health-care provider to formulate a treatment plan or management strategy for the patient.

When a definitive diagnosis has not been reached, the assessment should reflect the presenting symptom or complaint and should list some of the most likely differential diagnoses with the term "rule out" (R/O). This is useful to demonstrate the decision-making process; however, care should be taken to ensure that the documentation used in the assessment section and the ICD-9 codes assigned for the visit clearly reflect that these conditions are being considered but have not yet been established as diagnoses. Example 5.5 illustrates this. Coding is discussed in more detail in Chapter 1.

EXAMPLE 5.5

A: Left lower quadrant abdominal pain (789.04)
   R/O diverticulosis, ovarian cyst, ureterolithiasis
A: Right great toe pain (729.5)
   R/O gout, arthritis, fracture

A: Right ear pain (388.70)
   R/O otitis externa, otitis media, eustachian tube dysfunction
A: Calf pain (729.5)
   R/O deep vein thrombosis, cellulitis, muscle strain

Application Exercise 5.6

List several differential diagnoses for the following chief complaints:

Neck pain _____

Low back pain _____

Cough _____

Epistaxis _____

Shortness of breath _____

Application Exercise 5.7

Read the following note and answer the questions.

CC: Ms. Kearns has had chest pain for the past 24 hours.

1. Develop a differential diagnosis for chest pain without having any other information, keeping in mind that there are many conditions other than cardiovascular ones that can cause chest pain.

_____

_____

_____

_____

Now, consider the following information.

S: The chest pain started yesterday approximately 2 hours after she had vigorously cleaned the bathroom using a new cleaner. The pain worsened later in the day while she was gardening. Yesterday, the pain was in the substernal area; today, it radiates to the left anterior chest area. At rest, the pain is described as "aching," with a pain scale rating of 2/10; however, with moving about and taking a deep breath, the pain becomes sharp and shooting, with a rating of 7/10. She feels slightly feverish; has a dry, nonproductive cough; is short of breath at rest and has worsening dyspnea on exertion; has clear rhinorrhea; and has a slight frontal headache. The chest pain does not radiate to her arm, neck, or jaw. She denies sore throat, ear pain, nausea or vomiting, and abdominal or back pain. She has taken Advil, two tablets every 8 hours, with some relief of symptoms. No relief of cough with Robitussin DM.

PMH: Positive for allergic rhinitis, appendectomy, and tonsillectomy. Denies hypertension, heart disease, diabetes, or cancer. Has regular menstrual cycles every 28 days. Current medications: Allegra 180 mg/d PRN allergic rhinitis symptoms. NKDA.

FH: No cardiovascular disease, diabetes, or cancer.

SH: She has smoked cigarettes one PPD for the past 15 years. She denies alcohol or drug use.

2. Revise the differential diagnoses based on the subjective information and list in order of most likely to least likely.

_____

_____

_____

O: This 42-year-old woman appears mildly anxious but in no acute distress. She is alert and oriented.

Vital signs: BP 144/90, P 98, R 22, T 99.4 orally. Height is 5'6"; weight 150 pounds.

Skin: Warm, slightly diaphoretic. Turgor is good. There is no rash.

HEENT: TMs are intact with bony landmarks well visualized. The nose is slightly congested with pink turbinates and clear discharge. There is mild pharyngeal erythema without exudates.

Neck: Supple, nontender. No adenopathy, thyromegaly, or jugular venous distention (JVD) noted.

Heart: Rate is 98 and regular without murmurs, rubs, or gallop. Normal S1 and S2.

Chest/Lungs: Chest wall is tender to palpation in the left 4th to 7th costochondral area. No wheezes, rhonchi, or crackles heard on auscultation.

Extremities: Peripheral pulses are 2+ and equal bilaterally. There is no cyanosis, clubbing, or edema.

3. Revise the differential diagnoses based on the objective findings.

_____

_____

_____

4. What diagnostic testing, if any, would you order to further narrow the differential diagnoses?

_____

_____

In Application Exercise 5.7, think about how the patient's age and gender lead you to consider certain differential diagnoses. The DDX would probably be somewhat different if the patient was a 73-year-old man. Other factors such as vital signs and pertinent positives and negatives from the subjective and objective will help to narrow the differential diagnoses to one most likely diagnosis. Diagnostic studies may also help further refine the DDX. If you have not reached a definitive diagnosis for Mrs. Kearns when she leaves your facility, you can document the presenting complaint of chest pain as the assessment.

Plan

This section of the SOAP note includes documentation of diagnostic studies that will be obtained, referrals to other health-care providers, therapeutic interventions, education, disposition of the patient, and any planned follow-up visits. Each diagnosis or condition documented in the assessment should be addressed in the plan. The details of the plan should follow an orderly manner, which may vary depending on your practice setting. One suggested format is the following:

1. Additional laboratory and diagnostic tests.
2. Consults: referrals to specialists, therapists (physical, occupational), counselors, or other professionals.
3. Therapeutic modalities: pharmacological and nonpharmacological management.
4. Health promotion: address risk factors as appropriate and consider age-appropriate preventive health screening.
5. Patient education: explanations and advice given to patients and family members.
6. Disposition/follow-up instructions: when the patient is to return, the conditions or symptoms that indicate the patient should return sooner, and when to go to another facility such as an emergency department, urgent care center, specialist, or therapist.

Diagnostic Tests

Additional testing may be necessary to establish or evaluate a condition. Laboratory and imaging studies, physiological assessments, and other evaluations not performed during the patient encounter are components of the plan. Some tests, such as magnetic resonance imaging (MRI), may require prior authorization from the patient's insurance carrier. Documentation should establish the rationale for any testing ordered by the health-care provider.

Consults

Specialist consultations or referral to other health-care providers may be needed to establish a definitive diagnosis, to evaluate a known condition, or for treatment of an acute or chronic condition. For example, a patient with right lower quadrant (RLQ) pain may be referred to a surgeon to be evaluated for possible appendicitis. Pregnant women are often referred to an obstetrical-gynecological (OB/GYN) specialist for obstetrical management. A pediatric patient with speech difficulties could be referred to a speech therapist for evaluation and management. Physical therapists typically evaluate and treat injuries and musculoskeletal problems. Many insurance companies require an authorization for such consults. A copy of the medical record pertaining to the complaint is frequently reviewed to establish the "medical necessity" of the consultation. Thorough documentation is critical in justifying the need for service.

Therapeutic Modalities

Pharmacological Treatment

Patients are frequently prescribed medications to treat illnesses, conditions, or symptoms. Specific details of prescribed medication must be documented, such as name, dose, route of administration, frequency of administration, and duration. Prescription writing is covered in Chapter 10. Over-the-counter (OTC) medications are often recommended; the same details listed earlier for prescription medications should be documented for OTC medications. When prescribing or recommending a medication for use as needed (PRN), documentation should indicate what condition or symptom the medication is intended for, for example, diphenhydramine 25 mg 1–2 tablets at bedtime PRN sleep.

Documentation should also address any change in current medications, such as adjusting the dosage or frequency or discontinuing a medication. For example, Mrs. Jones has been taking amoxicillin for sinusitis for the past 5 days and is not improving. When issuing a new prescription for cephalexin, also document that she was instructed to discontinue the amoxicillin.

Nonpharmacological Treatment

A wide variety of nonpharmacological treatment modalities may be included in the patient's overall management plan. Behavioral and lifestyle changes, such as smoking cessation, weight loss, exercise, relaxation techniques, and dietary adjustments, are often recommended. Specific instructions may include "drink plenty of fluids and rest" or "rest, ice, compression, and elevation" (RICE) of an injured extremity. Dressing changes, activity modification, and monitoring parameters (e.g., blood pressure and blood glucose levels) are all nonpharmacological treatment modalities. Patient education is an important adjunct to therapeutic recommendations.

Health Promotion

The World Health Organization defines health promotion as "the process of enabling people to increase control over their health and its determinants, and thereby improve their health." One aspect of health promotion is education, which is discussed later. Another aspect is disease prevention through identification of risk factors and routine screening tests. Preventive care for adults is discussed in detail in Chapter 3, and preventive care for pediatric patients is discussed in Chapter 4.

Patient Education

Patient satisfaction surveys report that patient education is considered an important indicator of the quality of care received. When a patient has a positive encounter with a health-care provider, it is often because the provider took time to explain everything. Most patients want to know what is causing their symptoms, what their treatment options are, the expected outcome, and why or when to return to the office. When medication is prescribed or recommended, patients should be informed about the benefits and risks and potential side effects. Educating patients about their condition or disease enables them to take control of their health. Patients should be encouraged to be active participants in their own health care, which often improves compliance with treatment.

MEDICOLEGAL ALERT !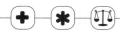

Documentation of patient education is not only good medical practice, it also may prevent a lawsuit. This applies to medications prescribed, tests performed, consents obtained, warnings, recommendations, patient education, and follow-up instructions.

Printed handouts are valuable tools to reinforce instructions given verbally to patients. There are many resources available on just about any condition you might encounter. Some books have tearout sheets to give to patients. Others have pages you can photocopy. There are software programs and websites that allow you to customize and personalize handouts with your office logo and information. Pharmaceutical companies may provide patient education materials; for example, a company that makes insulin will offer handouts related to care of a diabetic patient, such as dietary information, logbooks for patients to record blood glucose readings, and other educational materials for patients and their families. Documenting which handouts and materials you give the patient may prompt you to inquire about the patient's understanding of the material at a subsequent visit. Simply providing written material to the patient does not meet your obligation to provide education. You should determine the patient's ability to read and understand the material before distributing written materials. Figure 5-1 is an example of a patient education handout.

Follow-Up Instructions

It is important to document follow-up instructions at every patient visit, regardless of the reason for the visit. Specific information that should be documented includes when the patient should return for follow-up, signs or symptoms that could indicate worsening of the patient's condition, and what to do if those signs or symptoms develop. The patient may be advised to call the provider for further instructions. The provider may determine that the patient should return to the office for reevaluation or may instruct the patient to go to an urgent care center or emergency department if a serious problem may have developed.

The time frame for routine follow-up is usually determined by how soon you would expect a patient to exhibit a response to the treatment initiated. If a patient has been taking antibiotics for otitis media, you would expect the patient to improve within 48 to 72 hours; therefore, documentation would include "follow up if not improved in 2 to 3 days." Consider potential complications that could occur; in the case of otitis media, meningitis is a rare but serious complication. Document the specific symptoms that indicate the need for evaluation, such as persistent fever, headache, vomiting, or neck stiffness. This is especially important for pediatric patients and in situations in which the patient's condition could deteriorate rapidly. Failure to document your instructions to the patient is considered failure to provide those instructions.

Follow-up visits are an opportune time to ask patients whether they have any questions about what was discussed at previous visits. Encouragement and reinforcement will promote patient understanding of the condition and compliance with treatment, which, in turn, may lead to a more favorable outcome. Numerous studies indicate that communication between clinician and patient is the single most effective predictor of patient adherence to a treatment plan. If the clinician uses effective communication skills, the patient will become an educated participant in the treatment, thereby increasing the likelihood of compliance. The concept of effective clinician-patient communication is a necessity, not an option.

Sleep Hygiene Guide

- Take a hot bath to raise your temperature for 30 minutes within 2 hours of bedtime. A hot drink may also help you.

- Daily exercise at least 6 hours before bedtime is best.

- Consider purchasing a "noisemaker" to block out background noise. It plays soothing sounds of "white noise" or raindrops, ocean waves, etc.

- Limit naps to 10 or 15 minutes during the day. Short naps can be beneficial.

- Listen to tapes of relaxing music or soothing natural sounds if you have trouble falling alseep.

- Jot down problems and set aside a time the next day to focus on them.

- Eliminate intrusive sound and light from your bedroom so you won't be awakened accidentally.

- Sleep in a cool, well-ventilated room (ideal temperature 64° to 66°F).

- Limit caffeine use to no more than 3 cups consumed before 10 a.m.

- Do not smoke after 7 p.m. or quit smoking altogether. **Nicotine has the same effect as caffeine on sleep.**

- Use alcohol lightly. Alcohol can fragment sleep, especially the second half of your sleeping period.

- Avoid heavy meals and heavy spices in the evening. If you have regurgitation problems, raising the head of the bed should help.

- Develop a bedtime ritual. Bedtime reading, unrelated to work, may help relax you.

- If you wake in the night, don't try too hard to fall asleep; rather, focus on the pleasant sensations of relaxation.

- Avoid unfamiliar sleep environments.

- Quality of sleep is important. Too much time in bed can decrease the quality of the next night's sleep.

- Limit the bedroom to sleep and relaxation. Don't use it as a work area.

Figure 5-1 Sleep Hygiene Guide.

Application Exercise 5.8

Refer to Ms. Kearns' note from Application Exercise 5.7. Assume that your facility does not have the capability to perform any diagnostic testing. The assessment is chest pain. Write a plan for Ms. Kearns that addresses each of the components mentioned previously.

_____
_____
_____
_____
_____
_____
_____
_____
_____

Ms. Kearns returns for a follow-up visit 2 days later.

Here are her test results:

CBC: WBC 7.0, RBC 4.75, Hgb 15.1, Hct 47.3, MCV 98, MCH 31.8, MCHC 31.9, RDW 13.7, platelet count 326, neutrophils 55, lymphocytes 35, monocytes 7, eosinophils 3, basophils 1.

CXR: normal per radiologist.

ECG: normal sinus rhythm (NSR) without acute changes, per my interpretation.

Based on these results, what is your assessment and plan?

_____
_____
_____
_____
_____
_____

To reinforce the content of this chapter, please complete the worksheets that follow. Worksheets 5.5, 5.6, and 5.7 include SOAP notes for visits in different practice settings, written by various providers. Compare and contrast these notes and how they are adapted for the chief complaint and setting of care.

Part A

Read the following and answer the questions that follow:

A 45-year-old woman presents with a chief complaint of right hand pain.

List the seven cardinal aspects of the history of present illness that should be documented in the subjective information.

_____

_____

_____

List several pertinent aspects of the PMH that should be documented.

_____

_____

_____

What information about the patient's social history would be important to document?

_____

_____

_____

Part B

A patient presents with a chief complaint of back pain. Below are several statements from the HPI for a chief complaint of back pain. Number them in the order they should appear in the subjective paragraph.

1. _____ Pertinent negative associated symptom: The patient denies any trauma.

2. _____ Aggravating factor: The pain is worse after standing or walking for more than 20 minutes.

3. _____ Onset: The pain started 3 days ago after moving some heavy furniture.

4. _____ Pertinent positive associated symptom: The patient has had a tingling sensation in the right buttock area.

5. _____ Severity: The pain is described as a dull ache and is rated as a 4/10.

Part C

After the HPI, the past medical history (PMH) should be documented. Place a check beside all statements that are part of the PMH.

_____ There is no family history of heart disease.

_____ The patient smokes 1 pack per day.

_____ The patient is allergic to penicillin.

_____ The patient works as a mechanic.

_____ The patient has no chronic medical conditions.

_____ The patient takes Zantac daily.

Part D

Which of the following would be documented as subjective information? Circle all that apply.

vital signs

x-ray report

physical examination findings

history obtained from spouse

family history

review of systems

medications

complete blood count (CBC) results

onset of chief complaint

Part E

Number the following sentences in the order they should appear in the objective paragraph, according to "head-to-toe" order.

1. _____ The abdomen is soft and nondistended.

2. _____ The oropharynx shows some erythema of the posterior pharyngeal wall but no exudates.

3. _____ Auscultation of the lungs does not reveal any abnormal breath sounds.

4. _____ The neck is supple with full range of motion, and there are no signs of meningeal irritation.

5. _____ The skin is warm to touch and without cyanosis.

Medical Terminology

Next to each lay term, write an acceptable medical term and the ICD-9 code.

1. miscarriage _____

2. mole _____

3. nearsightedness _____

4. stiff neck _____

5. athlete's foot _____

6. hives _____

7. measles _____

8. tingling _____

9. loss of appetite _____

10. shingles _____

11. canker sore _____

12. stye _____

Assessment and Plan

S: This 6-year-old child presents with a sore throat times 3 days. His mother states that he has had a fever of 101.5 orally, seems to have difficulty swallowing, and complains of a headache. His appetite is decreased. He has a runny nose with clear discharge. Denies cough, abdominal pain, vomiting, or diarrhea. There are no known exposures to communicable diseases. Tylenol helps the fever and sore throat "a little." PMH is negative. Meds: none. NKDA. The child is generally healthy. He is up to date on his immunizations.

O: T 100.8 (oral), P 98, R 20, BP 100/64

General: WDWN Caucasian male in NAD.

Skin: No rash

HEENT: Canals and TMs are unremarkable. Nasal mucosa is slightly congested with pink turbinates and clear discharge. Pharynx shows 3+ injected tonsils with scant exudates.

NECK: Supple. Tender, moderately enlarged tonsillar lymph nodes.

HEART: Rate 98 and regular without murmur.

LUNGS: Clear to auscultation. No adventitious sounds. Nonlabored breathing.

Abdomen: Soft, nondistended. Mildly tender throughout without guarding, rebound, or change in facial expression. No organomegaly or masses. Bowel sounds are normoactive.

1. What is your assessment of the patient described in the preceding example?

_____

_____

_____

2. What tests, if any, would you order? How might the results affect your DDX?

_____

_____

3. Write a Plan for this patient using all of the components discussed.

_____

_____

_____

_____

Plan Components

Which of the following would be documented in the plan? Underline all that apply.

physical examination findings

information from medical records

patient education

CBC results

R/O ankle fracture

laboratory and x-ray orders

vital signs

recommended OTC medications

follow-up instructions

review of systems

referrals

Number the following sentences in the suggested order they should appear in the plan.

_____ Discussed the DDX with patient.

_____ Follow-up in 2 weeks.

_____ CT of chest if symptoms not resolved within 2 weeks.

_____ Refer to respiratory for pulmonary function testing.

_____ Go to the ED if shortness of breath worsens despite albuterol.

_____ Handout on monitoring peak expiratory flow readings given and explained..

_____ Albuterol inhaler 1–2 puffs every 4–6 hours PRN wheezing.

SOAP Note Analysis—Sandra Harris

Below is a SOAP note for patient Sandra Harris. Ms. Harris presented to an urgent care center with complaints of nausea and vomiting. She has not been seen at this urgent care before. The SOAP note was written by Jason Wilson, a physician assistant student who is on a rotation at the urgent care center. Please read the note and answer the questions that follow.

S:

CC: "I have been nauseated and throwing up."

HPI: Pt is a 41-year-old who presents with a 1-day hx of nausea. Nausea began yesterday morning, and she began vomiting in the afternoon. Since onset of vomiting, she is unable to keep down solid food or liquids. She initially vomited 2-3 times per hour and then less frequently. Pt denies diarrhea or constipation. Pt denies recent travel or camping trip. Pt states a coworker was sick last week with an unknown illness.

PMH: Lactose intolerance. No meds.

ROS: + N/V, negative SOB, palpitations.

O: General: A&O x 3, in moderate distress, lying on exam table with emesis basin.

Vital Signs: BP 116/62, P 104, R 20, T 101

CV: RRR, no murmur

Respiratory: No wheezing or crackles

Abd: + bowel sounds x 4. Negative Murphy's and McBurney's.

A: Food poisoning, R/O hepatitis A, R/O GERD

P: IV of normal saline fluid bolus
CBC, BMP
Ibuprofen

Jason Wilson, PA-S II

---

1. Analyze the subjective portion of the note. List additional information that should be included in the documentation.

2. Analyze the objective portion of the note. List additional information that should be included in the documentation.

3. Is the assessment supported by the subjective and objective information? Why or why not?

4. Did you consider other differential diagnoses than the ones documented? If so, list.

5. What condition/symptom/diagnosis would be most appropriate to document for this visit? Can you find an ICD-9 code for it?

6. Does the plan correspond to the assessment? Why or why not?

7. Did you consider other interventions that could be included in the plan? If so, list.

SOAP Note Analysis–David Tobin

David Tobin is a patient who presented to an emergency department. Jacqueline Mitchell, the resident working in the ED, saw him and wrote this SOAP note. Please read it and answer the questions that follow.

S:

CC: "My lips and tongue swelled up and I thought I was going to die."

HPI: Pt states that 6 hours ago he had sudden onset of swelling in his lips and tongue. He had a hard time breathing. His wife urged him to take some Benadryl and he took one 25 mg tablet. After approximately 1 hour, the swelling began to resolve, and the difficulty breathing also resolved. At this time, he is not experiencing any difficulty breathing, and he feels that the swelling is almost completely gone. He specifically denies any chest pain or heart racing associated with this episode. He did not notice any itching of the skin or hives. He had one similar episode many years ago after eating shrimp, and has avoided all shellfish since that time. He is certain that he has not ingested shellfish in the past 48 hours.

PMH: HTN for at least 10 years. He was in good control on HCTZ only until recently. He saw his primary care provider earlier this week and was given a prescription for a new medication. The prescription is labeled as lisinopril 10 mg. He has taken four doses of lisinopril but never developed any symptoms until today. No hx of asthma or urticaria. Denies any immune disorders. Has never had any surgery.

   Medications: HCTZ 12.5 mg once daily for "many years." Lisinopril 10 mg daily started in the past 4 days.

   Allergies: No drug allergies that he is aware of. States an allergy to shellfish, which caused swelling of the lips and a rash; did not have dyspnea associated with that episode.

FAMILY Hx: No hx of angioedema. Mother had HTN; deceased at age 72 from CVA. Otherwise noncontributory.

SOCIAL Hx: Denies tobacco use. He drinks 3-4 beers per week. Denies drug use.

O: General: Pleasant 47-year-old male sitting in chair talking comfortably. No respiratory difficulty or cyanosis. Does not appear anxious at this time.

   Vital Signs: BP 138/86; P 98; R 22; T 98.9; pulse oximetry 98% on room air.

   Skin: Intact without lesions, no urticaria.

   HEENT: Head normocephalic. No noticeable swelling of lips. Oropharynx without erythema. No swelling of the tongue or uvula.

   Neck: Supple, full ROM. No tracheal deviation.

   Chest: Heart RRR. No murmurs. Breath sounds clear in all fields without wheezing. Good air movement throughout without increased effort of breathing.

   Ext: No swelling of hands or feet.

A: 1. Angioedema, resolved, probably secondary to lisinopril.
   2. HTN, stable at present.

P: 1. Stop lisinopril and do not take again.
   2. Follow up with PCP regarding medication change, continue HCTZ as directed.
   3. Return to ED immediately if any recurrence of symptoms.
   4. May take Benadryl 25-50 mg every 6 hours PRN itching or return of swelling of lips or tongue.

Jacqueline Mitchell, MD

---

1. Analyze the subjective portion of the note. List additional information that should be included in the documentation.

2. Analyze the objective portion of the note. List additional information that should be included in the documentation.

3. Is the assessment supported by the subjective and objective information? Why or why not?

4. Did you consider other differential diagnoses than the ones documented? If so, list.

5. What condition/symptom/diagnosis would be most appropriate to document for this visit? Can you find an ICD-9 code for it?

6. Does the plan correspond to the assessment? Why or why not?

7. Did you consider other interventions that could be included in the plan? If so, list.

SOAP Note Analysis—Cassandra Fields

The following SOAP note is for patient Cassandra Fields. Ms. Fields presented to an internal medicine office with complaints of abdominal pain. She has been seen at this office before, although not by this provider. She is seen by Michael Worly, Physician Assistant, who writes the SOAP note. Please read the note (page 113) and answer the questions that follow.

1. Analyze the subjective portion of the note. List additional information that should be included in the documentation.

2. Analyze the objective portion of the note. List additional information that should be included in the documentation.

3. Is the assessment supported by the subjective and objective information? Why or why not?

4. Did you consider other differential diagnoses than the ones documented? If so, list.

5. What condition/symptom/diagnosis would be most appropriate to document for this visit? Can you find an ICD-9 code for it?

6. Does the plan correspond to the assessment? Why or why not?

7. Did you consider other interventions that could be included in the plan? If so, list.

S:

CC: "My stomach has been hurting, and it is getting worse."

HPI: Ms. Fields complains of LLQ abdominal pain that began 3 days ago. She describes the pain as "crampy" and intermittent, although she says the pain never entirely goes away but waxes and wanes. At the onset, the pain was 2/10; however, it has progressively worsened every day, and she now rates the pain as an 8/10. The pain does not radiate but stays in the LLQ. The pain does not seem to be related to food intake. She has not identified any aggravating factors. She did take some Tums yesterday, 2 tablets, but did not experience any relief or change in the pain. She has felt warm and has had chills, but has not actually taken her temperature. She has had some nausea that started yesterday, but has not vomited. Pt has had chronic constipation for "at least 10 years" and says that she normally takes a laxative 2-3 times a week to stimulate bowel movements; in the past 24 hours, she has had 4-5 loose stools. She specifically denies any blood in the stool.

PMH: No hx of GI problems in the past other than the chronic constipation, no colitis, ulcers, malabsorption problems. No abdominal surgery; only surgical history is a breast biopsy 5 years ago that was negative. No previous episodes of similar symptoms. Menopausal for about 12 years.

   Medications: Ex-lax 2-3 times weekly for "at least 10 years". Takes a multivitamin once daily. No regular prescription meds.

   Allergies: Sulfa drugs, which she says gives her a rash.

FH: No hx of colon or other cancer.

SOCIAL: Denies tobacco use; occasional cocktail "on special occasions" but does not consume alcohol on a regular basis. Married, cares for husband who has dementia.

O: General: 64-year-old obese black woman sitting on table. Alert and conversant; febrile, looks mildly ill but NAD. Good historian.

   VS: BP 132/78; P 99.2; R 18; T 100.8

   Heart: RRR

   Lungs: Clear to auscultation

   Abd: Soft, obese, nondistended. No surgical scars. Tenderness to palpation localized to LLQ. No guarding or rebound. No masses or organomegaly. Bowel sounds present throughout. No tympany to percussion.

   Rectal: Soft dark stool in rectal vault. No masses. Stool negative for occult blood.

   Flat and upright abdominal plain films do not show any air fluid levels and no free air in the peritoneum, per my interpretation. Blood work pending.

A: 1. LLQ pain, probably acute diverticulitis, R/O partial bowel obstruction.
   2. Chronic constipation.

P: 1. CBC, CMP, UA
   2. Stop Ex-lax for now.
   3. Discussed further workup; pt unable to stay overnight in hospital as she is sole caretaker for husband. Since patient is not vomiting, will manage as outpatient but discussed with pt the potential complications of ruptured diverticula, possible widespread infection requiring surgery, and need for her to contact me immediately if she worsens at all. If condition worsens, will likely need hospitalization with urgent CT scan of abdomen, surgical consult.
   4. Metronidazole 500 mg PO BID x 14 days + ciprofloxacin extended release 500 mg by mouth once daily for 14 days. Pt educated on reason for double-antibiotic therapy.
   5. Acetaminophen 500 to 1000 mg every 4 hours prn pain or fever. Pt offered narcotic analgesic but declined.
   6. Promethazine 25 mg tablet PO every 6 hours prn N/V; advised on possible drowsiness, should not drive or operate machinery while taking.
   7. Return for follow-up in 48 hours. If any increased pain or vomiting and unable to keep down antibiotics, call office immediately.
   8. Clear liquid diet until nausea and pain resolve, then slowly advance diet.
   9. Will need routine colonoscopy when asymptomatic because she has not had one in approx. 10 years.
   10 . Patient given handout on diverticular disease, questions answered.

Michael Worly, PA-C

Writing a SOAP Note from Narrative

Now that you have evaluated some sample SOAP notes, it is time to apply what you have learned. This worksheet will give you the opportunity to take subjective and objective data gathered during a patient encounter and document them as a SOAP note. The subjective data are presented in narrative form. Pertinent positive and negative findings are given to incorporate into the objective portion of the note. With this information, you should be able to formulate and document an assessment and plan. Critically analyze the information given and determine how much of it needs to be documented. Document the encounter as you would for one that takes place in a primary care outpatient setting.

Ms. Monica Jacobs is a 57-year-old woman who comes in because of "leaking urine." This has been an occasional problem for the past 6 months or so, mostly occurring when she coughs or sneezes. In the past week, the problem is worse, and she says, "I just can't seem to hold my urine." She has to go to the bathroom every 1 to 2 hours and only voids a small amount each time. She gets up at least once during the night to void. She reports feeling an urgency to void but does not have any burning or pain when she voids. The sense of urgency is great; she states, "I have to go immediately or I will wet myself." She has been limiting her fluid intake to see if it would help with the symptoms, and has quit drinking coffee and tea; this hasn't seemed to make a difference. The problem is frustrating, and she has "to plan my day around where bathrooms are located. If I'm at the mall or the grocery store or waiting for my kids at soccer practice, I know where every bathroom is located." Ms. Jacobs is very self-conscious about the problem and says, "It is embarrassing to walk around with a wet spot on my pants. I've started wearing those pads that old women wear; I can't stand the thought I might have to start wearing diapers!" She has noticed her urine is dark with a strong odor. She thinks this is due to limiting her fluid intake. She has not had any fever or chills and has not had any nausea or vomiting.

Ms. Jacobs is generally healthy and does not have any active or chronic diseases. She takes a multivitamin every day and calcium supplements as recommended by her OB/GYN. She is allergic to penicillin, which causes a rash and swelling in her lips. She last saw her OB/GYN about 9 months ago for her routine checkup and didn't mention this because it happened infrequently at the time and she thought is was all "normal since I'm getting older." She entered menopause at age 49 and says she hasn't really had any problems with menopausal symptoms. Her checkup with the OB/GYN did not reveal any abnormal findings. Ms. Jacobs is married and has 5 children; all births were vaginal deliveries without complications. She has never had any abdominal or gynecological surgery. She had surgery for "chronic sinus problems" at age 28 and carpal tunnel surgery on the right hand at age 46. Her only sexual partner is her husband. Intercourse is pleasurable as long as she uses a lubricant. She does not discuss her problem with her husband because she is embarrassed about it.

Ms. Jacobs' parents are both deceased. Her father died at age 61 of a heart attack. Her mother had diabetes, diagnosed around the age of 45. She died from complications of colon cancer. Ms. Jacobs has three siblings: an older brother with blood pressure problems, one sister who has diabetes, and a younger brother who does not have any health problems she is aware of.

Ms. Jacobs is a life-long nonsmoker. She drinks wine 2–3 times a month. She has never used any illicit drugs. She typically drinks 2–3 cups of coffee per day and 3–4 glasses of tea daily, but has cut out those beverages for the past week to see whether it improved her symptoms. Her daily exercise consists of taking her dogs for a walk, although she admits that she has not done that for the past week as she "can't even make it around the block without feeling the urge to urinate and having to go. I'd have to wear a diaper to make it through my usual route."

(*The only positive findings from the ROS are those above. As you write the SOAP note, consider whether you need to include any pertinent negatives in your documentation.*)

Ms. Jacobs is a well-developed, well-nourished woman who appears her stated age. She is not in any distress at the present time. She is alert and cooperative and interactive and answers questions appropriately.

Vital signs recorded in the chart are as follows:

BP 124/72, P 86, RR 18, T 99.1, height: 5'8", weight: 174 lb

The physical examination (excluding the pelvic exam) is essentially normal. (*Write in findings for a "normal examination" that you would conduct related to the patient's problem.*) Here are the findings for the pelvic and rectal examinations:

Pelvic: atrophic changes noted of the external genitalia, but no erythema, lesions, or masses. Vaginal mucosa pale, loss of rugae consistent with age-related changes. Cervix parous, pale, without discharge. Uterus anterior, midline, smooth, and not enlarged. No adnexal tenderness. Rectovaginal wall intact. Positive dribbling of urine with cough and bearing down.

Rectal: no perirectal lesions or fissures. External rectal sphincter tone intact; rectal vault with soft brown stool; without masses.

A voided urine sample is obtained and results of a urine dip are as follows:

Color: dark amber

Clarity: clear

Specific gravity: 1.022

pH: 6.5

Negative for nitrites, leukocyte esterase, protein, blood, glucose, urobilinogen, and bilirubin.

Write a SOAP note based on the subjective and objective information above, adding your assessment and plan. Assume that the urine dip is the only test that can be performed immediately in the office; any other diagnostic studies will have to be sent to an outside laboratory.

After writing the SOAP note, answer the following questions.

1. Did you decide not to include any subjective information given in your documentation? Why or why not?

2. Do you feel additional subjective information should be documented that was not provided? If so, list.

3. Do you feel additional objective information should be documented that was not provided? If so, list.

4. Are you able to establish a definitive diagnosis for Ms. Jacobs at this encounter? Why or why not?

5. List any assessments you included in your documentation and ICD-9 codes for any that would be billed as part of this visit.

6. How many elements of the plan, described earlier under Plan, are included in your documentation?

Writing a SOAP note is sometimes difficult for students or health-care providers with limited experience, especially formulating the plan of care. If you fall into one of these categories, we encourage you to compare your SOAP note with others and to seek feedback from faculty or other experienced providers.

Abbreviations

These abbreviations were introduced in Chapter 5. Beside each, write the meaning as indicated by the context in this chapter.

A&O _____

BID _____

BMP _____

cm _____

CT _____

CVA _____

DDX _____

DM _____

ED _____

FH _____

GERD _____

HgbA1c, HbA1c _____

HCTZ _____

HR _____

HX, Hx _____

IV _____

JVD _____

LLQ _____

MCH _____

MCHC _____

MCV _____

mg _____

MRI _____

NAD _____

NKDA _____

NSR _____

N/V _____

OB/GYN _____

PCP _____

PPD _____

PRN _____

RBC _____

RDW _____

RICE _____

RLQ _____

UTI _____

WDWN _____

Chapter 6

Outpatient Charting and Communication

OBJECTIVES

- Identify information that may be part of a patient's medical record other than documentation of medical encounters.
- Discuss how a problem list may be used.
- Discuss the rationale for maintaining a medication list.
- List conditions in which flow sheets are useful.
- Discuss the documentation that should be included in a noncompliance note.
- Describe the typical content of a letter from a consulting provider to a referring provider.
- Discuss the purpose of advance directives.
- Discuss the importance of documenting telephone communication with patients.
- Discuss the use of electronic mail communication in the outpatient setting.
- Discuss some of the challenges and benefits associated with health-care providers' use of social media sites.

As discussed in Chapter 5, SOAP notes may be used to document the details of a patient encounter in either an inpatient (hospital) or outpatient (office) setting. Documenting the medical encounter is just one component of a patient's medical record; other types of documents should be kept to ensure continuity of care and to preserve information used in overall patient management. A medical record is created for each patient and should be arranged in a consistent, uniform manner. The contents and organization of the record will vary depending on the needs of the practice. Some providers may use forms such as a problem list, medication list, or flow sheet for some of their patients. Patients may not always be compliant with recommended treatment or follow a provider's recommendation. From a medicolegal standpoint, it is important to document noncompliance when it occurs. Other information that may become part of the patient's medical record includes demographic and billing information, communication with other providers, results of laboratory or other diagnostic studies, records from other health-care providers

or hospitals, information related to advance directives, and documentation of telephone and electronic communication with patients.

Problem List

To promote continuity of care by identifying key elements of the patient's health history, information from parts of the medical records is often summarized on a problem list, such as the one shown in Figure 6-1. The list is usually prominently displayed in the chart for easy access and reference. Problems are listed as either active or inactive. Active problems include current or chronic conditions that require ongoing management or further workup. The date of onset and the *International Classification of Diseases, 9th Revision* (ICD-9) code for each problem is documented. Inactive problems are those that occurred in the past but are now resolved and can be either medical or surgical. It is important to update the list

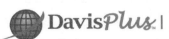 **DavisPlus** | Visit **http://davisplus.fadavis.com** for complete learning activities on actual EMR software at, Keyword: Sullivan

Vernon Scott, MD, PC
Health History / Problem List

Name:	S.S.# ____-____-_____	Male ____		Adv. Directives Yes __ No __
DOB:	Tel.# ____-____-_____	Fem ___ G __ P __ Ab __	Organ Donor Yes __ No__	

PROBLEM LIST	ALLERGIES:	
1.	Hospitalizations:	Surgeries:
2.	Date:	Reason:	Date:	Reason:
3.				
4.				
5.				
6.				
7.				
8.				
9.				
10.				

Social History	Family History	CANCER: colon ___ breast ___ other ___
S ____ M ____ D ____ W ____	Father:	HTN: CAD: CVA:
Smoking: ETOH:	Mother:	DM:
Caffeine: Exercise:	Siblings:	Osteoporosis:
Occup:	Children:	Other:

Breast	Date / Result							
Pap/Pelvic Exam	Date / Result							
Mammogram	Date / Result							
Prostate/Testicular	Date / Result							
PSA	Date / Result							
Colonoscopy/Sigmoid	Date / Result							
FOBT Cards	Date / Result							
CBC	Date / Result							
CMP	Date / Result							
TSH	Date / Result							
Total Cholesterol	Date / Result							
HDL	Date / Result							
LDL	Date / Result							
Triglycerides	Date / Result							
CXR	Date / Result							
ECG	Date / Result							
DEXA	Date / Result							

Figure 6-1 Sample problem list.

by entering pertinent data as soon as it is received. For example, if a bone density report confirms the diagnosis of osteoporosis, this diagnosis should be added to the problem list. Upon receiving a hospital discharge summary, any newly diagnosed conditions or surgeries should be added to the list. The organization and content of the problem list will vary depending on the needs of the practice or facility.

Application Exercise 6.1

Refer to the comprehensive history and physical examination shown in Figure 2-1. Use the data from the figure to create a problem list for Mr. Jensen, and then compare it with the problem list shown in Figure 6-2.

Medication List

A medication list provides a quick and easy format to document all the medications a patient is taking at any given time. All prescription and nonprescription medications should be listed. It is important to include herbal products, vitamins, minerals, dietary supplements, or other regularly used over-the-counter (OTC) products. A comprehensive list will alert the provider to possible drug-drug or drug-herb interactions. It will also help to avoid duplication, such as prescribing too many agents containing acetaminophen. The list should include the name of the medication, indication, strength, and dosing directions, as shown in Figure 6-3. The prescriber may wish to include the quantity written for and number of refills authorized on the medication list in order to have this information easily located in one place. This is helpful to office staff who may take messages from patients requesting refills. If a patient takes more than one prescription drug for a condition, such as antihypertensive medications, it is helpful to list them together. When a medication is discontinued, it is helpful to indicate the date and reason why directly on the medication list. Medication allergies should be noted prominently in the chart, and the specific reaction to each should be documented on the medication list. Allergies to food or other substances, such as nickel, latex, or tape, may be included on the medication list. If the patient has had adverse reactions to any medications, such as a cough from an angiotensin-converting enzyme (ACE) inhibitor or severe nausea from codeine, document this information on the medication list as well. Providers may wish to include information about the patient's insurance plan if use of a specific formulary is required. It is convenient to include the name, location, and phone number for the pharmacy that the patient uses to fill prescriptions.

It is imperative that the provider review and update the medication list at every visit.

MEDICOLEGAL ALERT !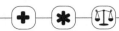

Although the medication list is helpful as a quick reminder of medications a patient is taking, you should never assume that it is a complete and accurate record. Patients may start taking medications on their own or prescribed by another provider, or they may discontinue a medication and forget to tell you. It is your responsibility as the provider to determine what medications the patient is taking at every visit before writing any prescriptions.

Application Exercise 6.2

Refer to the comprehensive history and physical examination (see Fig. 2-1) for Mr. William Jensen. Using the blank form in Figure 6-3, complete a medication list for Mr. Jensen. Compare it with the form shown in Figure 6-4.

Flow Sheets

Many chronic medical conditions require regular monitoring of certain parameters. The frequency of monitoring depends on whether the patient is stable or unstable. For conditions in which monitoring of a laboratory test or some other parameter is needed, a flow sheet is helpful. Flow sheets are commonly used to track results of coagulation studies, such as the international normalized ratio (INR) and prothrombin time (PT) for a patient on anticoagulant therapy, blood pressure readings of the patient with hypertension, blood glucose and hemoglobin A1c levels of patients with diabetes, and results of lipid studies of patients with dyslipidemia. Another use of flow sheets is to track periodic interventions or treatments for certain conditions, such as a patient with anemia who receives monthly vitamin B_{12} injections or a patient who receives Depo-Provera injections every 3 months for contraception. Figure 6-5 shows an example of a flow sheet that is used to monitor anticoagulation therapy.

Noncompliance with Medical Treatment

Health-care providers are obligated to educate and inform patients about their medical conditions, the treatment options available and the risks and benefits of each, and the risks and benefits of no treatment at all. Despite the best efforts of health-care providers,

Vernon Scott, MD, PC
Health History / Problem List

Name: William R. Jensen	S.S.# ____-____-_____	Male _X_		Adv. Directives Yes _X_ No __
DOB: March 30, 19XX	Tel.# ____-____-_____	Fem ___ G __ P __ Ab __		Organ Donor Yes _X_ No__

PROBLEM LIST		ALLERGIES: PENICILLIN			
1. Hypertension, diagnosed at age 53		Hospitalizations:		Surgeries:	
2. Dyslipidemia, diagnosed at age 58		Date:	Reason:	Date:	Reason:
3.				1988	right rotator cuff repair
4.				1981	left inguinal herniorrhaphy
5.					
6.					
7.					
8.					
9.					
10.					

Social History	Family History	CANCER: colon ___
		breast _M_
		other ___
S ____ M _X_ D ____ W ____	Father: died at age 74, complications of COPD, alcoholism	HTN: X CAD: X CVA:
Smoking: pipe 3 x wk ETOH	Mother: died at age 70, breast cancer	DM:
Caffeine: 2-3 per day Exercise: walk	Siblings: brother, age 71, HTN	Osteoporosis:
Occup: retired electrician	Children:	Other:

Breast	Date						
	Result						
Pap/Pelvic Exam	Date						
	Result						
Mammogram	Date						
	Result						
Prostate/Testicular	Date						
	Result						
PSA	Date						
	Result						
Colonoscopy/Sigmoid	Date						
	Result						
FOBT Cards	Date						
	Result						
CBC	Date						
	Result						
CMP	Date						
	Result						
TSH	Date						
	Result						
Total Cholesterol	Date						
	Result						
HDL	Date						
	Result						
LDL	Date						
	Result						
Triglycerides	Date						
	Result						
CXR	Date						
	Result						
ECG	Date						
	Result						
DEXA	Date						
	Result						

Figure 6-2 Problem list for Mr. Jensen.

MEDICATION LIST

Last name:		First:		Middle Initial:

Date of birth:	Contact Number:

DRUG ALLERGIES:

Preferred Pharmacy:	Pharmacy Phone:

Location:	Insurance plan:

Drug Name and Dose	Schedule	Date Started	Reason

Regular OTC Medications	Dosage	Frequency	Reason

Supplements/Vitamins	Dosage	Frequency	Reason

Figure 6-3 Sample medication list.

MEDICATION LIST

Last name: Jensen		**First:** William		**Middle initial:** R.

Date of birth: March 30, 19XX		**Contact Number:** 555-987-6543

DRUG ALLERGIES: penicillin - rash

Preferred Pharmacy: MedMart		**Pharmacy Phone:** 555-780-4444

Location: Poplar St at 12th Ave.		**Insurance plan:** Medicare

Drug Name and Dose	**Schedule**	**Date Started**	**Reason**
Lotensin HCT 20/12.5	every am	4/10/20XX	HTN
Mevacor 20 mg	1w/evening meal	10/2/20XX	dyslipidemia

Regular OTC Medication	**Dosage**	**Frequency**	**Reason**

Supplements/Vitamins	**Dosage**	**Frequency**	**Reason**
One-A-Day for Men	1 tablet	daily	general well-being
Fish oil supplement	1 tablet	a.m. and p.m.	CVD prophylaxis

Figure 6-4 Medication list for Mr. Jensen.

patients will not always follow their advice. There are many reasons why a patient may be noncompliant with recommended treatment; some are unintentional, and some are intentional. Some unintentional barriers to compliance may be the patient's culture, language, religious practices or beliefs, or socioeconomic factors. Every attempt should be made to identify barriers and assist the patient in becoming compliant if the patient desires to do so. Even when fully informed about the possible consequences of noncompliance, patients may choose not to follow a recommended treatment plan.

COUMADIN/ANTICOAGULANT FLOW SHEET

Name _____   Date Coumadin Started _____

Phone _____   Diagnosis _____

DATE	Coumadin Dose (mg)	INR	Protime	Coumadin New Dose	When to Recheck	Remarks

Figure 6-5 Coumadin/anticoagulant flow sheet.

If a patient's medical condition fails to improve, the health-care provider must determine why. Failure to improve could mean that the patient has not been correctly diagnosed, the correct treatment has not been initiated, or the patient has not been compliant with the recommended treatment. It is important to have a conversation with the patient, and perhaps family members or caregivers, to determine whether noncompliance is a factor. The patient should be asked whether he or she is taking any prescribed medication; if so, is the patient taking it appropriately? Has the patient instituted recommended lifestyle changes? Is the patient getting diagnostic tests done, or going to therapy? Has the patient consulted and followed up with the specialist? After exploring these considerations, try to ascertain the patient's understanding of the ramifications of noncompliance. If the patient simply refuses to follow treatment recommendations, even when he or she understands the potential consequences of not following treatment, then the patient is considered to be noncompliant. The information discussed with the patient, including the potential consequences of continued noncompliance, and the patient's response must be documented in detail. "Noncompliance" should be documented in the assessment and on the problem list. Any advice or education provided should be documented in the plan. The ICD-9 code V15.81 may be used for noncompliance with medical treatment.

EXAMPLE 6.1 NONCOMPLIANCE NOTE_____

S: Mr. Graham, age 49, is here for follow-up on hypertension. He has not been taking the hydrochlorothiazide 12.5 mg that was prescribed for him at the last office visit 2 weeks ago. He states, "I feel fine. I don't need to take any medicine." He denies chest pain, shortness of breath, swelling in the feet or ankles, visual changes, or headache. He has been counseled on smoking cessation but continues to smoke a pack of cigarettes daily. At the last visit, I recommended that he try to exercise 20 to 30 minutes 3 days of the week, but he has not yet initiated any exercise. His mother died of a stroke at age 59, and his father died at age 51 years from a myocardial infarction. He has a younger brother with hypertension that is controlled with medication.

O: Mr. Graham is a well-developed, obese man in no acute distress (NAD). He appears agitated.

Ht 6 ft, 2 in, Wt: 265 lb, BP right 168/102, left 172/104, T 98.2 orally, pulse is 94 and regular, respirations 20 per minute.

Eyes: Pupils are round and reactive to light bilaterally. Discs are sharp with normal cup-to-disc ratio. Fundi are unremarkable without AV nicking or exudates.

Neck: No carotid bruits or jugular venous distention (JVD).

Heart: Regular rate and rhythm (RRR) without murmur, clicks, or gallops. Normal S1 and S2.

Chest: Breath sounds clear to auscultation (CTA) all fields. There is no increased anteroposterior (AP) diameter of the thorax.

Abdomen: Soft, nontender, no organomegaly or masses, physiological bowel sounds.

Extremities: No edema. Pedal pulses are 2+ and equal bilaterally.

Urinalysis (UA): Specific gravity 1.012, no proteinuria or hematuria.

Electrocardiogram (ECG): normal sinus rhythm (NSR) without acute ischemic changes.

AP and lateral chest x-ray (CXR): No active disease, no cardiomegaly.

A: (1) Uncontrolled hypertension
(HTN), recently diagnosed.   401.9
(2) Noncompliance; patient has
refused treatment up to this point.   V15.81
(3) Obesity with body mass index
(BMI) of 34.   278.01
(4) Tobacco use disorder   305.1

P: Had 15-minute discussion with patient regarding hypertension, its historical course with and without treatment, importance of taking prescribed medication daily, and potential complications of nontreatment, including stroke, heart attack, and death. Discussed his personal and family risk factors for these conditions. Also discussed HTN as the "silent killer" and explained possible end-organ damage despite not having symptoms or feeling bad. He stated his understanding and had no questions. He expressed reservations about "starting a pill that I will have to take forever" but stated he will consider starting the medication. He did agree to have the nurse at work check his blood pressure daily, and he will get the fasting blood work done. He agreed to follow up here in 2 weeks.

MEDICOLEGAL ALERT !

It is crucial to document noncompliance in a patient's medical record. If it is not documented and the patient has a poor outcome, the patient or a family member may file a malpractice suit against you claiming that you were negligent or did not care for the patient appropriately. You must document that you counseled the patient about the medical condition, discussed the risks and benefits of the recommended and alternative treatment options, and warned the patient about potential morbidity and mortality complications. Whenever possible, use direct quotes from the patient. Refrain from making any judgment statements about the patient; document objective observations only.

Demographic and Billing Information

It is necessary to collect some demographic information about patients. At a minimum, you should document the patient's full legal name, address, telephone number, and date of birth. If the patient is a minor, document who is authorized to make health-care decisions for the patient. In the case of a minor when the parents are unmarried or divorced, it is prudent to document who is the custodial parent. Because of concerns about identify theft, it is recommended that the patient's Social Security number (SSN) not be used as an identification number or medical record number. Include the SSN in the medical record only if it is needed for billing purposes or another specific reason.

Billing information is important to document in the record. If the patient has insurance, identify the policyholder and his or her relationship to the patient. Make a copy of the insurance identification card and keep it in the chart. It is generally recommended that billing information and any correspondence regarding billing and payment issues be kept separate from clinical data.

Results of Laboratory Studies and Other Diagnostic Tests

Evaluation of a patient's condition often requires ordering laboratory tests, ECGs, imaging studies, and other diagnostic tests. Some electronic medical record (EMR) systems are designed to integrate with outside laboratories or other vendors that provide diagnostic testing so that results are communicated from the vendor directly into the patient's medical record. In a paper chart, it is helpful to have a section of the medical record specifically for the results of such tests. These are usually filed in chronological order, with the most recent results accessed first. Diagnostic imaging reports, rather than the actual images, are usually kept in the patient's record if the images were done at another location. Even when imaging studies are done on site, the actual images are often stored in a specific location, and just the reports are kept in the medical record.

Communication with Other Providers

A referral is when one health-care provider advises the patient to see another provider. Often, a referral or request for consultation is made when evaluation or management of a condition is beyond the scope of the referring provider's training or experience. The consultant's role may be to recommend further diagnostic testing, make a diagnosis, recommend a plan of treatment, or manage the patient's condition, or a combination of these. To clarify the role of each provider, reference may be made to the *referring provider* and the *consulting provider*. It is the referring provider's responsibility to specify the reason for the referral and the action desired so that the consulting provider knows whether to provide an opinion only or to manage the patient's condition actively. Any information pertinent to the referral must be transmitted to the consulting provider for review and may include a written summary, progress notes, problem list, medication list, flow sheets, test results, other consultants' notes, and sometimes hospital records. This communication between providers helps to avoid duplicating tests that have already been done or prescribing treatment that may have been previously tried but was not effective.

The primary care provider maintains responsibility for the overall health of the patient even when the patient is under a specialist's care. Consulting providers are expected to communicate with the referring provider in a timely manner. Patient authorization is not needed for communication between providers; it is implied with the referral. The initial consultation note typically consists of a comprehensive history; a complete or focused physical examination; impression, or assessment; and recommendations for care, management, or further workup. If the patient is to remain under the care of the consulting provider, the referring provider should be updated periodically on the patient's condition and response to treatment.

A comprehensive history and physical examination for Mr. William Jensen was provided in Figure 2-1. Part of the plan for the visit was to refer the patient to Dr. Michael Bennett for colonoscopy and biopsy. Figure 6-6 shows a letter from Dr. Scott to Dr. Bennett requesting assistance in the workup of this patient. Figure 6-7 shows a letter from Dr. Bennett to Dr. Scott with the results of the workup.

Prior Medical Records

When available, medical records from other providers and specialists should be reviewed. These records may be invaluable in filling in details and providing insight into the patient's past medical history, especially when the patient has a chronic condition that requires ongoing care. It is particularly helpful to evaluate what treatments have been tried in the past

Vernon Scott, MD
2000 Oak Street, Suite 311
Phoenix, AZ 85005
602-537-2000

Michael W. Bennett, MD
Southwest Gastrointestinal Specialty Group
5700 E. VanHorn St. Suite 25
Phoenix, AZ 85002

RE: William R. Jensen   DOB: March 30, 19XX

Dear Dr. Bennett,

Thank you for agreeing to see Mr. William R. Jensen. Mr. Jensen is a pleasant 67-year-old man who is a new patient to my practice. He presented to my office with complaints of fatigue and feeling weak. He also gave a history of a 10-pound unintentional weight loss over the past 2 months. His PMH is significant for hypertension and dyslipidemia, which have been stable with medical management. He is presently taking Lotensin HCT 20/12.5 once daily and Mevacor 20 mg once daily. He is allergic to penicillin, which gives him a rash. During workup at my office, he was found to have hemoccult-positive stools. His WBC is 5.8 and H&H 13 and 46. There is a family history of breast cancer. Mr. Jensen has had one colonoscopy approximately 15 years ago and no screening since.

Considering the fatigue, weight loss, and hemoccult-positive stool, I recommended to Mr. Jensen that he undergo colonoscopy with biopsy. He is scheduled to see you within the next 2 weeks. I have enclosed a copy of his CBC, CMP, and ECG for your review. Should you need additional information, please do not hesitate to contact me.

Sincerely,

Vernon Scott, MD

Encl: 3

Figure 6-6 Referral letter to Dr. Bennett.

and the efficacy of the treatments; this will avoid prescribing an ineffective treatment and may save time and money for both the provider and the patient. Results of prior laboratory tests or diagnostic studies can be used for comparison purposes. If a patient has been hospitalized, it is helpful to have a copy of the admission history and physical examination and the discharge summary in the medical records. Especially in instances in which the patient is managed by a hospitalist and not the patient's regular health-care provider, having access to such documents helps to ensure continuity of care and to provide accurate information pertaining to the patient's condition. In some instances, the admitting physician will indicate that a copy of the records should be sent to the primary health-care provider. At times, the patient may need to request a copy of these records from the hospital and give them to the provider. To ensure compliance with Health Insurance Portability and Accountability Act (HIPAA) regulations, a signed release of information is required to release any medical records from one facility or provider to another.

All staff should be aware of this requirement and should know the proper procedures for releasing medical records.

Advance Directives

Health-care advance directives are documents that communicate a person's wishes about health-care decisions in the event the person becomes incapable of making health-care decisions. Often, patients communicate their wishes to their health-care providers, but when a person can no longer communicate sufficiently, another process for decision making is needed. With the growing ability of medical technology to prolong life, decision making about medical care is of great concern. Patients may have strong feelings that death is preferable to perpetual dependence on medical equipment or having no hope of returning to a certain quality of life. Others feel just as strongly that heroic measures and technology should be used to extend life as long as possible. Advance directives

Michael W. Bennett, MD
Southwest Gastrointestinal Specialty Group
5700 E. VanHorn St., Suite 25
Phoenix, AZ 85002

Vernon Scott, MD
2000 Oak Street, Suite 311
Phoenix, AZ 85005

RE: William R. Jensen   DOB: March 30, 19XX

Dear Dr. Scott,

It was a pleasure to see Mr. William Jensen for consultation regarding his weight loss and fatigue. Prior to the colonoscopy, Mr. Jensen sent in three stool sample cards, two of which were positive for blood. A colonoscopy was performed at the outpatient surgical center; he tolerated the procedure well. GI prep was adequate. Several suspicious polypoid lesions were visualized at the hepatic flexure area. Multiple biopsies were obtained, and there were no complications.

The pathology report confirms the diagnosis of adenocarcinoma of the colon. I met with Mr. Jensen and his wife yesterday to discuss the diagnosis and usual course of surgical management. I recommended that he see Dr. David Sanders for more information on the various surgical approaches. Mr. Jensen was agreeable to this and will call for an appointment.

I have enclosed a copy of the pathology report for your records. Thank you for allowing me to participate in the care of this patient. If he elects surgery, I would be happy to follow him with you. Please call me if any questions.

Respectfully,

Michael W. Bennett, MD

Encl: 1

Figure 6-7 Consultation letter from Dr. Bennett.

are important for younger as well as older adults. Unexpected end-of-life situations can happen at any age.

There are two basic kinds of advance directives: living wills and health-care power of attorney. Both of these have been researched and written about in detail elsewhere; only a brief discussion of each is provided here with the intention that health-care providers will talk with their patients about advance directives and encourage them to make these important decisions before being in a situation in which the directives are needed. Once the decisions are made, the patient should complete the necessary forms and submit a copy to the health-care provider so that it becomes a permanent part of the medical record.

A living will expresses a person's preference for medical care. In some states, the document is called a directive to doctors or a declaration. Living wills become effective only when the patient has lost capacity to make health-care decisions and that patient has a particular condition, such as a terminal illness or permanent unconsciousness. Specific issues usually covered in a living will include cardiopulmonary resuscitation, mechanical ventilation, and artificial nutrition and hydration. Health-care providers often need to explain the details involved in each of these issues so that the patient is able to make informed decisions. To be valid, a living will must comply with state law. A living will should be signed, dated, and witnessed by two people. Some states require a notary or permit a notary in lieu of two witnesses. The executed living will should be kept as a permanent part of the patient's medical record.

A health-care power of attorney (POA) is a document in which one person (the patient, or principal) names another person (the agent, attorney-in-fact, or proxy) to make decisions about health care. A POA differs from a living will in that it focuses on the decision-making process and not on a specific decision. The POA can cover a far broader range of health-care decisions. The health-care POA is different from a durable power of attorney, which authorizes someone to make financial transactions for the principal; it is specific to health-care decision making. The health-care POA can include a living will provision, but should do so only as guidance for the agent, rather than as a binding selection. An ideal agent has the ability to talk effectively with health-care providers and act as a strong advocate. The principal should discuss the details of possible future medical choices with the agent because the agent should be guided by the principal's preferences. The law of each state prescribes the essential formalities for a valid POA for health care. Most states require two witnesses; a few permit notarization as an alternative. Forms specific to each state are readily available from a variety of Internet sites. Once executed, a copy of the health-care POA document should be submitted to the health-care provider and made a permanent part of the medical record.

Documenting Communications with Patients

Communication with patients frequently occurs outside the office visit. Telephone communication is a common means of exchanging information between patients and health-care providers. The scope of telephone calls extends beyond the basic call to the provider's office to arrange an appointment. Calls are often requests for medical advice or are a means of providing other information, such as results of diagnostic tests. Therefore, the conversation that occurs by telephone is still an important part of the patient-provider relationship and, as such, is subject to documentation in much the same way as other medical visits.

Each practice should develop protocols delineating which calls must be transferred to the provider immediately, which calls may be returned at a later time, and which calls may be handled by another professional or office staff. If members of the professional staff are authorized to give telephone advice, written protocols should define the scope of the professional staff member's authority to give such advice in order to minimize the likelihood of staff practicing medicine without a license by giving advice that is outside of their scope of training.

Some offices use a telephone call log to document every call. If used, such logs should be retained as long as medical records are retained. Others may use specific forms for documenting telephone calls. Regardless of how the documentation is done, the same information should be consistently documented. This includes the date and time of the call, patient's name, name of caller and relationship to the patient, the complaint, advice given, follow-up plan, and disposition. The advice should be documented in detail, and ideally the caller should be asked to repeat it so that the provider can verify that the advice was understood. Failure to document may lead to liability related to failure to diagnose, delay of treatment, improper treatment, failure to follow up, and breach of confidentiality.

If the provider attempts to reach a patient by phone but is unable to do so, the attempts should be documented, including the date and time of each attempt. Before leaving messages on an answering machine or with someone other than the patient, consent should be obtained from the patient. The consent should specifically indicate with whom messages might be left and if messages may be left on an answering machine. Document in the patient's record that a message was left. The provider should never leave clinical information or advice on an answering machine; instead, leave only a name (without title) and phone number, and request a call back.

Telephone communication between provider and patient is not without its frustrations. Providers often view calls as unnecessary interruptions. Patients express frustration that they may have to wait by the phone to receive a call back from the provider. Several studies have shown that patients would prefer communicating with providers by electronic mail (e-mail); in one study (Stouffer, 2008), 90% of respondents wanted their providers to use e-mail communication. Like other modes of communication, there are advantages and disadvantages to using e-mail.

One of the greatest advantages is the convenience for patients. A patient can send an e-mail and receive a response without staying on hold or waiting by the phone. Patients believe that requesting prescription refills, obtaining routine test results, and scheduling appointments by e-mail saves time (Rajecki, 2009). Zhou and colleagues (2007) found that the use of e-mail and electronic messaging decreased the amount of time that providers spent on the telephone. Another advantage is that e-mail creates a documentation trail that can be used to record activity and conversation, providing a transcript of all that is said, and not said, in an electronic format.

There are perceived and real disadvantages to using e-mail. One of the most frequently cited disadvantages is related to revenue. A study at one large health maintenance organization (HMO) reported a decrease in annual office visit rates among patients who had online access to their provider (Zhou et al., 2007). A decrease in office visits could mean decreased income for the provider because office visits are billable visits. Only a few private insurance plans reimburse the provider for "e-visits" or "virtual visits" conducted by e-mail. According to the American Health Information Management Association (AHIMA), the lack of reimbursement from Medicare is a limiting factor in the number of providers using e-mail. If the Medicare policy were to change, it is likely that e-mail communications between provider and patient would increase.

Confidentiality and protected health information (PHI) are another concern with e-mail or electronic messaging. State and federal laws vary when it comes to patient privacy, particularly for patient conditions such as sexually transmitted diseases (STDs), HIV, substance abuse, and treatment for mental health conditions. Laws about e-mailing patients who seek care for these conditions are very stringent and may cause confusion for providers. HIPAA requires that electronic PHI, including e-mail, be communicated in a secure way, that is, through an encrypted system. There are many commercial services available that allow encrypted communication, but providers may be unwilling to pay for these services. In addition, patients may be unwilling to use encryption services to communicate with providers when their unencrypted e-mail system is quick and simple to use. Safeguarding the confidentiality of e-mail messages is difficult. Confidentiality can be breached by outsiders (hackers) or by patients and providers themselves who reply to or forward e-mails to individuals outside the patient-provider relationship. E-mails may be intercepted, altered, or delivered to the wrong address, resulting in people other than the intended recipients having access to the e-mail communication.

Many providers have concerns about potential legal problems. E-mails are still provider-patient communication and are discoverable—even deleted ones. A poorly written e-mail may be used to portray a provider as unprofessional. E-mails should be checked for accuracy and appropriate language. Flippant or humorous messages may look disrespectful when viewed later, out of context. There have not been any law suits yet over provider-patient e-mail consultations, but providers predict this will occur.

Other concerns about the use of e-mail have been identified. Providers may fear being bombarded by e-mails or having patients abuse the privilege. It may be difficult to confirm the identity of the patient in an e-mail request. Messages can be delayed by hours or even days, and not receiving a response in a timely manner may have adverse health consequences. Patients may e-mail about multiple complaints or problems. Viruses may be transmitted through attachments that may cause serious damage to computer systems. Patients may come to expect a quick response to e-mail. Limiting e-mails to English only may cause problems for patients with limited English proficiency. A certain level of patient literacy is required for the e-mail exchange to be beneficial and efficient.

If the decision is made to communicate with patients by e-mail, specific actions must be taken. Obtain written permission from patients to communicate with them by e-mail. Set expectations and limitations with patients about what they can e-mail and how long it will take to respond. Develop policies for the use of e-mail, including how e-mail messages will be incorporated into the patient's medical record. Most EMR systems have a feature that will archive e-mails in the patient's record. If this feature is not available, or if an EMR system is not used, e-mails should be printed and saved in the patient's medical record. Provider-patient e-mails are considered health-care organization business records and are therefore subject to the same storage, retention, retrieval, privacy, and security and confidentiality provisions as any other patient-identifiable health information. Confirm that you have the correct e-mail address for the intended recipient. Ensure that PHI sent by e-mail is encrypted with access provided only to authorized individuals who have an access code. Add a confidentiality disclaimer to e-mail messages that states the content is confidential and only intended for the stated recipient. It should also state that anyone receiving the e-mail in error must notify the sender, and return or destroy the e-mail as per the request of the sender. Never use e-mail distribution lists to send personal information.

The American Medical Association and American Medical Informatics Association have adopted guidelines for providers who choose to communicate with patients by e-mail. These associations stress that e-mail is best used as an *extension* of the patient-provider relationship and not a *replacement* for the relationship. Both sets of guidelines are available online for review. Unfortunately, a study done in 2006 (Brooks & Menachemi, 2006) found that few providers who communicated with patients by e-mail routinely used these guidelines, despite their availability for several years. A separate study (White et al., 2004) found that most patients involved with regular provider e-mail communication do follow guidelines when they are educated about their nature and importance. Providers should also be familiar with and follow state laws governing the use of e-mail communications.

Social Networking

Patients often use the Internet to educate themselves about medical conditions and treatment options. Information obtained from websites may have tremendous influence on patients, whether or not that information is credible or supported by medical research.

A portion of the medical encounter may be spent discussing information the patient brings to the visit, especially when the provider may have to educate patients on the inaccuracy of information. Disease-specific sites on conditions from asthma to Zollinger-Ellison syndrome are plentiful. Many health-care providers visit medical websites regularly. For years, providers have used the Internet to seek out clinical information about diseases, participate in continuing education programs, and collaborate with other providers across the country and around the world. Although the Internet continues to be used in these "traditional" ways, it is increasingly used as a means of social networking.

Social networking sites, such as Facebook, MySpace, and Twitter, have evolved from a preoccupation of high school and college students to the mainstream of social interaction that spans divisions of age, profession, and socioeconomic status. Several provider-only sites, such as Sermo, Ozmosis, PA-CLife, and Nurse LinkUp, offer providers the chance to connect with others in their profession for knowledge sharing, networking, and support. Access to these sites is controlled so that providers are able to share opinions and interact in a safe, guarded environment. Providers may be required to disclose their name and credentials, preventing users to hide behind a cloak of anonymity. Registered users of many online medical communities can flag information they believe is inappropriate, which enhances the quality of the information posted on the site.

Although these types of professional sites are growing in number and popularity, many providers are also turning to social media for professional reasons or networking. Hospitals and health-care systems use social media to communicate with colleagues and patients. Bennett (2010) reported that more than 1000 hospitals have accounts on a social media site, and a number of hospitals have blogs authored by the chief executive officer in an effort to personalize their message. Proponents of social networking cite benefits such as an increased presence in the community, the ability to promote certain services, and marketing to attract new patients. Others indicate that the use of social networking offers a way to stay abreast of medical news, share practice management tips, and build consensus on issues important to them. The ease of facilitating communication is also an advantage, particularly when communicating findings from research.

New findings can be disseminated through social media the minute they are learned, putting useful information in the hands of clinicians more quickly than the traditional dissemination through professional journals. Clinical research is often sponsored by industry, and few people may evaluate the content before it is published in a journal. In an online community, review by potentially thousands of professionals may promote superior credibility.

Despite the benefits of social networking, there are also concerns and challenges. Perhaps the greatest concern—and the reason to include the topic of social networking in a text on documentation—is the permanence of information posted on sites. Of equal concern is that there is no anonymity on the Web. Information posted on most social sites is indexed on Google and can be found by patients, supervisors, potential employers, attorneys, and others. Even when information is removed from a site, it is usually archived somewhere and accessible in the future. A study published in the *Journal of the American Medical Association* (Chretien et al., 2009) found that 60% of U.S. medical schools reported incidents of students posting inappropriate or unprofessional content on blogs, social networking sites, or other places on the Internet. Before posting information on a social site, health-care providers should consider how the content would likely be interpreted in various settings, such as an interview, a departmental meeting, or during a trial. The information, whether in written form or photographs, should be considered permanent documentation that can be accessed by anyone at any time. The tourism industry in Las Vegas launched a successful campaign based on the idea that "what happens in Vegas stays in Vegas." Health-care providers who participate in social networking should have the premise that "what happens in Vegas shows up on the Internet the rest of your life."

Another concern related to social networking is the potential to breach patient confidentiality. Even with the best of intentions, it is easy to divulge protected health information when posting a case and seeking input from colleagues. Information shared should be generic enough that no one can identify a patient in the course of reading a post. Another challenge is the blurring of the boundaries of the patient-provider relationship and the merging of professional and personal lives. Providers must decide whether they will accept a "friend" request from patients. Although many websites allow users to choose higher privacy settings and to control which personal content is available to whom, once information is posted on a social networking site, there is no longer any control over that information. Providers should also realize that information could be posted on other sites and could be viewed as providing medical advice, resulting in a liability risk.

Social networking is likely here to stay. Healthcare professionals need to carefully consider whether or not to participate in social networking. If the decision is made to do so, it is recommended that separate sites be used for professional and personal purposes in order to maintain appropriate boundaries. On any site that patients have access to, a disclaimer should be used to state clearly that the provider is not giving medical advice to individuals. Guidelines for postings should be established, as should guidelines for dealing with "friend" requests. Students in professional programs and licensed providers should take extra precautions to ensure they are not in violation of school, employer, or professional liability carrier policies, or hospital or professional societies' ethics codes. Remember that social networks are not HIPAA compliant and should never be used for any patient-provider communication. By applying these commonsense principles, providers should be able to realize the benefits and protect themselves from the perils of social networking.

To reinforce the content of this chapter, please complete the worksheets that follow.

Worksheet 6.1

1. In addition to a SOAP note, identify at least four types of documentation that could be kept in a patient's medical record.

_____

_____

_____

_____

2. Explain the rationale for using a medication list.

_____

_____

3. Figure 6-5 shows a flow sheet used to track information for a patient who is on anticoagulation therapy. Identify at least three other conditions for which a flow sheet might be used and the information that could be included.

_____

_____

_____

4. Identify the two basic kinds of advance directives.

_____

5. Describe the purpose of a living will.

_____

_____

_____

6. Describe the purpose of a durable power of attorney.

_____

_____

7. Caring Connections is a program of the National Hospice and Palliative Care Organization. Visit their website at www.caringinfo.org and find your state's requirements for a living will and power of attorney.

8. Identify at least four components of a telephone call that should be documented and placed in the patient's medical record.

9. Identify three advantages to using e-mail to communicate with patients.

_____

_____

_____

10. Identify three disadvantages to using e-mail to communicate with patients.

_____

_____

_____

11. Visit the websites of the American Medical Association (AMA) and the American Medical Informatics Association (AIMA). Identify at least four guidelines for providers who choose to communicate with patients by e-mail.

_____

_____

_____

_____

12. Identify three benefits that providers, hospitals, or health systems can realize with social networking.

_____

_____

_____

13. List three concerns related to providers having pages on social networking sites.

_____

_____

_____

14. Identify at least three recommendations to providers who choose to have a presence on a social networking site.

_____

_____

_____

Jennifer Erwin

Refer to Worksheet 3.2, the sexual history for Jennifer Erwin. Using the information provided in the history and the answers to the questions for the worksheet, identify the areas of a problem list that could be completed for this patient.

Ms. Monica Jacobs

Refer to Worksheet 5.8 and review the information given for Ms. Monica Jacobs. Complete a problem list and medication list based on the information.

Worksheet 6.4

Recording Telephone Calls

The narrative of a phone conversation between Mariel Novak, FNP, and Cindy Florinda, mother of a 15-month-old boy, is shown below. After reading the narrative, complete the telephone log form provided.

MN: Hello, may I speak with Cindy?

CF: This is Cindy.

MN: Hi, Cindy. This is Mariel, the nurse practitioner at Peoria Pediatrics. I'm returning your phone call. How may I help you?

CF: I'm calling about my son Tyler. He is running a fever, and he has a rash. I'm concerned.

MN: How old is Tyler?

CF: He is 15 months old.

MN: Is Tyler on any regular medications?

CF: No.

MN: Is he allergic to any medications?

CF: No.

MN: When did he start running a fever?

CF: Last night around 8 p.m. I've been giving him Children's Advil, but his temperature goes back up.

MN: How much does Tyler weigh?

CF: He's about 22 pounds.

MN: And how much Advil did you give him?

CF: I think it is 200 mg. Let me check on the bottle. (Pause) Yes, it is 200 mg. Is that OK?

MN: Yes, that is the correct dose for his weight. Is Tyler having other symptoms, like runny nose, coughing, vomiting, or diarrhea?

CF: He has had a runny nose for a few days. Nothing else except the rash.

MN: When did you notice the rash?

CF: He had it when he woke up this morning.

MN: Does he scratch or seem to be bothered by the rash?

CF: No, he doesn't.

MN: Is he eating and drinking fluids?

CF: He doesn't seem to be as hungry as he normally is, but he is drinking OK.

MN: When was the last time he wet his diaper or urinated?

CF: About 4 hours ago.

MN: Is anyone else in the household ill?

CF: No, everyone else is fine.

MN: How would you describe his activity?

CF: When his temperature is up, he acts grumpy, but when it comes down, he seems to be fine. He did take a longer nap today than usual.

MN: When was the last time Tyler was at the office?

CF: I took him in about a week and a half ago for a nurse visit. They gave him a shot. I think it was the MMR vaccine.

MN: Has Tyler ever had reactions or problems after other vaccines?

CF: No.

MN: Let me be sure I've got everything. Tyler started running a fever last night and had a rash this morning. He doesn't have runny nose, cough, or vomiting, and he is drinking fluids OK and urinating. He got the MMR vaccine about a week and a half ago. He is a little grumpy when his temperature is up but otherwise seems to be OK. Is there anything else you can think of?

CF: No, that's all.

MN: Does he have any swelling or redness where they gave him the shot?

CF: No.

MN: Cindy, I think Tyler's symptoms are related to the MMR vaccine he got. It is fairly common for children to develop a fever and sometimes a rash 1 to 2 weeks after getting the vaccine. This doesn't necessarily mean that he is having a reaction to the vaccine. It is more likely that the measles part of the vaccine is starting to work. I think it is OK to continue giving him the Advil for fever. You can give it every 6 hours, and keep the dose at 200 mg. His appetite might be decreased for a few days, but as long as he is drinking fluids OK, he should be fine. You want to keep an eye on his urine output. If he goes longer than 6 hours without wetting a diaper or urinating, he could be getting dehydrated, and I want you to call back if that happens. Do you feel comfortable with this plan?

CF: Yes. I just hope his fever doesn't last too long.

MN: If he has fever for more than 48 hours, you should bring him in to the office so we can have a look at him, OK? Also, if he starts to get real drowsy and you have a hard time waking him up, you should call right away.

CF: OK.

MN: Do you have any questions?

CF: No. I appreciate you calling me back so soon. Thanks.

MN: You're welcome. I hope Tyler is feeling better soon. Remember to call if his fever lasts for more than 48 hours, if he goes more than 6 hours without urinating, or if he gets really drowsy or lethargic and you can't wake him up.

CF: OK, I will. Goodbye.

MN: Goodbye.

Peoria Pediatrics Telephone Log Form

Date: ___/___/___   Time _____

Caller/Relationship: _____

Patient: _____ Age: _____

Reason for call: _____

HPI/PMH: _____

_____

_____

Medications: _____

Allergies: _____

Diagnosis: _____

Recommendations/Rx: _____

Disposition: _____

Follow-up: _____

_____

Pharmacy: _____ Phone: _____

Billing:

Brief (99371)   Intermediate (99372)

Abbreviations

These abbreviations were introduced in Chapter 6. Beside each, write the meaning as indicated by the context of this chapter.

ACE, ACEI _____

AHIMA _____

AMIA _____

AP _____

CTA _____

INR _____

MMR _____

N/V/D _____

POA _____

PT _____

SSN _____

Chapter 7

Admitting a Patient to the Hospital

OBJECTIVES

- Identify components of an admission history and physical examination for a medical and a surgical admission and compare these to the comprehensive history and physical examination.
- List specific components of typical admit orders.
- Define Computerized Physician Order Entry (CPOE) and Clinical Decision Support System (CDSS).
- Discuss the benefits and challenges of using a CPOE/CDSS system.
- Identify components of an admit note.

According to the 2008 National Hospital Discharge Survey, there were about 34.9 million hospital admissions in the United States in 2006.* The average length of stay for hospitalized patients was 4.8 days. Using a conservative estimate of 25 orders per patient, this amounts to 872.5 million orders generated annually. This estimate gives an indication of the enormity of the work associated with managing hospitalized patients and may help you appreciate the need for accuracy and attention to detail when authoring documents that relate to patient care.

Regulatory agencies such as The Joint Commission (formerly the Joint Commission on Accreditation of Healthcare Organizations) and the Centers for Medicare and Medicaid Services (CMS) have standards for the content of medical records for hospitalized patients. Although it is rather lengthy, CMS Section 482.24 of Title 42 from the Code of Federal Regulations (2004) deserves inclusion because it serves as the basis for much of the content of this chapter:

(c) The medical record must contain information to justify admission and continued hospitalization, support the diagnosis, and describe the patient's progress and response to medications and services. (1) All entries must be legible and complete, and must be authenticated and dated promptly by the person (identified by name and discipline) who is responsible for ordering, providing, or evaluating the service furnished. (i) The author of each entry must be identified and must authenticate his or her entry. (ii) Authentication may include signatures, written initials or computer entry. (2) All records must document the following, as appropriate: (i) Evidence of a physical examination, including a health history, performed no more than seven days prior to admission or within 48 hours after admission. (ii) Admitting diagnosis. (iii) Results of all consultative evaluations of the patient and appropriate findings by clinical and other staff involved in the care of the patient. (iv) Documentation of complications, hospital acquired infections, and unfavorable reactions to drugs and anesthesia. (v) Properly executed informed consent forms for procedures and treatments specified by the medical staff, or by Federal or State law if applicable, to require written patient consent. (vi) All practitioners' orders, nursing notes, reports of treatment, medication reports, radiology and laboratory reports, and vital signs and other information necessary to monitor the patient's condition. (vii) Discharge summary with outcome of hospitalization, disposition of case, and provisions for follow-up care. (viii) Final diagnosis with completion of medical records within 30 days following discharge.

---

*Most current data available at time of publication.

Since publication of the first edition of this text, much has changed about the way certain documents may be generated. At that time, the adoption of electronic medical record (EMR) systems within hospitals was limited. Early EMR use in the hospital focused on nursing functions at the point of care, or the bedside, such as medication administration, monitoring of vital signs, and other direct care tasks. EMR use by medical staff providers was fairly limited; orders were typically handwritten, and documents such as admission history and physical examinations (H&Ps) and discharge summaries were dictated, and then transcribed copies were placed in the patient's chart. (See Appendix C for suggestions on dictating records.) Recently, EMR and Computerized Physician Order Entry (CPOE) systems have become more widely used and, where implemented, have greatly reduced or replaced handwritten orders. EMR systems were discussed in Chapter 1, and CPOE will be discussed in more detail later in this chapter. Regardless of *how* these tasks are now completed, the requirement of what should be documented in an admission H&P or admission orders has not changed significantly.

Admission History and Physical Examination

One of the most important documents generated during a patient's hospital stay is the admission H&P. Numerous members of the health-care team use information from the H&P as the cornerstone of their interactions with and management of the hospitalized patient. There are some differences between medical and surgical admissions. A medical admission indicates that the patient has a condition that will be managed with medical therapies, often by administration of various medications, rather than requiring surgery; pneumonia, deep vein thrombosis, sepsis, or altered mental status are conditions that are medically managed. A surgical admission is one in which an operative procedure treats the condition, such as an appendectomy for acute appendicitis, joint replacement for advanced arthritis, or surgical repair of a torn anterior cruciate ligament.

Medical Admission History and Physical Examination

Refer to Table 2.1 to review the components of a comprehensive H&P; the content of an admission H&P will be much the same. Identification information will include a unique numerical or alphanumerical identifier assigned to every hospitalized patient.

The terminology of such an identifier may vary, but it is often referred to as the medical record number. The same identifier is used throughout the hospital stay and is often used for the same patient for each interaction at the hospital, whether there is an actual admission, outpatient testing, or an emergency department visit. Policies on how to identify patients will vary from hospital to hospital; it is the provider's responsibility to know the policy for each institution at which they have privileges.

The chief complaint should reflect the primary reason for the hospitalization and is best recorded in the patient's own words. The same CMS Documentation Guidelines for Evaluation and Management (E/M) of Services discussed in Chapter 2 pertain to the admission H&P; therefore, the same elements of the history of present illness (HPI) should be documented. The past medical history (PMH) section of an admission H&P may be more abbreviated or focused than that of the comprehensive H&P. If a patient were admitted for pneumonia, it would be important to document any respiratory conditions the patient currently has or has had because the admitting problem is a respiratory system problem. Document any chronic conditions the patient is being treated for that would have an impact on the patient during the hospitalization, especially diabetes, cardiovascular disease, or cancer. If the patient has had any type of surgery involving the respiratory system, it would be important to include that in the PMH; otherwise, a list of all the surgeries the patient has had in the past may not be important to document because these would have little if any bearing on managing the patient's pneumonia.

It is *always* important to document all medications a patient has been taking up to the time of admission. Complete drug information, including the dosing unit, frequency of administration, and route of administration, should be documented. Because additional medications are likely to be prescribed during the hospitalization, the prescriber and pharmacy staff must be able to determine whether drug-drug interactions or drug-disease interactions could occur. Likewise, it is *always* important to document any drug allergies. In some hospitals, patients with drug allergies are given a special armband to wear that alerts all caregivers to their allergies. The chart is often flagged or marked in some way to call attention to any known allergies in an attempt to avoid prescribing or administering a medication that the patient is allergic to or a closely related medication.

It is usually not necessary to document health maintenance information in an admission H&P because the focus of the hospitalization is to treat and resolve the current medical condition, and health maintenance is better addressed on an outpatient basis when the patient is not acutely ill. It may be important to include immunization status; in the case of a patient admitted for pneumonia, you should document whether the patient has had pneumococcal vaccination and when that was done.

The amount of family history that needs to be documented in an admission H&P will vary according to the reason for admission. If a patient is admitted for pneumonia, family history is not likely to affect management of the patient. If a patient is admitted because of acute substernal chest pain and the plan is to rule out myocardial infarction, a family history of cardiovascular disease would be an important risk factor that providers would want to be aware of because the number of risk factors could affect patient management.

Documentation of the psychosocial history should contain information about who is responsible for medical decision making, especially if the patient is not able to make his or her own decisions. A hospitalization can be a major stressor, not only for the patient, but also for families or other social units as a whole. If the patient is a caregiver for someone else, such as a spouse with dementia or a special needs child, the concern about who will care for that person often adds additional stress that can affect the patient's course of recovery. Other psychosocial history to document includes what kind of help the patient may need at the time of discharge; what support system, if any, is available to the patient; what religious practices are important to the patient and if they can be observed in the hospital setting; and if there are dietary considerations that may affect the patient's nutritional needs during the hospital stay. Ancillary personnel, such as social workers, discharge planners, nutritional counselors, and chaplains or clergy, are typically available to help address psychosocial concerns on the patient's behalf. At some hospitals, a specific order may be needed to initiate these services.

Language and cultural barriers could have a dramatic impact on a patient's hospital course. The Department of Health and Human Services (HHS), Office for Civil Rights (OCR) is responsible for enforcing Title VI of the Civil Rights Act of 1964, which prohibits discrimination on the basis of race, color, and national origin, and Section 504 of the Rehabilitation Act of 1973, which prohibits discrimination on the basis of disability by recipients of financial assistance from HHS. OCR is also responsible for ensuring compliance with Title II of the Americans with Disabilities Act as it applies to health and human services, activities of state and local governments. Under these laws, hospitals must communicate effectively with patients, family members, and visitors who are deaf or hard-of-hearing and with persons who have limited English proficiency. The OCR has determined that effective communication must be provided at "critical points" during hospitalization. Critical points include those points during which critical medical information is communicated, such as at admission, when explaining medical procedures, when an informed consent is required for treatment, and at discharge. Documenting the need for interpretive services in the psychosocial history section of the admission H&P helps support hospitals' compliance with these regulations and helps ensure the best care for the patient.

Providers need to be aware of the CMS Guidelines for E/M services when deciding how much of the review of systems (ROS) to document. This decision will also be influenced by the patient's overall medical condition, the reason for the hospitalization, and the level of acuity. The higher the level of complexity of the E/M, the greater the need for detailed documentation. These factors will also determine how much physical examination should be documented.

The patient's progress—or lack thereof—will be gauged by change from their baseline at admission; therefore, documentation of the general assessment is important to allow for this comparison. Describe the patient's level of alertness; orientation to person, place, and time and ability to comprehend their situation; and reliability to provide the history or document who provided the history if it was someone other than the patient. Describe the patient's overall state of health, such as well-developed, well-nourished; frail and emaciated; or appears older than stated age. Documentation of the general appearance should paint a picture of the patient at the time of admission so that someone reading the H&P who has not seen the patient would be able to formulate an image of the patient.

Multiple sets of vital signs may be documented in the admission H&P. If a patient presents to the medical floor at 3:00 p.m. and the H&P is performed at 5:00 p.m. the following day, it is appropriate to document the first set of vital signs that were obtained the afternoon of admission and the most recently obtained vital signs. Document the date and time that each set was obtained. Because care is provided around the clock during a hospitalization, military time is typically used to avoid confusion between morning and evening times.

Documentation of laboratory data should support the need for the hospitalization. Not every test result obtained is documented in the admission H&P because these results can be found elsewhere in the medical record. Results that are most pertinent to the reason for hospitalization should be included. If multiple problems are identified in the assessment section, the abnormal results correlating to each problem are typically documented. Using the example of a patient admitted with pneumonia, it would be important to document that the chest radiograph confirms the presence of a right lower lobe (RLL) infiltrate and that the complete blood count (CBC) shows an elevated white blood cell count (WBC) of 13.7 and the differential indicates a left shift. Normal results are typically not documented in this section.

Two of the most important sections of the admission H&P are those that contain the problem list, assessments, and differential diagnoses and that outline the treatment plan. The problem that necessitated hospital admission is listed first as the admitting diagnosis. When a patient presents with a symptom, such as chest pain, and a definitive diagnosis has not yet been reached, the problem or symptom is stated, followed by a brief overview or explanation of why the patient needs admission. Consider these two examples:

1. Chest pain, strong risk factors for cardiac etiology. Initial cardiac enzymes are within normal limits (WNL). There is ST-segment elevation in the anterior leads; however, it is unclear whether these are acute changes.
2. Acute mental status change. Patient transferred from long-term care facility because of confusion, hypotension, and elevated WBC. Indwelling catheter in place with cloudy urine. Cultures are pending; urosepsis is likely as a cause for these symptoms.

After the initial problem or diagnosis, document any significant comorbid conditions or other problems that may affect the patient's course of treatment in the hospital. In the previous example of a patient with acute mental status change, a decrease in creatinine clearance signifying renal insufficiency would be significant because renal insufficiency would affect the choice of antibiotics and could create problems with volume status. Comorbid conditions typically documented in this section include hypertension, diabetes, renal disease, any hematologic or oncologic problems, and any medical conditions that would require ongoing monitoring and treatment.

The plan portion of the H&P briefly outlines what care the patient will receive during the hospitalization. It is not necessary to document every intervention that will be initiated because these will be detailed in the admission orders, but rather to provide a cursory overview of treatment. The plan

corresponding to the two previous examples could be documented as follows:

1. Admit to telemetry. Continue thrombolytic therapy that was started in the ED. Continue serial ECG and cardiac enzymes. Old records to the floor to see if previous ECGs available for comparison.
2. Begin empirical broad-spectrum antibiotic therapy. Will closely monitor patient's intake and output and daily weights. Will hold off on vasopressor therapy at this time, but it may be needed if patient becomes more hypotensive.

Procedures that will be done during the hospitalization are sometimes documented in the plan, especially if more than one is needed and there could be scheduling conflicts. If the admitting physician plans to obtain consultations with specialists, this is often mentioned in the plan as well. At times, the assessment and plan sections may be combined into one section. Examples of this will be shown in some of the worksheets used in this chapter. It is usually personal preference of the provider to document as one section or to combine; both ways meet CMS guidelines.

Surgical Admission History and Physical Examination

When a patient presents for elective (or scheduled) surgery, the admission H&P is often done during a preoperative office visit. Federal guidelines state that an H&P completed up to 7 days before admission is acceptable. Advances in surgical techniques allow for many procedures to be performed on an outpatient basis that previously would have required hospitalization, such as cholecystectomy and arthroscopic procedures. Many hospitals operate outpatient or same-day surgery centers, and some may use specially developed templates to document the admission H&P, such as the one shown in Figure 7-1. Complex surgical procedures, or procedures performed on patients with complex medical conditions, often necessitate hospital admission to ensure adequate preoperative preparation and monitoring of the patient's postoperative progress.

The surgical admission H&P is documented similarly to a comprehensive H&P and a medical admission H&P; however, there are some important differences. The chief complaint may be stated as a condition ("I have gallstones"), or the patient's statement may reflect what operative procedure is planned ("I am being admitted to have my gallbladder removed"). The HPI documents key events or findings that indicate the need for surgical intervention.

Central Medical SurgiCenter
1333 N. 30th St.
Central City, US
Phone: 802-555-4400 Fax: 802-555-4801

Same-day surgery history and physical form

Patient's name: _____ MR#: _____

DOB: _____ Gender: ☐ Male ☐ Female

Diagnosis: _____

Surgical procedure: _____

Surgeon: _____

Anesthesia: ☐ General ☐ Local ☐ Other _____

Pertinent HPI: _____

Medications: _____

Allergies: _____

Chronic medical conditions: _____

Preop labs: (check box for desired tests)

☐ HGB ☐ HCT ☐ CBC ☐ UA ☐ ECG

☐ CXR ☐ CMP ☐ Glucose ☐ PT ☐ INR (International Normalized Ratio)

☐ Other: _____

Vital signs: _____ BP _____ pulse _____ resp. _____ temp

EXAM: ☐ Well developed, well nourished ☐ A&O x 3 ☐ No distress

HEENT: ☐ Normal   ☐ Abnormal _____

Neck: ☐ Normal   ☐ Abnormal _____

Lungs: ☐ Normal   ☐ Abnormal _____

Heart: ☐ Normal   ☐ Abnormal _____

Abd: ☐ Normal   ☐ Abnormal _____

Ext: ☐ Normal   ☐ Abnormal _____

Neuro: ☐ Normal   ☐ Abnormal _____

Cleared for surgery?   ☐ Yes ☐ No

Consent to read: _____

Consent signed?   ☐ Yes ☐ No   NPO?   ☐ Yes ☐ No

Figure 7-1 Sample same-day surgery H&P.

The PMH should document pertinent medical conditions that would affect the hospitalization. Specifically, document whether the patient has hypertension, diabetes, or any condition that is being treated with corticosteroids or antiplatelet therapy because any of these will require careful perioperative management. A detailed surgical history should be documented, including any previous procedures, what type of anesthesia was used, and if any complications resulted from those procedures, such as bleeding, malignant hyperthermia, or anesthetic complications. Document whether the patient required transfusion of blood or blood products. A complete medication list and documentation of any drug allergies would be included as discussed previously in the medical admission H&P section.

Documentation of the family history should include any known bleeding disorders that are genetic or have a familial tendency. If the surgery were for a condition that has a familial predisposition, such as certain types of cancers, those conditions and the family members affected would be documented as well. The same details of the psychosocial history discussed in medical admission H&Ps should be documented in a surgical H&P.

If not fully explored in the HPI, the ROS should focus on the system most closely related to the planned surgical procedure. In the example of a patient being admitted for cholecystectomy, a detailed gastrointestinal ROS should be documented. Inclusion of other systems or the level of review of other systems will be influenced by the complexity of the planned procedure as well as the type of anesthesia planned and any comorbid conditions the patient may have.

Documentation of the physical examination should clearly establish the patient's baseline preoperative condition because postoperative assessment will focus on return to preoperative functioning. Careful attention should be given to examination of the body area involved in the surgery. Many inpatient surgeries will be done with the patient under general anesthesia; therefore, pulmonary functioning is especially important to document. Examination of the upper respiratory system should include the mouth, noting any loose teeth or dental work such as partial or full dentures. Lower respiratory system assessment should include chest shape, symmetry of expansion with respiration, diaphragmatic movement, respiratory effort, and the quality of breath sounds in all lung fields. How much additional examination is done is influenced by the presence of comorbid conditions, overall patient health status, complexity of the planned surgical procedure, estimated operative time, and anticipated postoperative course.

Laboratory or other diagnostic studies are sometimes completed on an outpatient basis before the patient's hospital admission. When this is the case, it is important to document pertinent results in the H&P, and a copy of all results should be made part of the permanent medical record. The need for baseline preoperative testing is correlated to the patient's age, overall medical condition, and type of surgery the patient will have. Some facilities have set policies, such as obtaining an electrocardiogram (ECG) in every patient 40 years of age or older and a chest radiograph in any patient who smokes or who is 50 years of age or older. It is important to document

the patient's willingness to accept transfusion of blood or blood products and whether the patient's blood has been typed and cross-matched or if preoperative autologous blood donation has been done.

The condition necessitating surgical intervention is typically listed first in the assessment and problem list section, followed by any comorbid conditions that would require perioperative monitoring or that could potentially give rise to postoperative complications. Documentation of the plan includes the planned operative intervention and may also include specific preoperative preparation, patient education, consultations, and a general outline of postoperative care.

Chapter 2 contains a sample comprehensive H&P for Mr. William R. Jensen (see Fig. 2-1) who presented in an outpatient setting to Dr. Scott and was evaluated for fatigue and blood in the stool. Subsequent evaluation by a gastroenterologist and surgeon led to the diagnosis of adenocarcinoma of the colon. Using a case study format, we will follow this patient's care as he is admitted for surgical management. Figure 7-2 shows a sample admission H&P for Mr. Jensen who presents for surgical management. Compare Figures 7-2 and 2-1 to see how the comprehensive H&P is modified for a surgical admission H&P. Two sets of admit orders will be written for Mr. Jensen: his initial preoperative admit orders and the initial postoperative orders. Documentation of an admit note will be discussed in this chapter. In Chapter 8, we will follow Mr. Jensen's care through documentation of the operative report, an operative note, daily progress notes, and orders, and conclude the hospitalization with documentation of discharge orders and the discharge summary in Chapter 9.

Admit Orders

When a patient is admitted to the hospital, the orders written at the time of admission direct the healthcare team in caring for the patient. It is important that the orders are completed in a timely manner and are unambiguous. Once written, an order is considered to be in effect until another order is written to change or stop the original order, unless a time limit is provided in the original order. An order to record intake and output would be carried out until an order is written to discontinue intake and output. For example, an order for *Ancef 1 g IV q 24 hr × 3 days* will be given only for 3 days; thus, it is not necessary to write an order to stop Ancef.

At some facilities, it is acceptable to use prewritten order sets. These order sets are developed for conditions that require hospital admission so often that the same orders would be written over and over, such as

Mr. Jensen's Surgical Admission

PATIENT NAME: William R. Jensen

ADMIT DATE: XX/XX/XX

SEX: Male

Billing #: 5728431

DOB: XX/XX/XX

MEDICAL RECORD #: 35-87-26

Dictating Physician/PA/NP: Sanders, David K., MD

Primary Care Physician: Vernon Scott, MD

CHIEF COMPLAINT: "I have cancer, and I'm going to have surgery."

HISTORY OF PRESENT ILLNESS: This is a 67-year-old Caucasian male who was referred to me by his primary care physician, Vernon Scott, MD, after being diagnosed with colon cancer. Mr. Jensen initially presented to Dr. Scott's office with complaints of fatigue and "feeling weak." During a routine workup, he was found to have hemoccult-positive stool. At this time, Mr. Jensen was referred to a gastroenterologist, Michael Bennett, MD. Dr. Bennett performed a colonoscopy on Mr. Jensen and found several suspicious polypoid lesions at the right hepatic flexure area. Biopsies were obtained and sent to pathology. Pathology reports confirm adenocarcinoma. Dr. Scott and Dr. Bennett consulted, and they referred Mr. Jensen to me for surgical evaluation. I saw Mr. Jensen in my office on XX/XX/XX and discussed with him options for treatment. I recommended that we proceed with a right hemicolectomy. I discussed with Mr. Jensen and his wife the likely benefits of the surgery. I discussed specific risks of surgery, including infection, bleeding, perforation of bowel or vessel, possible anesthetic complications, and death. I answered questions to their satisfaction and believe Mr. Jensen competent to give informed consent. He stated his wish to proceed, and his wife is agreeable; therefore, Mr. Jensen is admitted now for elective surgery.

PAST MEDICAL HISTORY:
  Medical: Mr. Jensen has a history of hypertension, dyslipidemia, and left inguinal hernia. Hypertension and dyslipidemia are medically managed by Dr. Scott and are stable at this time.

  Surgical: Mr. Jensen had repair of a torn rotator cuff, right shoulder (Dr. Rodriquez, Grand Rapids, MI), approximately 24 years ago. He had a left inguinal herniorrhaphy approximately 15 years ago (Dr. Simmons, Grand Rapids, MI). All surgical procedures tolerated well; no complications with bleeding or infection postoperatively. He did not have any complications from anesthesia. He has never had any blood transfusions but is agreeable to receive blood or blood products if needed. Since the likelihood of significant bleeding is fairly low, he did not arrange for autologous donation.

  Medications: Lotensin HTC 20/12.5, once daily; Mevacor 20 mg once daily. Occasional acetaminophen.

  Allergies: Mr. Jensen states an allergy to PENICILLIN DRUGS and breaks out in a rash when he takes anything containing penicillin.

FAMILY HISTORY: Mother deceased, age 70, breast cancer. No other family history of cancer. No history of bleeding disorders.

PSYCHOSOCIAL HISTORY: Mr. Jensen is a retired electrician. He is married and lives in a single-story home with his wife. They have three adult children who all live nearby. Mr. Jensen smokes a pipe about 3 times a week. He does not drink alcohol or use any recreational drugs. He is still active and walks approximately 2 miles 4 of 7 days per week. He also bicycles occasionally. He is competent to make his own decisions regarding health care. He has designated his wife as medical power of attorney. Advance directives and living will have been discussed, and both were present at time of admission. Mr. Jensen desires full resuscitation and any heroic measures indicated. His wife and children are available to help care for him at home after discharge. They have a good support system. He denies any specific dietary considerations. No particular religious practices that he desires to participate in while in the hospital.

REVIEW OF SYSTEMS:
  General: Easily fatigued, feels weak. Denies any near-syncope or lightheadedness. Overall mood is positive, and he believes having the surgery is his best chance for cure.

  HEENT: Denies previous nasal or sinus surgery. Denies dental problems.

  Respiratory: Denies cough or shortness of breath.

  Cardiovascular: Specifically denies chest pain, angina, and pleuritic pain. Denies any heart palpitations or irregularities in rhythm. No history of heart murmur.

  Gastrointestinal: Biopsy-proven adenocarcinoma per HPI. Hemoccult-positive stool at initial presentation to Dr. Scott, along with 10-pound unintentional weight loss over past few months. Weight has been stable since. Denies abdominal pain, nausea, vomiting, diarrhea. Denies any difficulty swallowing or chewing.

  Genitourinary: Denies nocturia or dysuria.

  Hematologic: Denies easy bruising or bleeding from gums.

(Continued)

PHYSICAL EXAMINATION:
   Vital Signs: BP 142/80; P 86 and regular, R 16 and regular; Temp 97.8 orally. His current weight is 174 pounds.

   General: Mr. Jensen is a well-developed, well-nourished Caucasian man who is alert and cooperative. He is a good historian and answers questions appropriately.

   Skin: Intact, no lesions noted. Turgor is good.

   HEENT: Nose patent bilaterally. No polyps noted. Oropharynx without erythema or exudate. Buccal mucosa intact without lesions. Full dentition in good repair, no loose teeth.

   Neck: No carotid bruits. No tracheal deviation noted. No masses palpated.

   Cardiovascular: Regular heart rate and rhythm. No murmurs, gallops, or rubs.

   Respiratory: Breath sounds clear to auscultation in all lung fields. Diaphragmatic excursion is symmetrical. No increased AP diameter.

   Abdomen: Soft, nontender. No masses or organomegaly. Bowel sounds physiological in all four quadrants. No guarding or rebound noted. Well-healed left inguinal scar from previous surgery.

   Rectal/GU: Soft brown stool in rectal vault, guaiac positive.

   Musculoskeletal: No clubbing, cyanosis, or edema.

   Neurological: CN II-XII grossly intact. No focal neurological deficits.

LABORATORY DATA:
   CBC: WBC 5800; Hct 48; Hgb 16. Peripheral smear shows normochromic, normocytic cells, differential unremarkable.

   CXR: No consolidations or effusions.

   UA: WNL.

   PT, PTT (partial thromboplastin time): 12.4 and 31.

   ECG: Normal sinus rhythm with rate of 84. No ectopy, no ischemic changes.

ASSESSMENT:
   1. Adenocarcinoma of the colon.
   2. Hypertension. Stable on current medications. Will be monitored closely postoperatively.
   3. Dyslipidemia.

PLAN:
   1. Mr. Jensen is admitted for elective right hemicolectomy. Admission orders written. Consent form completed and on chart.
   2. Routine postoperative care.
   3. Will have Dr. Scott follow for medical management of hypertension.

   David K. Sanders, MD

   DD: XX/XX/XX 0927

   DT: XX/XX/XX 1132

Figure 7-2 Mr. Jensen's surgical admission H&P.

chest pain, rule out acute myocardial infarction (AMI); cerebrovascular accident (CVA); or preoperative care. In facilities where prewritten orders are used, there is usually an established protocol for development, review, and acceptance of the order sets that involves medical staff members from various disciplines, nursing staff, pharmacists, and sometimes other health-care team members. An example of a prewritten order set is shown in Figure 7-3. There are several mnemonics that may be used to help you remember what admission orders should be written. One mnemonic is AD CAVA DIMPLS, which stands for Admit, Diagnosis, Condition, Activity, Vital signs, Allergies, Diet, Interventions, Medications, Procedures, Labs, and Special instructions. Each component is described in more detail, and an example of each is provided. Figure 7-4 presents the mnemonic in a condensed form.

Preadmission Orders

Tests:

☐ Preadmission Labs: _____

_____

Other Tests:

☐ _____ Medical Necessity _____

☐ _____ Medical Necessity _____

☐ _____ Medical Necessity _____

☐ _____ Medical Necessity _____

☐ _____ Medical Necessity _____

Orders are per anesthesia guidelines

RN Sign/RN Initials	Date	Time

Preoperative Orders

☐ Start Intravenous (IV) Fluid _____ 1000 mL at to keep open rate.

☐ May use lidocaine/prilocaine (Emla) Cream for IV site discomfort

☐ May use Pain Ease for IV site discomfort

☐ Lidocaine 1%: give 0.1 mL intradermal for IV site prep.

☐ Other IV: _____

Tests:

Preoperative Labs: _____

Other Tests:

☐ _____ Medical Necessity _____

☐ _____ Medical Necessity _____

☐ _____ Medical Necessity _____

Treatments:

☐ Arterial Line:

☐ Small-volume Nebulizer orders: _____

Additional Orders:

_____
_____
_____
_____

Physician Name - Print and Sign	Date	Time

Figure 7-3 Preoperative order set.

Admission Orders Mnemonic

AD CAVA DIMPLS

Admit: admitting physician and type of unit or hospital floor

Diagnosis: chief reason for the patient's admission

Condition: usually a one-word description

Activity: level of activity allowed depending on age, diagnosis, medications, etc.

Vital signs: frequency with which vital signs should be obtained

Allergies: list any medication allergies

Diet: what type of diet patient is allowed

Interventions: IV therapy, respiratory therapy, etc.

Medications: medications related to reason for admission and any chronic medications the patient may be taking

Procedures: wound care, ostomy care, etc.

Labs: any laboratory or diagnostic tests needed

Special instructions: notify if certain parameters are exceeded, or conditional orders (if this occurs, do this)

Figure 7-4 Admission orders mnemonic.

Admit: Specify the admitting physician and the hospital unit to which the patient should be admitted. *Admit to Dr. Johnson to the orthopedic floor* or *Admit to Dr. Myers to telemetry unit.*

Diagnosis: State the admitting diagnosis and, in the case of a surgical admission, include the name of the procedure to be performed. When a patient has more than one admitting diagnosis, the problem most responsible for admission should be listed as the primary diagnosis. Comorbid conditions that should be monitored during the hospital stay are documented as additional diagnoses. *Primary diagnosis: pneumonia. Secondary diagnosis: type 2 diabetes.*

Condition: This reflects the patient's condition at the time of admission. If the patient has terminal cancer and is likely to die within a few hours, the condition should reflect that. Words commonly used to describe condition are *stable, unstable, guarded, critical, morbid,* and *comatose.*

Activity: Indicate the level of activity the patient is permitted to have. There are several activity orders commonly used; the condition of the patient (including mental alertness) and the overall health condition of the patient determine which order is most appropriate. Common activity orders include the following:
- Up ad lib (the patient may be out of bed as he or she wishes)
- Activity as tolerated (whatever the condition allows the patient to do)
- Bedrest with bathroom privileges, abbreviated as BR with BRP (allowed out of bed to go to the bathroom; otherwise in bed)
- Out of bed (OOB)
- Ambulate a certain number of times a day
- Ambulate with assistance
- Non–weight-bearing

Vital signs: This order reflects how often the standard vital signs (T, P, R, and BP) should be obtained and will vary according to the patient's condition. Some hospitals have standing orders for vital signs depending on the type of unit or floor to which the patient is admitted. Critical or intensive care units almost always have their own standing orders. Some vital signs are monitored continuously as the patient's condition warrants; for instance, BP and HR are monitored continuously in a patient who recently had a myocardial infarction. Typical orders for medical admissions are *VS q8h while awake* (if the patient is very stable and if it is not necessary to awaken a patient to obtain vital signs) and *VS q4h.*

Weight is generally obtained at the time of admission only. If a patient's condition necessitates monitoring of volume status or renal function, as in the case of heart failure, edema or fluid retention, write an order to *weigh daily.*

Allergies: This is not actually an order but rather a specific notation of allergies the patient may have to any medication, food, or other substance. It is customary to include the specific agent the patient is allergic to and what reaction the patient has to the agent. One way to note this is *Allergic to penicillin (rash) and aspirin (dyspnea)*. Some providers document the details of the reaction in the PMH section of the admission H&P and list the drugs only in the orders; this is an acceptable practice. If it is hospital policy to identify patients with allergies by a special armband or other designation, a specific order for this is not necessary.

Diet: The first step in determining which diet order to write is usually to determine whether it is safe to allow the patient to eat. If the patient is going to have surgery or a procedure that requires sedation and therefore carries a risk for aspiration, or if a patient is not mentally alert enough or physically able to eat and swallow, it is safer for the patient not to receive any nourishment by mouth. The order for this is *NPO*, an abbreviation for the Latin phrase *nil per os*, interpreted as *nothing by mouth*. If allowing the patient to eat does not pose a threat to safety, there are many dietary orders that can be written. It is not possible to include all the dietary orders in this text; some of the more common types of diets are shown in Table 7-1. Consultation with a dietitian or nutritional support personnel is usually an option. Hospitals will often have a dietary manual available for review as well.

Interventions: This refers to interventions by nursing or other ancillary staff, such as physical therapy or respiratory therapy. One example of an intervention is *single volume nebulizer (SVN) with 0.5 cc albuterol in 2.5 cc normal saline (NS) q4h*. Another example is *Physical therapist (PT) to instruct on bed to wheelchair transfers*. Intravenous (IV) therapy is also considered an intervention. An order for IV therapy should specify the type of fluid and the rate of administration, such as *D_5NS (5% dextrose in NS) at 80 cc/hr*. (Consult the References section for suggested readings related to principles of IV therapy.)

Medications: A study by Bobb and colleagues (2004) looked at the etiology of prescribing errors in the hospital setting. They found that almost two thirds of verified prescribing errors identified in the study period were made on the day of admission. Many of the errors were due to incomplete patient medication histories. Dosing errors were the most common preventable medication error; health-care providers should be cognizant of the potential for serious adverse drug events if medication orders are not carefully and completely written. Always specify the name of the medication, the dose, the route of administration, and the frequency. It is common to write orders first for any medications that are given for the condition necessitating hospitalization, then orders for any medications taken before hospitalization that need to be continued, and then orders for any symptomatic medications.

Symptomatic medications are those that may or may not be needed. During a hospitalization, patients experience sleeplessness, constipation, pain, and nausea with such frequency that orders are typically written at the time of admission so that medications are available to treat these symptoms if they develop. Not only will these orders reduce discomfort for the patient, they will also prevent nursing staff from having to call a prescriber at 2:00 a.m. to request a sleep aid. These medications would be ordered on a prn basis and are given only as requested by the patient. If you write an order for a prn medication, you always want to include the indication for giving the medication. An order written as *morphine 2 mg IV prn* is open for interpretation. Although the nursing staff would recognize that morphine is a narcotic analgesic and would know that it is given to relieve pain, the order is ambiguous. Instead, it should be written with

Table 7-1	Common Diets for Oral Intake

Condition	**Dietary Intervention**	**Typical Order**
Diabetes	Restrict sugars and fats; follow recommendations of the American Diabetes Association (ADA)	1400-calorie ADA diet
Hypertension Kidney disease	Salt restriction	Low sodium diet, 2 g Na$^+$ diet
Coronary artery disease or hypercholesterolemia	Fat and cholesterol restriction	Cardiac diet; low-fat, low-cholesterol diet National Cholesterol Education Program (NCEP) Step Two diet
Unable to chew well, ill-fitting dentures	Allow soft foods only	Soft mechanical diet

specific dosing, frequency, and indication instructions, such as *morphine 2 mg IV q2h prn pain*. This prevents the medication from being administered for reasons other than pain and establishes a safe time frame in which the medication may be administered. A specific dose should always be ordered, rather than a range of dosing such as *morphine 2–6 mg IV q2-3h prn pain*. This helps prevent inappropriate administration of the medication.

Procedures: Many routine procedures are part of a patient's daily care, and it may seem intuitive that these procedures should be performed. However, writing an order for such procedures as daily catheter care, wound or ostomy care, and dressing changes provides justification for performing these procedures and allows the hospital to charge for the necessary supplies. The order should specify how frequently the procedures should be carried out.

Labs: It may be necessary to monitor certain laboratory values or obtain diagnostic studies as part of a patient's care. For instance, when a patient is on an anticoagulant medication, you monitor the bleeding time. If a patient develops fever and a cough, you might order a chest x-ray (CXR). You should always have a rationale for ordering laboratory or other diagnostic studies. If a patient had surgery but had very little intraoperative bleeding, it is unnecessary to order *H&H* (hematocrit and hemoglobin) *qam;* you would not expect the values to change because there was little blood loss. When ordering radiographic studies, the indication for the study should be included, not only to aid the radiology staff in interpreting the study, but also to establish the relevance of the study to the patient's overall care. An example is *AP (anteroposterior) & lateral CXR to R/O atelectasis*.

Special instructions: The rationale for special instruction orders is to ensure that nursing staff informs the provider of changes in a patient's condition that may require some intervention. For instance, results of glucose monitoring above or below a certain level may require withholding, increasing, or decreasing insulin doses. You would write an order to *Notify Dr. Williams if blood sugar is <100 mg/dL or >350 mg/dL*. If a patient was admitted 2 days ago for AMI and now has new onset of atrial fibrillation, you want to be alerted to that fact. You should never assume that the nursing staff will automatically notify you of such developments. As a general rule, they probably would; however, the responsibility of managing changes in the patient's condition rests on the attending medical staff—not the nursing staff—and you can only manage what you are aware of. Writing the special instruction order protects you as a clinician and helps to ensure the best treatment for the patient.

Perioperative Orders

When a patient is admitted for surgery, the initial preoperative orders are in effect until the patient goes to surgery. Preoperative orders for Mr. Jensen are shown in Figure 7-5. After surgery, the patient goes to the postanesthesia care unit (PACU), sometimes referred to as the recovery room. While there, the staff generally follows prewritten PACU orders, like those shown in Figure 7-6. Once the patient is awake, maintaining an airway with adequate respirations, and has stable vital signs, the patient is essentially readmitted to the hospital, and a new set of postoperative orders must be written. We will use the same mnemonic provided earlier, AD CAVA DIMPLS, to write the postoperative orders for Mr. Jensen.

Admit: The patient is typically admitted to the surgeon.

Diagnosis: The postoperative admitting diagnosis is usually the surgical procedure. For instance, Mr. Jensen's admitting diagnosis could be written as *hemicolectomy*. You may see *S/P hemicolectomy*, meaning "status post."

Condition: Condition refers to how the patient is immediately after surgery when the postoperative orders are written.

Activity: When writing the activity order, keep in mind that postoperative patients usually require at least some narcotic pain relief, which may impair judgment or function. Safety precautions may be indicated, such as *side rails up at all times* or *ambulate only with assistance*. To prevent complications associated with immobility, patients are usually encouraged to be out of bed immediately after surgery, but the activity level must take into consideration the type of surgery and the patient's overall condition. An activity order for Mr. Jensen could be *OOB tid with assistance*.

Vital signs: In the immediate postoperative period, vital signs are obtained progressively. A common postoperative order is *VS qh x 4;* if stable, then *q2h x 4, then q4h*. An order such as this reflects the possibility that a patient's condition might

---

Preoperative Admit Orders for Mr. Jensen

XX/XX/XX 2030

1. Admit to Dr. Sanders, surgical floor

2. Dx: colon cancer

3. Condition: good

4. Activity: up ad lib

5. Vital signs q4h while awake

6. Allergic to PENICILLIN

7. Clear liquid diet now; NPO after midnight

8. Instruct on use of incentive spirometry

9. IV D$_5$ NS at 80 mL/hr

10. Restoril 15 mg at bedtime prn for sleeplessness

11. Valium 5 mg IM on call to operating room

12. Hold routine meds at present

Signature, title: _____

Countersignature: _____

Figure 7-5 Preoperative admit orders for Mr. Jensen.

change in the immediate postoperative period and that more frequent assessment is needed initially, but if the patient's vital signs remain stable, less frequent assessment is permitted.

Allergies: Any allergies should be noted in the orders.

Diet: Surgical patients usually have special dietary needs in the preoperative and postoperative periods. The type of surgery and the type of anesthesia usually determine the type of diet ordered. As a general rule, patients who have general anesthesia should be NPO for 8 hours or longer before surgery to avoid gastric distention and to reduce the risk for postoperative vomiting and aspiration. When a patient undergoes surgery involving the gastrointestinal tract, paralyzing agents are often used to prevent peristalsis during surgery. Various factors such as age, mobility, and overall health status affect how quickly bowel function returns after surgery. Patients are kept NPO until bowel function returns. Once bowel function resumes, indicated by the return of bowel sounds or passing of flatus, the diet is advanced from liquids to solids as tolerated. Typically, the initial diet order is *clear liquids*. If the patient is able to tolerate clear liquids without any nausea or vomiting, the diet is advanced to *full liquids*, then to a *regular diet* or any special diet indicated for specific medical conditions. Table 7-2 provides information about the liquids and foods allowed on clear and full liquid diets. Some practitioners might prefer to write an order to *advance diet as tolerated* and not specify when to advance the diet or what type of diet to follow, leaving the details to the judgment of the nursing or dietary staff.

Interventions: Like any patient who has had abdominal surgery, Mr. Jensen is likely to have shallow respirations postoperatively, which puts him at risk for pulmonary complications. To prevent such complications, an important intervention order for Mr. Jensen is *incentive spirometry* (ICS) *q4h while awake*. In some institutions, the nursing staff will instruct the patient on spirometry; in others, a respiratory therapist does this. Another important intervention is maintaining hydration and nutrition. Until adequate oral intake is possible, IV fluids should be administered. For Mr. Jensen, we will order *D$_5$NS @ 120 cc/hr.*

☐ Oxygen 2–6 L with nasal cannula or 6–10 L/min flow with simple mask. Titrate to maintain saturation above 93%.
☐ Small-Volume Nebulizer - _____ for bronchospasm.
☐ Remove oropharyngeal / nasopharyngeal airway when patient maintains airway. May reinsert as needed for airway obstruction.

Medications:	**Hold and Notify Physician of Allergy to Any Ordered Medication**
☐ Morphine sulfate:	2 mg IV every 5 minutes for moderate pain (pain scale 4–7)
	2 mg IV every 2 minutes for severe pain (pain scale 8–10); **MAX DOSE:** _____ **mg**
☐ Hydromorphone:	0.2 mg slow IV push every 5 minutes for moderate pain (pain scale 4–7)
	0.2 mg slow IV push every 2 minutes for severe pain (pain scale 8–10); **MAX DOSE:** _____ **mg**
☐ Fentanyl:	_____ mcg IV every 5 minutes for moderate pain (pain scale 4–7)
	_____ mcg IV every 2 minutes for severe pain (pain scale 8–10); **MAX DOSE:** _____ **mg**
☐ Ketorolac:	_____ mg IV one time for moderate pain; **do not use with moderate renal impairment**
☐ Acetaminophen 325 mg:	2 tablets orally for mild pain (scale 1–4) every 4 hours as needed.
☐ Hydrocodone/Acetaminophen 5 mg/500 mg:	1 tablet orally as needed every 4 hours for moderate pain (pain scale 5–7)
	2 tablets orally as needed every 4 hours for severe pain (pain scale 8–10)
☐ Oxycodone/Acetaminophen 5 mg/325 mg:	1 tablet orally as needed every 4 hours for moderate pain (pain scale 5–7)
	2 tablets orally as needed every 4 hours for severe pain (pain scaled 8–10)
☐ Midazolam:	_____ mg IV as needed for anxiety; **MAX DOSE:** _____ **mg**
☐ Lorazepam:	_____ mg IV as needed for anxiety; **MAY REPEAT** _____ **times**
☐ Droperidol:	0.625 mg IV every 15 minutes for nausea; maximum dose of 1.25 mg in 1 hour.
☐ Ondansetron:	4 mg slow IV push over 2 minutes for nausea; to be given as a one-time dose only on the day of surgery
☐ Prochlorperazine:	5 mg slow IV push over 2 minutes every 6 hours as needed for nausea; may repeat dose after 15 minutes if no relief. Maximum dose of 10 mg in 6 hours. Total maximum dose in 24 hours is 40 mg.
☐ Metoclopramide:	10 mg IV one time for nausea
☐ Meperidine:	12.5 mg slow IV; push every 15 minutes as needed for treatment of postanesthetic shivering; **MAX DOSE:** _____ **mg**

Hypotension for Blood Pressure less than _____ **systolic**	☐ **Call Anesthesia**
☐ Ephedrine _____ mg IV every _____ minutes	☐ 5% Albumin 250 mL IV over _____ minutes
☐ Fluid Bolus 500 mL Ringers Lactate IV over 30 minutes	☐ Other: _____

Sinus Bradycardia: defined a heart rate below 40	☐ Atropine 0.5 mg IV every 5 minutes until a heart rate greater than or equal to 60 or a maximum dose 3 mg is achieved.
☐ **Call Anesthesia**	<u>**CAUTION: Doses less than 0.5 may be associated with paradoxical bradycardia.**</u>
☐ Other: _____	

Hypertension for Blood Pressure greater than _____ **systolic** ☐ **Call Anesthesia**

<u>**PREFERRED AGENTS FOR SAME-DAY SURGERY (SDS)**</u>	<u>**PREFERRED AGENTS FOR INPATIENT USE**</u>
☐ Esmolol (Brevibloc): Give 500 mcg/kg IV over 1 min. if inadequate response, give 50 mcg/kg IV—repeat every minute as needed for hypertension and/or tachycardia. Maximum of 4 doses. **Do NOT give if heart rate less than** _____	☐ Labetalol (Trandate) 5 mg IV every 5 minutes. Maximum 20 mg IV. **Do NOT give if heart rate less than** _____
☐ Oral Agent: _____	☐ Oral Agent: _____
☐ Other: _____	☐ Other: _____

Discharge when criteria of Aldrete score greater than or equal to 8 is met or per physician order.

Other:

☐ Fingerstick for glucose as needed

☐ Other: _____

** DISCONTINUE MEDICATION ORDERS ON THIS PAGE WHEN TRANSFERRED TO NURSING UNIT **		
Physician Name - Print and Sign - To Activate Only Orders Checked Above	Date	Time

Figure 7-6 PACU orders.

Table 7-2 Diets Commonly Used in the Postoperative Period

Type of Diet	Foods Allowed
Clear Liquid Diet Often prescribed for a short period after surgery to give gastrointestinal tract a rest	Broth Gelatin Tea Popsicles Clear juices, such as apple, cranberry, or grape Clear sodas, such as lemon-lime or ginger ale Coffee may be allowed with physician approval
Full Liquid Diet Prescribed as a transition from clear liquid to a soft or regular diet	All the foods shown for clear liquid diet plus: Milk Yogurt Pudding Milkshake, ice cream, sherbet Smooth cream soups Oatmeal, cream of wheat, grits, gravy Dark sodas, such as colas Juices with pulp, such as orange, grapefruit, pineapple
Soft Diet May be prescribed if patient has a sore throat following endotracheal intubation or dental problems	Oatmeal Mashed or baked potatoes Bananas Scrambled eggs Soft bread or rolls (not toasted) Applesauce Gelatin Puddings
Regular Diet Similar to what most patients would consume at home	Most foods are allowed; moderate in salt, sugar, and fat Specific foods not allowed will vary by facility; consult with dietary and nutritional support personnel

Medications: Mr. Jensen will require some medications. Medications administered orally are withheld until bowel function returns. Symptomatic medications are indicated, especially for pain and nausea. Specify not only the name of the medication but also the dose, route, and frequency, and for any prn medications, the indications for them. Some hospitals require the use of generic drug names, whereas others accept generic or trade names. Check with the hospital pharmacy to be sure which you should use. A common option for managing postoperative pain is a patient-controlled analgesia (PCA) system. This refers to an electronically controlled infusion pump that delivers a prescribed amount of intravenous analgesic to a patient when the pump is activated. Use of PCA has been shown to reduce the time between when a patient feels pain and when the analgesia is delivered. It also reduces the chances for medication errors because the PCA is programmed per the physician's order for specific doses and time intervals between doses. There is also a "lock-out" feature that prevents overdosing. Figure 7-7 shows a prewritten order set for PCA.

An antiemetic drug is usually ordered as a prn medication. Nausea is fairly common in the postoperative period, and antiemetics can reduce nausea and prevent vomiting. Most antiemetics potentiate the action of narcotic analgesics, so they are frequently administered together. The analgesics and antiemetics should be ordered separately, however, so that they may be administered individually if both are not needed.

Once bowel function returns, Mr. Jensen's preoperative medications should be ordered. It is also desirable to change from parenteral analgesics to oral analgesics when the patient is able to tolerate oral intake. In fact, the patient's ability to obtain effective pain relief from oral analgesics and return to oral intake of liquids and foods are often considered criteria for discharge.

Procedures: One procedure indicated for Mr. Jensen is *daily wound care*. Order *daily*

ADULT PATIENT-CONTROLLED ANALGESIC (PCA) ORDER FORM

Contact the following physician for orders, questions, or inadequate pain relief: _____

Choose one item	Morphine Sulfate 1 mg/mL	HYDROmorphone 0.2 mg/mL	Fentanyl 20 mcg/mL
Loading Dose	_____ mg (**2–4 mg**) IV every 15 minutes until patient comfortable. Not to exceed 3 doses.	_____ mg (**0.2–0.6 mg**) IV every 15 minutes until patient comfortable. Not to exceed 3 doses.	_____ mcg (**10–40 mcg**) IV every 15 minutes until patient comfortable. Not to exceed 3 doses.
PCA Demand Dose	_____ mg (**1–2.5 mg** [1 mg*])	_____ mg (**0.2–0.4 mg** [0.2 mg*])	_____ mcg (**10–25 mcg** [10 mcg*])
Lockout Interval	_____ mins (**6–15 mins** [12 mins*])	_____ mins (**6–15 mins** [8 mins*])	_____ mins (**4–8 mins** [6 mins*])

*Ranges marked with * are recommended for opioid-naive patients*

4-hour Limit	_____ mg (**15–30 mg**)	_____ mg (**4–8 mg**)	_____ mcg (**100–200 mcg**)
Bolus Dose	_____ mg every _____ hours	_____ mg every _____ hours	_____ mcg every _____ hours
Basal Rate *(optional)*	*Restricted to opioid-tolerant patients*		
	_____ mg/hr (**0–2 mg/hr** [1 mg/hr*])	_____ mg/hr (**0–0.3 mg/hr** [0.2 mg/hr*])	_____ mcg/hr (**0–25 mcg/hr** [10 mcg/hr*])

Doses shown in parentheses are for reference only—patient's needs may require more or less than shown

Supplemental PCA administration instructions:
- ☐ When patient begins to use oral pain medication, increase lockout to _____ minutes
- ☐ Continuous pulse oximetry, except when ambulating.
- ☐ Nasal oxygen administration: 1–4 liters as needed to maintain oxygen saturation greater than or equal to _____ %.
- ☐ Contact physician for oxygen saturation less than _____ %.
- ☐ Other: _____
- ☐ Notify physician for:
  - Respiratory rate less than 8 per minute **AND** initiate naloxone (Narcan) protocol.
  - Uncontrolled pain
  - Persistent itching

Adjunct medications (may continue for 24 hours following discontinuation of PCA)
- ☐ If no continuous IVF ordered, infuse 0.9% saline IV or _____ IV at 20 mL/hr to maintain IV site patency.
- ☐ Ondansetron (Zofran) 4 mg slow IV over 2 minutes one time day of surgery only as needed for nausea.
- ☐ Prochlorperazine (Compazine) 5 mg slow IV over 2 minutes every 6 hours as needed for nausea. May repeat in 20 minutes. May give orally. 24-hour Max. dose is 40 mg.
- ☐ Metoclopramide (Reglan) _____ mg slow IV over 2 minutes every 4 hours as needed for nausea. (Do not give for colorectal surgery.) May give orally.
- ☐ Diphenhydramine (Benadryl) _____ mg slow IV over 2 minutes as needed for itching. May give orally.
- ☐ Hydroxyzine (Vistaril/Atarax) 25 mg IM or orally every 4 hours as needed for itching.
- ☐ Nalbuphine (Nubain) _____ mg slow IV over 2 minutes every 6 hours as needed for itching *(recommended range 2.5–5 mg dose).*
- ☐ Bowel care of choice:
  - ☐ Bisacodyl (Dulcolax) _____ mg orally every _____ as needed
  - ☐ Docusate sodium _____ mg orally every _____ as needed
- ☐ Other: _____

Figure 7-7 PCA order set.

catheter care if the patient has an indwelling urinary catheter.

Labs: Laboratory studies are not indicated for Mr. Jensen, because he did not have any significant abnormalities from the preoperative laboratory studies and because he did not have any significant blood loss during surgery.

Special instructions: Some special instruction orders might be prudent for Mr. Jensen. Because he has a history of hypertension and usually takes antihypertensive medication, you would want to know whether his blood pressure was elevated above an acceptable level. Likewise, development of a fever would be important, and you would want to be notified if that occurred. A complete set of postoperative orders for Mr. Jensen is shown in Figure 7-8.

Computerized Physician Order Entry

As stated earlier in this chapter, the *content* of admission orders has not changed greatly; however, the process by which orders are documented is very different in hospitals that have adopted the Computerized Physician (or Provider) Order Entry (CPOE). Even before the publication of the Institute of Medicine's report *To Err is Human: Building a Safer Health System* (Kohn et al., 2000) identified an unexpectedly high error rate in medical care, health-care providers recognized that the rate of medication errors and adverse drug events (ADEs) in hospitalized patients was unacceptably high. Since the report, awareness of the potential for severe harm from medication errors and of the frequency of ADEs has increased dramatically. Studies conducted after publication of the report concluded that a great number of medication errors and ADEs were preventable. One step that can be taken to reduce errors is to avoid using certain dangerous abbreviations, acronyms, and symbols when writing orders; in fact, since 2004, The Joint Commission has required organizations to have a "Do Not Use" list. The Institute for Safe Medical Practice (ISMP) also provides a list of Error-Prone Abbreviations, Symbols and Dose Designations, which is shown in Appendix D. The increasing concerns for safety and the desire for reducing and preventing medication errors have resulted in adoption of CPOE in some hospital systems.

Osheroff and associates (2005) define CPOE as "the portion of a clinical information system that enables a patient's care provider to enter an order for a medication, clinical laboratory or radiology test, or procedure directly into a computer that then

---

XX/XX/XX

0723

1. Admit to Dr. Sanders, surgical floor

2. Dx: adenocarcinoma of colon; S/P right hemicolectomy

3. Condition: stable

4. Bedrest

5. VS q1h x 4; if stable q2h x 4; if stable q4h

6. Allergic to PENICILLIN

7. NPO

8. Incentive spirometry q4h while awake

9. I&O

10. D5$\frac{1}{2}$ NS 150 mL/hr

11. Morphine sulfate 1 mg/mL by PCA; demand dose 1 mg, lockout every 12 minutes

12. 4-hour Dose limit; 20 mg

13. Phenergan 25 mg IM q4h prn for nausea

14. Routine wound care

15. Routine catheter care

16. Notify if systolic pressure >150 mm Hg or HR >130

Signature, Credential: _____

Countersignature: _____

Figure 7-8 Postoperative orders for Mr. Jensen.

transmits the order to the appropriate department, or individuals, so it can be carried out." Bobb and colleagues (2004) found that of 1111 prescribing errors confirmed in their study, 65% were likely preventable with a basic CPOE system. Other studies report preventable errors in the range of 43% to 72%. The number of potential preventable errors identified increased when basic CPOE was used in conjunction with the Clinical Decision Support System (CDSS). CDSS consists of automated checking to identify potential drug dose, allergy, and interaction errors; notify of duplicate orders; recommend preadministration or postadministration tests; provide access to clinical reference information, research, and guidelines; and substitute medication and test recommendations. Some CDSSs can also monitor patient treatment, ensuring, for example, that the right drug is administered to the right patient at the right time, and can issue an alert or reminder and suggest a different course of treatment if a patient's condition changes or if test results are abnormal. Most CDSSs can provide health-care professionals with immediate electronic access to their orders and comprehensive views of patient clinical data and laboratory test results, allowing providers to make more informed decisions about medications. Studies of CPOEs in major hospitals have found cost savings, increased use of preventive care interventions, and improved clinical care.

Many of the same challenges discussed in Chapter 1 related to widespread adoption of EMRs apply to CPOE use within hospitals. The most significant challenges are cost of purchasing and implementing CPOE (specifically systems with CDSS); lack of interoperability with ancillary departments, especially in hospitals where some form of CPOE may already have been implemented; and disrupted workflow for physicians, pharmacists, and nurses, leading to provider resistance, particularly if actions to try to ensure ready adoption have not been carried out. Although CPOE has been shown to decrease errors and improve quality, hospitals have been slow to adopt it. Classen and colleagues reported in 2007 that about 15% of U.S. hospitals have fully implemented systems. Even where available, it is not uniformly adopted, with reported use rates as low as 25% and as high as 90%.

The literature supports the beneficial effect of CPOE in reducing the frequency of a range of medication errors, including serious errors with the potential for harm. Few data are available regarding the impact of CPOE on ADEs, with no study showing a significant decrease in actual patient harm. Further research should be conducted to compare "homegrown" with commercially available systems.

Such comparisons are particularly important because the institutions that have published CPOE outcomes have generally been those with strong institutional commitments to their systems. Whether less committed institutions purchasing "off-the-shelf" systems will see comparable benefits remains to be determined. Studying the benefits of such complex systems requires rigorous methodology and sufficient size to provide the power to study ADEs. Further research also needs to address optimal ways for institutions to acquire and implement computerized ordering systems.

Admit Notes

Records such as the admission H&P and the discharge summary are often dictated, resulting in a 24- to 48-hour delay between the time of dictation and when the transcribed record appears on the chart. Because of this delay, it is customary to write a brief admit note in the chart. The purpose of the admit note is to summarize the admission H&P and to provide information that will be needed to care for the patient until the dictated records get to the chart. Document that an admission H&P has been performed and dictated, indicating the date and time it was done. This informs other medical staff members that the H&P has been done so that it will not be duplicated. It also serves as documentation that the H&P has been completed in the required time.

The admit note is a permanent part of the medical record. As such, it should be thorough enough to communicate the reason for the patient's hospitalization and should include the presumptive diagnosis and treatment plan, but keep in mind that it is a brief summary of the H&P. An admit note typically contains the patient's identifying information, reason for admission, pertinent past medical history, medications, allergies, pertinent physical examination findings, pertinent laboratory data, admitting diagnosis, and a summary of the treatment plan. It is usually written as a narrative paragraph. Here is one example of an admit note.

EXAMPLE 7.1

Admit note: Ms. Blanchard is a 72-year-old woman who developed symptoms of fever and cough 2 days ago and has had progressive dyspnea. Her past medical history is significant for COPD and hypertension. She takes Accupril 10 mg daily and uses a Combivent inhaler twice daily. On physical examination, she is febrile and dyspneic but not cyanotic. Crackles are heard in the right posterior lung. Heart is tachycardic but regular, with a rate of 112. Chest x-ray reveals a right lower lobe (RLL) infiltrate. Presumptive diagnosis is RLL pneumonia. Ms. Blanchard is admitted to the medical service for IV antibiotic therapy and supportive respiratory care.

Application Exercise 7.1

Referring to the information found in the H&P for Mr. Jensen (see Fig. 7-2), write an admit note in the space provided. Label it as an admit note, record the date and time of the entry, and provide the information as indicated in the previous paragraph. Admit notes for surgical admissions do not vary greatly from those for medical admissions. The plan of treatment is the surgical procedure the patient is scheduled to have.

_____

_____

_____

_____

_____

Once you have completed your admit note, compare it with Example 7.2.

EXAMPLE 7.2

Admit Note: Mr. Jensen is a 67-year-old Caucasian man who has colon cancer. Mr. Jensen originally presented with complaints of fatigue and on workup was found to have blood in the stool. Colonoscopy revealed adenocarcinoma. Past medical history is significant for hypertension and hypercholesterolemia. He is taking Lotensin HCT 20/12.5 once daily in the morning and Mevacor 20 mg once daily in the afternoon. He is allergic to penicillin medications, which cause a rash. Laboratory studies done at time of admission reveal that the CBC is normal; the chemistry panel reveals triglyceride of 178; LDL of 208; total cholesterol of 267; CEA of 17; otherwise WNL. CXR shows borderline cardiomegaly but no effusion. The ECG is WNL. Mr. Jensen will be admitted for elective right hemicolectomy. Routine preoperative orders are written. H&P done and dictated.

To reinforce the content of this chapter, please complete the worksheets that follow.

Admission H&P for Mr. Carl Hunter

Read and critically analyze the admission H&P for Mr. Carl Hunter shown in Figure 7-9. Answer the questions that follow.

1. Is this a medical or surgical admission?

_____

2. The medication listed for this patient is aspirin. Based on the documented PMH, what is the indication for this medication?

_____

3. What additional information should be documented about the medication?

_____

_____

4. Do you feel that the information documented in the social history is sufficient? Why or why not?

_____

_____

_____

5. List the systems explored in the ROS and the total number of systems reviewed.

_____

_____

_____

_____

6. Does the ROS meet CMS guidelines for documentation? Why or why not?

_____

_____

_____

7. Do you think the H&P contains enough information to justify hospital admission? Why or why not?

_____

_____

Admission H&P for Mr. Carl Hunter

Patient: Carl Hunter   MRN: 14-28-75

Sex: male   DOB: 8/1/19XX   Billing #: M49223-7

Admitting Physician: Samuel Mason, MD   Date of Admission: XX/XX/20XX

CHIEF COMPLAINT: Urinary frequency and urgency

HISTORY OF PRESENT ILLNESS: This is a pleasant 76-year-old man who has been having urinary urgency and frequency for the past week. Two days ago, he developed a fever. He remains febrile now and has experienced nausea but no vomiting. He denies abdominal pain, chest pain, shortness of breath, or diarrhea. He does have a history of benign prostatic hyperplasia.

PAST MEDICAL HISTORY:
      1. Status post-TURP for benign prostatic hyperplasia.
      2. Inguinal hernia status post repair.
      3. Carpal tunnel with repair

ALLERGIES: NO KNOWN DRUG ALLERGIES.

MEDICATIONS: Aspirin only.

FAMILY HISTORY: Father and brother both had BPH.

SOCIAL HISTORY: The patient is a former smoker, quit many years ago. Denies drug use. He drinks alcohol socially.

REVIEW OF SYMPTOMS: The patient denies any palpitations, chest pain, weakness, headaches, vision changes, nausea, vomiting, abdominal pain. He did say that he had a history of blood clots due to an injury. This happened many years ago, he doesn't recall the specific date or his age at the time but says it was when he was in his 40s. He has never had any problems since.

PHYSICAL EXAMINATION:
    Vital Signs: Blood pressure is 128/69, pulse is 84, temperature is 100.3ºF with 02 sats 93% on room air, weight is 184 lb.

    General: He is alert, awake, pleasant and in no acute distress.

    Head: Head is atraumatic, normocephalic. EOMs are intact. No scleral icterus.

    Neck: No lymphadenopathy noted.

    Cardiovascular: Regular rate. Normal S1, S2 without any murmurs or JVD.

    Abdomen: Soft, nontender, nondistended. No pain in the hypogastric area. No costovertebral angle tenderness. No rebound tenderness or guarding.

    Extremities: Nonedematous. Peripheral pulses present. No clubbing or cyanosis.

    Neurologic: The patient is alert and oriented to time, place, and person. He responded to all questions appropriately. No focal neurologic deficits.

LABORATORY DATA:
    CBC: WBC 12.9, hemoglobin 12.8, hematocrit 36.4 with neutrophils 83%. INR 1.2. Creatinine 1.4, BUN 25, sodium 134, potassium 3.9, chloride 99, bicarbonate 24. The CT scan of the abdomen revealed diverticulosis of the colon with thickening of the sigmoid colon suspicious of intramural diverticulitis. No abscess or free air. No hydronephrosis or stones.

ASSESSMENT:
      1. Febrile.
      2. Urine frequency, urgency.
      3. Leukocytosis.
      4. Hematuria.
      5. Bacteriuria.
      6. Acute renal failure.
      7. CT scan of abdomen showed diverticulosis and thickening of the sigmoid colon; intramural diverticulitis.
      8. History of TURP.

PLAN:
      1. Obtain urine cultures, stain, sensitivity.
      2. Blood cultures.
      3. IV fluid resuscitation.
      4. Start IV Flagyl.
      5. Check PSA. Urology consultation and possible cystoscopy if urology recommends.
      6. GI prophylaxis with Nexium.
      7. Further plans depending on the hospital course.

Figure 7-9 Admission H&P for Mr. Carl Hunter.

8. Read the assessment section and then the laboratory data section. Identify any additional information that you think should be recorded in the laboratory data section.

_____

_____

_____

9. After reading and critically analyzing the H&P, identify strengths and weaknesses of the document.

_____

_____

_____

Admit Orders for Mr. Carl Hunter

Read the admission H&P for Mr. Carl Hunter shown in Figure 7-9. Using the mnemonic AD CAVA DIMPLS shown in Figure 7-4, write admission orders to reflect the assessment and plan.

A: _____

D: _____

C: _____

A: _____

V: _____

A: _____

D: _____

I: _____

M: _____

P: _____

L: _____

S: _____

Worksheet 7.3

Admit Note for Mr. Carl Hunter

Read the admission H&P for Mr. Carl Hunter shown in Figure 7-9. Write an admit note based on the information documented in the H&P and using the notes in Examples 7.1 and 7.2 as a reference.

_____

_____

_____

_____

_____

_____

_____

_____

_____

_____

_____

_____

Admission H&P for Mrs. Gladys McLaughlin

Read and critically analyze the admission H&P for Mrs. Gladys McLaughlin shown in Figure 7-10. Answer the questions that follow.

1. Is this a medical or surgical admission?

_____

2. Review the PMH and identify strengths and weakness as documented.

_____

_____

_____

_____

3. The author states, "10-point review of systems is negative." Identify any information you find in other parts of the document that could be counted as ROS. List the systems reviewed and the total number of systems reviewed.

_____

_____

_____

_____

4. Based on the discussion of documenting the psychosocial history in Chapter 2, what elements could be added to the social history to make it more complete?

_____

_____

_____

_____

5. The assessment and plan in this admission H&P is a slightly different format compared with other H&Ps you have seen in this chapter. Do you feel the assessment and plan sections, as documented, sufficiently reflect a reason for hospitalization for this patient? Does the H&P meet CMS guidelines for documentation? Why or why not?

_____

_____

_____

_____

Patient: Gladys McLaughlin

MRN: 68-25-71

Sex: female   DOB: 1/29/19XX

Billing #: M452941-2

Admitting Physician: JoAnn Brooks, MD

Date of Admission: XX/XX/20XX

Primary Care Physician: Dr. Charles Rosenberg

CHIEF COMPLAINT: "Feeling lightheaded."

HISTORY OF PRESENT ILLNESS: The patient is a very pleasant 74-year-old woman who came to see Dr. Rosenberg today for a routine office physical examination and was noted to have a rapid heart rate. ECG obtained in his office showed atrial fibrillation with a rate in the 150s. No prior history of palpitations. The patient states that she felt lightheaded most of the day yesterday, and intermittently today. She denies syncope, headache, or visual changes. No chest pain or pressure, no shortness of breath. No other dizziness, focal numbness or weakness, speech difficulties, trouble swallowing, or difficulty moving extremities. No abdominal pain, recent diarrhea, or constipation. She does not exercise regularly but does do her own housework without any chest pressure or exertional dyspnea.

PAST MEDICAL HISTORY:
1. Diabetes mellitus, type 2.
2. Peripheral neuropathy due to diabetes.
3. Osteoporosis with vertebral compression fracture requiring kyphoplasty.
4. Kyphosis.
5. Hypertension.
6. 1–2+ mitral regurgitation.

ALLERGIES: PENICILLIN AND SULFA MEDICATIONS.

MEDICATIONS:
1. Lantus 22 units in the morning subcutaneously
2. Lisinopril 5 mg daily
3. Omeprazole 40 mg daily
4. Celebrex 200 mg daily
5. Xanax 0.25 mg twice daily
6. Aspirin 81 mg PO daily
7. Boniva 150 monthly
8. Mirtazapine 30 mg nightly

FAMILY HISTORY: Family history is remarkable for both parents dying in their early 40s. Her mother had uncontrolled hypertension, died from a stroke. Her father died from complications of long-standing diabetes.

SOCIAL HISTORY: The patient has been widowed since 2003. She has three daughters, one of whom lives nearby. She is a former smoker but quit in 2000. No significant alcohol intake.

REVIEW OF SYSTEMS: 10-point review of systems is negative.

PHYSICAL EXAMINATION:
Vital Signs: Blood pressure is 109/67, pulse 110 and irregular. Weight is 147 lb. Respiratory rate is 16. She is afebrile.

General: She is alert and fully oriented.

Skin: No pallor or jaundice noted.

HEENT: No evidence of head trauma. Oropharnyx is clear.

Neck: Supple. No increased jugular venous distention or carotid bruits are noted.

Heart: Heart rate is irregular, slightly tachycardic with an intermittent 2/6 systolic murmur.

Lungs: Clear to auscultation bilaterally. She has marked kyphosis.

Abdomen: Abdomen is soft, nontender, nondistended.

Extremities: There is no peripheral edema. Distal pulses are present and normal. She has normal strength in both upper and lower extremities.

Neurologic: Cranial nerves II–XII are intact.

LABORATORY STUDIES: ECG does show atrial fibrillation with rate of 150 with a right bundle branch block. WBC 9, Hgb 13.2, platelets 264,000, sodium 131, potassium 4.6, chloride 93, bicarb 25. BUN 17, creatinine 1.2, normal creatinine 0.9. Glucose 481.

(Continued)

Urinalysis had 6 WBCs. Hepatic function panel is within normal limits. TSH is within normal limits. Troponin was normal. Chest x-ray shows no active infiltrates.

ASSESSMENT: This is a very pleasant 74-year-old woman who presents with new-onset atrial fibrillation with rapid ventricular rate. She otherwise is fairly asymptomatic. Of note, she did have a recent 2-D echo in June of this past year, and it was essentially normal. There was some mild diastolic cardiac dysfunctions and 1–2 mitral regurgitation.

PLAN:
1. Atrial fibrillation. Will continue IV Cardizem, start on oral beta blocker and monitor heart rhythms. Will ask cardiology to consult. Continue to rule out myocardial infarction. Will give once-daily Lovenox.
2. Hypertension. Hold the ACE inhibitor at this time.
3. Osteoporosis. On treatment.
4. Diabetes mellitus, uncontrolled at this time. Will continue Lantus and institute insulin protocol.

Figure 7-10 Admission H&P for Mrs. Gladys McLaughlin.

Admit Orders for Mrs. Gladys McLaughlin

Read the admission H&P for Mrs. Gladys McLaughlin shown in Figure 7.10. Using the mnemonic AD CAVA DIMPLS shown in Figure 7-4, write admission orders to reflect the assessment and plan.

A: _____

D: _____

C: _____

A: _____

V: _____

A: _____

D: _____

I: _____

M: _____

P: _____

L: _____

S: _____

Admit Note for Mrs. Gladys McLaughlin

Read the admission H&P for Mrs. Gladys McLaughlin in Figure 7-10. Write an admit note based on the information documented in the H&P and using the notes in Examples 7.1 and 7.2 as a reference.

_____
_____
_____
_____
_____
_____
_____
_____
_____
_____
_____
_____

Abbreviations

These abbreviations were introduced in Chapter 7. Beside each, write the meaning as indicated by the content of this chapter.

ADA _____

AD CAVA DIMPLS _____

ADE _____

AP _____

BPH _____

BR _____

BRP _____

BUN _____

CDSS _____

CEA _____

CPOE _____

D5NS _____

H&H _____

ICS _____

ISMP _____

LDL _____

NCEP _____

NPO _____

NS _____

OCR _____

OOB _____

PACU _____

PCA _____

PT _____

RLL _____

SDS _____

S/P _____

SR _____

SVN _____

TID _____

TURP _____

Chapter 8

Documenting Daily Rounds and Other Events

OBJECTIVES

- Identify specific content that should be documented in daily progress notes.
- Document daily progress notes using the SOAP note format.
- Write orders that reflect continuous monitoring of a patient's condition and changes in the patient's care.
- Identify elements of an operative report.
- Discuss the difference between an operative report and an operative note.
- Identify elements of a procedure note.
- Identify elements of a delivery note.

Daily Progress Note

Whenever a patient is in the hospital, the admitting physician or a designee must visit the patient daily. This is often referred to as "making rounds" or "rounding on a patient." The purpose of the daily visit is to see how patients are responding to treatment and to determine whether any new problems have arisen. The SOAP note format introduced in Chapter 5 is frequently used to record information gathered during the daily visit. Some of the content documented in a daily progress note will be determined by whether the hospitalization is for a medical or surgical condition (discussed later); however, there are commonalities that would apply to either.

Subjective information includes the patient's comments or complaints and comments made by family members or health-care providers. Objective information includes a general assessment, physical examination findings, and review of laboratory or diagnostic test results and may include measurements such as vital signs or intake and output (I&O). Assessment documents the patient's response to therapy, indicates how the patient is progressing, and identifies any new problems. When applicable, documentation must also include any complications, hospital-acquired infections, and unfavorable reactions to drugs, including

anesthesia. The plan outlines any changes needed in the present care or initiates therapy for any new problems.

MEDICOLEGAL ALERT !

You may be responsible for rounding on more than one patient. Before making any entries in a patient's chart—either electronically or manually—take the time to verify that you have the correct chart. You should always check the name on the chart and check individual pages within the chart to be sure the identification data match the patient whose information you want to document. Making an entry in the wrong chart could result in a variety of problems, ranging from mere inconvenience to something much more serious. A good practice is to "make sure it's right before you write!"

Content of a Daily Progress Note
Medical Admissions

Remember that documentation of an admission history and physical examination (H&P) is required within 48 hours of hospitalization, as recommended by the Centers for Medicare and Medicaid Services (CMS) guidelines. The daily progress note does not need to contain information already documented in the H&P; instead, it focuses on any changes that have occurred in the condition of the patient from one day to the next. It is sometimes helpful to ask the patient a general question, such as, "Do you feel better, worse, or about the same?" The answer to this question provides the patient's perspective on his or her response to treatment and also allows for comparison of how you think the patient is progressing. Document the continued presence or resolution of any symptoms that the patient had at the time of admission. For example, if a patient was admitted for treatment of urosepsis and had fever and dysuria at the time of admission, document whether the patient still has these symptoms. To assess the patient's response to treatment or a procedure, you should anticipate what changes would be expected. The patient with urosepsis who is treated with antibiotics should become afebrile, and the urinalysis should show clearing of the infection. The patient should be monitored for development of symptoms that might indicate an adverse reaction to treatment. In the case of antibiotic administration, development of rash and difficulty breathing might indicate an adverse reaction, so the presence or absence of these symptoms is a pertinent positive or negative. In addition to information that is obtained directly from the patient, subjective information could also include review of notes from nursing staff, ancillary services personnel, or consulting providers and comments from staff or family members.

At least some physical examination is done during each daily visit. The general assessment is always important to document, providing a comparison to when you last saw the patient. Vital signs are monitored and recorded at different intervals during a 24-hour period, depending on what was ordered. The results are often plotted on a graphic sheet, such as the one shown in Figure 8-1, that can be easily referenced; therefore, only abnormal vital signs are typically documented in the daily progress note. Sometimes, a range of results (e.g., pulse 80 to 104 in past 24 hours) may be summarized in the note. Examination of the heart and lungs should be documented in every daily progress note, regardless of the reason for hospitalization; how much other examination is done depends largely on the reason for admission. A patient being treated for a cerebrovascular accident who has comorbid conditions would require more extensive examination, and therefore documentation, than a patient admitted for pneumonia who is otherwise healthy.

It is essential to document review of all test results in a timely manner because missing an abnormal result could have a negative impact on the patient's condition. "Shorthand" for documenting results of a complete blood count (CBC), electrolytes, or basic metabolic panel (Fig. 8-2) is sometimes used in the daily progress note. This provides an easy way to compare the newest results with previous ones.

The assessment should reflect evaluation of all the data available and any conclusions that can be drawn from them. The assessment should indicate whether the patient's condition is better, worse, or about the same since the last visit. If a patient was febrile at the time of admission but is now afebrile, the entry might read, "Patient now afebrile; improved."

The plan section of the daily visit note outlines changes that will be made in the treatment regimen already in effect, either stating or inferring the rationale for these changes. This may include procedures or diagnostic tests to be done and management of any new problems or complications.

Surgical Admissions

The main differences in the documentation of a daily visit to a postoperative patient rather than a medical patient will be in the subjective and objective sections of the note. When documenting the daily visit note of a patient who has had a surgical procedure, it is customary to label the note as "POD (postoperative day) #___," indicating what number postoperative day it is. This is helpful when trying to determine whether the patient is progressing as expected after surgery because there is a fairly well-established time frame of certain events, such as when bowel function returns, when drains are removed, and healing of a surgical incision.

When rounding on postoperative patients, answering routine questions can guide your evaluation of the patient each day. Is the patient getting adequate pain relief? Has bowel function returned? Can the activity level be advanced? Can the diet be advanced? Can any sutures, staples, tubes, or drains be removed? You should also determine whether any postoperative complications have occurred. You can anticipate what complications are likely based on the type of surgery that was done and then document enough information in the subjective and objective portions of the note to convey that such complications have or have not occurred.

Postoperative complications that can develop after almost any type of surgery include fever, urinary retention, fluid imbalance, and wound infection. More serious complications include hemorrhage, respiratory depression, and pulmonary or fat embolism. Fever is the most common postoperative complication and usually has one of five etiologies: respiratory, wound, or urinary tract infection, thromboembolic event, or

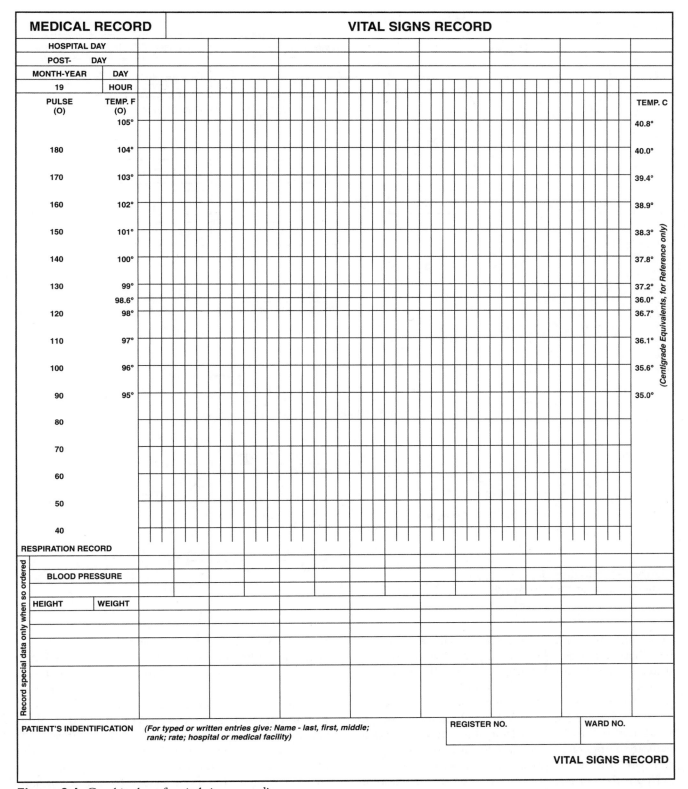

Figure 8-1 Graphic sheet for vital signs recording.

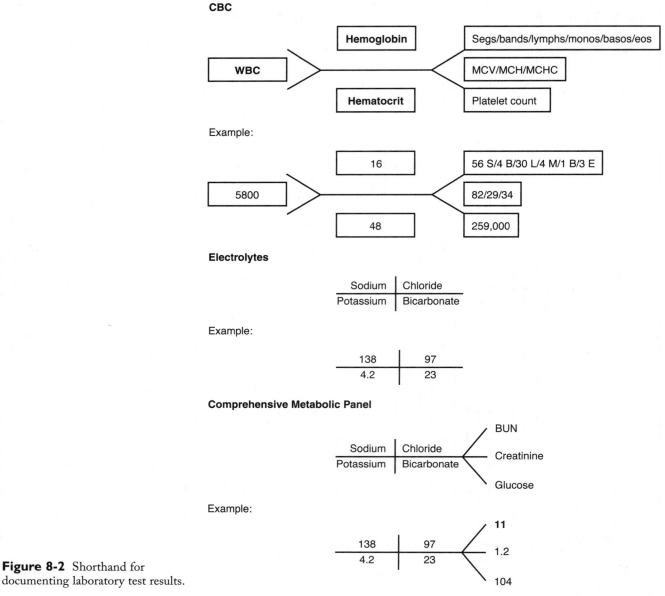

Figure 8-2 Shorthand for documenting laboratory test results.

drug side effect or adverse reaction. You can remember these etiologies by thinking of "wind, wound, water, walk, and wonder drug" (the *five Ws*, explained in Table 8-1). This should prompt you to ask the patient about any symptoms that could indicate development of these complications, such as fever, cough, shortness of breath or difficulty breathing, increased pain at the operative site, and swelling of the legs or calf pain. You would document the answers as pertinent positives or negatives in the subjective portion of the note.

Examining the cardiovascular and respiratory systems is part of the objective evaluation of every postoperative patient. Additionally, the surgical incision

or operative site should be inspected, and the appearance should be described in the note. Document the presence of any drains and the amount and color of any drainage. If the patient had general anesthesia, it is important to determine return of peristalsis. Document whether there is any abdominal distention and if bowel sounds are absent or present; if present, document the character of bowel sounds. Tailor the rest of the examination to the type of surgery that was performed. Do not neglect to assess for and document any pertinent findings related to preexisting or comorbid conditions the patient may have. A sample postoperative day #1 progress note for Mr. Jensen is shown in Figure 8-3.

Table 8-1		The Five Ws of Postoperative Fever		
Category	**System**	**When Fever Is Likely to Occur**	**Potential Problems**	**What to Assess**
Wind	Respiratory	Within first 48 hr after surgery	Hypoventilation, atelectasis, pneumonia	Respiratory rate and effort, breath sounds
Wound	Integumentary	Postoperative days 4 to 7	Wound infection, abscess	Amount and character of drainage, erythema, induration, increased tenderness at operative site
Water	Urinary	Anytime	Urinary tract infection (UTI), sepsis	Fever, chills, flank pain, urgency, dysuria; amount, color, and smell of urine
Walk	Vascular	Postoperative days 5 to 14	Deep vein thrombosis (DVT)	Calf tenderness, swelling, temperature of extremities
Wonder drug	Multisystem		Drug adverse reaction or drug-drug interaction	All medications patient has had since surgery

---

Date   XX/XX/XXXX POD #1
Time   0823

S: Mr. Jensen states that he rested fairly well last night. He has had adequate pain relief with PCA dosing and had only one bolus dose. The nurse indicates that Mr. Jensen has been using the incentive spirometer every 4 hours when awake. He denies any N/V, fever, or chills. He does not have any complaints at this time.

O: Vital signs: BP 136/86, P 92, R 16, temp is 98.8. Maximum temp since surgery has been 99.1. I&O is 1870 mL and 1710 mL. On exam, Mr. Jensen is awake, alert, and cooperative.

Heart: RRR

Resp: Breathing somewhat shallow, but breath sounds are without any wheezing or crackles.

ABD: Soft, nondistended. No bowel sounds audible. Minimal tenderness to palpation around operative incision. There is a small amount of serosanguineous drainage noted on dressing. The wound edges are dry and intact, and there is no erythema or warmth around the incision.

EXT: Lower extremities reveal no calf tenderness or swelling, no warmth to touch. Distal pulses are intact and equal bilaterally.

GU: Urinary catheter in place with 75 mL of clear yellow urine in drainage bag.

A: S/P hemicolectomy, POD #1. Progressing as expected without complications.

P: Remove catheter. May have BRP. Advance activity to OOB at least TID.

Signature, Credentials: _____

Countersignature: _____

Figure 8-3 First postoperative day progress note for Mr. Jensen.

Daily Orders

Any time there is a change in the plan of care for a hospitalized patient, corresponding orders must be written to reflect that change. Remember that in Chapter 7 we said that an order stays in effect until another order is written to modify or discontinue it. Once you have assessed the patient and recorded the daily progress note, you should write orders that correspond to any changes addressed in the plan. You might want to refer back to Figure 7.8 to review the postoperative orders that are currently in effect for Mr. Jensen. Now, look at the plan portion of the SOAP note shown in Figure 8-3. You will notice that an order should be written to remove the urinary catheter and another order written to change Mr. Jensen's activity level to allow for bathroom privileges and for him to be out of bed at least three times a day. As with any entry in the medical chart, you should indicate the date and time, write the necessary orders, and then add your signature and title.

Any time a change is made in the patient's management, the response to that change should be evaluated during the next visit. For instance, based on the plan documented in the POD #1 note, an order was written to remove the urinary catheter. The next time you round on Mr. Jensen, you should assess his response to removal of the catheter. Was he able to void after it was removed? Did he experience any urinary retention? The response is then documented in the progress note.

Application Exercise 8.1

Based on the plan section of the note in Figure 8-3, write orders that reflect the changes needed.

_____

_____

_____

Application Exercise 8.2

The subjective and objection portions of the POD #2 daily progress note are shown below. Use this information to write the assessment and plan. After you have completed the SOAP note for this visit, write any orders necessary.

Date, Time. POD #2

S: Mr. Jensen states that he rested fairly well last night. He is having adequate pain relief. He was able to void after the catheter was removed. He experiences minor discomfort at the incision site when he gets out of bed but otherwise is comfortable. He denies any chest pain, SOB, or difficulty breathing. He denies nausea or vomiting and states that he feels hungry. He continues to use the ICS every 4 hours when awake. He does not have any complaints at this time.

O: Maximum BP in the past 24 hours recorded as 152/94 with systolic consistently above 130 and diastolic consistently above 90. Maximum temperature since surgery has been 99.7°F. I&O is 1855 cc and 1635 cc. On physical examination, Mr. Jensen is awake and cooperative. Heart exam reveals a regular rate and rhythm; normal S1 and S2; no gallop, murmur, or ectopy. There is no JVD and no peripheral edema. Respirations are nonlabored, and there are normal breath sounds on auscultation of the lungs. The abdomen is soft, nondistended. Faint hypoactive bowel sounds heard throughout the abdomen. There is minimal tenderness to palpation around operative incision. Dressing is dry. Wound edges

are intact, and there is no erythema or warmth around the incision. No calf tenderness to palpation. No swelling of lower extremities. Distal pulses are intact and equal bilaterally.

_____

_____

_____

_____

_____

_____

_____

Application Exercise 8.2 Answer
Here is one possible way to document the assessment and plan for the POD #2 daily progress note:

A:

1. S/P hemicolectomy, POD #2. Progressing as expected.
2. Return of bowel function.
3. Wound healing without signs of infection.
4. Hypertension, previously stable on medication.

P:

1. Increase diet to clear liquids.
2. Continue routine wound care.
3. Resume prehospital medications of Lotensin and Mevacor.
4. Activity as tolerated.

Orders to correspond to your plan would read as follows:

1. Increase diet to clear liquids.
2. Activity as tolerated.
3. Lotensin HCT 20/12.5 mg one tablet PO daily.
4. Mevacor 20 mg one tablet PO daily.

MEDICOLEGAL ALERT !

Problems might arise when an intervention that should be done is omitted or when an intervention is performed longer than is necessary. An example is a patient who needs to have regular treatments with a bronchodilator, but the order is never written. The patient develops respiratory difficulty because an intervention was warranted but not done. There might also be problems if an intervention is done longer than necessary. An example of this is when a patient has a urinary catheter that could be removed, but the order is not written. The catheter remains in place longer than necessary, and the patient develops a urinary tract infection. Always remember to assess on a daily basis what interventions are indicated and which ones may be discontinued.

Full Operative Report and Operative Note

A full operative report, which provides a detailed narrative of the surgical procedure, must be documented for every patient undergoing a surgical procedure. The surgeon dictates this report. A full operative report for Mr. Jensen is shown in Figure 8-4. Because there could be a significant time lapse between the time the operative report is dictated and the time it is transcribed and placed in the chart, a brief operative note is often written. This is similar to writing an admit note to summarize the admission H&P and indicating that it has been done and dictated. The operative note (or "op note") is typically handwritten in the chart immediately after surgery and remains part of the medical record even after the full transcribed operative report is placed in the chart. The operative note includes the following information:

- Date of procedure
- Name of procedure
- Indication: reason for the procedure
- Surgeon
- Surgical assistants, if any
- Anesthesia: local, general, regional; name of person administering anesthesia
- Preoperative diagnosis: presumptive diagnosis before surgery
- Postoperative diagnosis: most likely diagnosis based on surgical findings
- Descriptions
  1. Specimens: what tissue was removed and what studies were done
  2. Estimated blood loss (EBL)
  3. Drains: types of drains, if any, and where placed
- Complications, if any (such as a nicked artery, punctured bowel, or complications from anesthesia)
- Disposition

Application Exercise 8.3

Review the full operative report for Mr. Jensen shown in Figure 8-4. Use the information from this report to compose an operative note in the space provided.
Date of procedure:
Name of procedure:

Continued

DATE OF PROCEDURE:	XX/XX/XXXX
PROCEDURE:	Right hemicolectomy
INDICATION:	Adenocarcinoma diagnosed by tissue biopsy
SURGEON:	David K. Sanders, MD
SURGICAL ASSISTANT:	Debbie Sullivan, PA-C
ANESTHESIA:	General, by Paul Bartlett, MD

PREOPERATIVE DIAGNOSIS:
    Adenocarcinoma, right colon

POSTOPERATIVE DIAGNOSIS:
    Adenocarcinoma, right colon

DESCRIPTION:
    Under endotracheal anesthesia, the patient's abdomen was prepped and draped. A midline incision was made. The liver was normal, except for a small cyst of the lateral aspect of the left lateral segment. The stomach, spleen, small bowel, and retroperitoneum were normal. There were no stones in the gallbladder. The colon was remarkable for a mass in the right colon. The right colon was mobilized and the ureter identified and preserved. The gastrocolic ligament was divided along its right side. The ileocolic vessels were transected near their takeoff from the SMA, and ligated with absorbable suture. The remaining mesentery was divided between clamps and ligated. The bowel ends were transected using a stapler. The resection included the right branch of the middle colic artery, and resection margins were in the distal ileum and transverse colon. Two tissue samples were obtained, one from the distal ileum and one from the transverse colon. An ileotransverse colostomy was performed using staples. The mesenteric defect was closed with staples. Hemostasis was checked, and the incision was irrigated. The fascia was closed with a single layer of running #1 PDS. The subcutaneous tissues were irrigated, and the skin was closed with Vicryl. Estimated blood loss was 80 mL.

COMPLICATIONS:
    None

DISPOSITION:
    The patient was transferred to the postanesthesia care unit in stable condition.

Figure 8-4 Full operative report.

Indication:
Surgeon:
Surgical assistant:
Anesthesia:
Preoperative diagnosis:
Postoperative diagnosis:
Description:
Complications:
Disposition:

Application Exercise 8.3 Answer
Here is one way the operative note for Mr. Jensen could be documented.

Date of procedure: xx/xx/xxxx
Name of procedure: Right hemicolectomy
Indication: Adenocarcinoma of the colon
Surgeon: D. Sanders, MD
Surgical assistant: D. Sullivan, PA-C
Anesthesia: General
Preoperative diagnosis: Adenocarcinoma, right colon
Postoperative diagnosis: Adenocarcinoma, right colon
Description: No unexpected findings, no evidence of metastasis, two tissue samples obtained for pathology; EBL 80 cc
Complications: None
Disposition: To recovery in stable condition

Other Types of Documents

In addition to admission H&Ps, admit notes, daily progress notes, and op notes, other types of documents are frequently created during the course of a patient's hospital stay. Procedure notes and delivery notes are discussed in this chapter. Discharge summaries and discharge orders will be discussed in Chapter 9, as will documentation related to patient elopement and a patient leaving the hospital against medical advice.

Procedure Note

The purpose of the procedure note is to document why and how a procedure was done and the patient's response to the procedure. The usual format includes the following elements:

• Name of the procedure
• Indication for the procedure
• Consent (if required, including risks and benefits, potential complications, and name and relationship of person giving consent)
• Anesthesia (if applicable)
• Details of the procedure
• Findings (if relevant)
• Complications

Suppose that, while he was in the hospital, Mr. Jensen fell and sustained a laceration to the scalp. You are called to evaluate him and, after examination, you determine that the laceration requires closure. After the laceration is repaired, you document the procedure. This could be documented using the SOAP note format; however, a procedure note is often written instead. Following is a procedure note documenting the repair of Mr. Jensen's scalp laceration.

xx/xx/xxxx   Procedure Note
1845   Procedure: Laceration repair
Indication: 2-cm full-thickness scalp laceration of the right occipital area.
Consent: Discussed with Mr. Jensen the need for laceration repair; possible complications of infection, bleeding; oral consent given by Mr. Jensen.
Anesthesia: Local with 1% lidocaine with epinephrine
Procedure: The area was prepped and draped in the usual sterile fashion. After local anesthesia, the wound was explored; no foreign bodies or step-offs were palpated. The wound was cleansed with Hibiclens and sterile water. The laceration was repaired with 3.0 nylon suture with a total of four interrupted sutures. Good approximation and hemostasis were achieved. Topical antibiotic ointment was applied.
Complications: None
Signature, title

The procedure note may be used in other settings for various types of procedures. The note could be used to document a biopsy done at a dermatology office, removal of a toenail at a primary care clinic, or thoracentesis done in the emergency department.

MEDICOLEGAL ALERT !

The issues related to consent are complex. Consent is not merely a form that needs to be completed; obtaining the patient's consent means obtaining the patient's authorization for diagnosis and treatment. It is the responsibility of the physician or the physician's representative to discuss with the patient the indications for a procedure, the risks and benefits associated with the procedure, and any alternative forms of treatment. Courts have consistently held that it is not the responsibility of the hospital or health-care organization or any of its employees to obtain consent. The person making the consent decision must be legally and actually competent and must be informed. A potential pitfall exists when there is more than one physician attending a patient and there may be confusion about which physician is responsible for obtaining consent. Generally, the burden to obtain consent rests with the person who will be performing the procedure for which consent is necessary. State laws may regulate who is responsible for obtaining consent and who may give consent. You are encouraged to consult the references provided at the end of this unit for more information regarding consent.

Delivery Note

A delivery note is used to document the outcome of an obstetrical admission. In many hospitals, the physician in attendance at the time of delivery is responsible for dictating a complete delivery record. A delivery note serves much the same function as the admit or operative note: to document at least some details of the delivery until the dictated record is transcribed and placed in the patient's chart.

The key information that should be documented in a delivery note includes the following:

- Type of delivery (vaginal, cesarean)
- Estimated gestational age of the fetus
- Viability of the fetus
- Sex of the fetus
- APGAR scores at 1 and 5 minutes (see Table 8-2 for criteria for Apgar score)
- Weight of the fetus
- Delivery of the placenta, including number of vessels in the umbilical cord and whether the placenta was intact
- If any lacerations or episiotomies, what extent and how repaired
- Estimated blood loss
- Condition of mother immediately after delivery

An example of a delivery note is provided here:

xx/xx/xxxx   Delivery note: 1028

Normal, spontaneous vaginal delivery (NSVD) of a full-term viable male infant, Apgar scores of 7 and 9. Weight 7 pounds, 2 oz., delivered over a second-degree central episiotomy. Intact placenta expelled spontaneously, three-vessel cord. No vaginal, cervical, or external genital lacerations. Episiotomy repaired with 2.0 chromic. EBL of 40 cc. Patient in good condition, no complications.

To reinforce the content of this chapter, please complete the worksheets that follow.

Table 8-2 Apgar Scoring Criteria*

Clinical Sign	Criteria for Assigned Points		
	0 Points	*1 Point*	*2 Points*
Heart rate	Absent	<100	>100
Respiratory effort	Absent	Slow and irregular	Good; strong
Muscle tone	Flaccid	Some flexion of the arms and legs	Active movements
Reflex irritability (reaction to suction of nares with bulb syringe)	No response	Grimace	Vigorous cry, sneeze, or cough
Color	Blue, pale	Pink body, blue extremities	Pink all over

*Score of 0 to 4 at 1 minute after birth indicates severe depression, requiring immediate resuscitation; score of 5 to 7 indicates some nervous system depression, and score of 8 to 10 is normal. Score of 0 to 7 at 5 minutes after birth indicates high risk for subsequent central nervous system and other organ system dysfunction; score of 8 to 10 is normal.

Worksheet 8.1

1. List several questions that should be answered daily for postoperative patients.

_____

_____

_____

_____

2. A postoperative patient has been on a full liquid diet for the past 24 hours. He now has full bowel sounds and says he is hungry. Write an order for a change in diet.

_____

_____

3. List seven components of a procedure note.

_____

_____

_____

_____

_____

_____

_____

_____

4. List at least five components of an operative note.

_____

_____

_____

_____

_____

_____

5. List at least five components of a delivery note.

_____

_____

_____

_____

_____

_____

6. List the five Ws that could be sources of postoperative fever.

_____

_____

_____

_____

_____

Mrs. Karen Stevens is a 50-year-old woman who presents for elective right carpal tunnel release. After reading the operative report shown in Figure 8-5, write an operative note.

PATIENT: Karen A. Stevens
Medical Record Number: 87-420-65
Same-Day Surgery Unit

DATE OF PROCEDURE: XX/XX/XXX

PROCEDURE: Right carpal tunnel release

INDICATION: Chronic right hand with intractable pain, numbness, and tingling

SURGEON: Ralph Benedict, DO

SURGICAL ASSISTANT: Susan Carmichael, PA-C

ANESTHESIA: Distal wrist block; Wendy Falconetti, CRNA

PREOPERATIVE DIAGNOSIS:
Carpal tunnel syndrome, right hand

POSTOPERATIVE DIAGNOSIS:
Carpal tunnel syndrome, right hand, severe

OPERATIVE INDICATIONS:
A very active 50-year-old right-hand-dominant woman has had pain, numbness, and tingling in the right hand for more than 8 months. She had conservative medical management with splinting and exercises and did not improve. She has noticed increasing pain and night awakening over the past 2 months, interfering with her activities of daily living. Electromyography and nerve conduction studies confirmed median nerve compression. She failed nonoperative management. We discussed the risks, benefits, and possible complications of operative and continued nonoperative management, and she gave her fully informed consent to the following procedure.

OPERATIVE REPORT IN DETAIL:
The patient was brought to the operating room and placed in the supine position on the operating room table. After adequate anesthesia, extremity was prepped and draped in usual sterile manner using a standard Betadine prep.

The right hand was elevated and exsanguinated using an Esmarch bandage, and the tourniquet was inflated to 250 mm Hg for about 25 minutes. Volar approach to the carpal ligament was performed incising the skin with a knife and using cautery for hemostasis. Tenotomy and forceps dissection carried out through the superficial palmar fascia, carried down to the volar carpal ligament, which was then transected sharply with a knife and carried proximal and distal under direct vision using the scissors and being careful to avoid the neurovascular structures.

Cautery was used for hemostasis. The nerve had an hourglass appearance where it was constricted as a result of the compression from the ligament, and so a small amount of Celestone was dripped onto the nerve to help quiet it down. The patient tolerated this portion of the procedure very well. The hand was then irrigated and closed with Monocryl and Prolene, and sterile compressive dressing was applied and the tourniquet deflated.

ESTIMATED BLOOD LOSS:
Less than 40 mL

COMPLICATIONS:
None

DISPOSITION:
To recovery room awake, alert, and in stable condition

Figure 8-5 Operative report for Mrs. Karen Stevens.

Worksheet 8.3

Mr. Dewayne McKay is a 54-year-old man who was admitted for cirrhosis of the liver. An abdominal paracentesis was done earlier today, and the following procedure note was written. After reading the note, answer the following questions.

Name of procedure: abdominal paracentesis
Indication for procedure: ascites
Consent: form signed by patient before procedure
Anesthesia: local, total of 4 cc
Procedure: area was prepped and draped in usual sterile fashion. A 20-gauge needle was inserted and approximately 1840 cc of fluid was removed. Fluid sent to lab for analysis.

Chris Reeder, MS-IV

1. What additional information about consent should be documented in the procedure note?

_____

_____

_____

2. After critically analyzing the note and comparing it to the one presented in the chapter, what additional information should be documented in the note?

_____

_____

_____

Information about paracentesis was not specifically presented in this chapter; however, you are encouraged to read about this procedure and answer the following questions.

3. List at least two laboratory values that are typically evaluated and documented before a paracentesis is performed.

_____

_____

4. List at least three tests that are typically ordered to evaluate ascitic fluid.

_____

_____

_____

Daily Visit SOAP notes

Refer to Figure 7.9, Admission H&P for Mr. Hunter. After reviewing the H&P, answer the questions below.

1. List at least three problems, symptoms, or complaints documented in the H&P that should be followed up when rounding on Mr. Hunter the day after his admission and documented in the subjective portion of the daily visit note. State your rationale for including each one.

_____

_____

_____

_____

2. List at least three findings that should be documented in the objective portion of the daily visit note and state your rationale for including each one.

_____

_____

_____

_____

Refer to Figure 7.10, admission H&P for Mrs. McLaughlin.

After reviewing the H&P, answer the questions below.

3. List at least three problems, symptoms, or complaints documented in the H&P that should be followed up when rounding on Mrs. McLaughlin the day after her admission and documented in the subjective portion of the daily visit note. State your rationale for including each one.

_____

_____

_____

_____

4. List at least three findings that should be documented in the objective portion of the daily visit note and state your rationale for including each one.

_____

_____

_____

_____

Abbreviations

These abbreviations were introduced in Chapter 8. Beside each, write the meaning as indicated by the content of this chapter.

CRNA _____

EBL _____

I&O _____

IM _____

NSVD _____

POD _____

SMA _____

SR _____

Chapter 9

Discharging Patients from the Hospital

OBJECTIVES

- List specific components of discharge orders.
- Discuss the content that should be included in a discharge summary.
- Define leaving against medical advice and the documentation of this event.
- Discuss patient elopement and documenting the event.

Discharge Orders

In Chapter 7, we saw that specific orders are written when a patient is admitted to the hospital. Likewise, specific orders are written at the time of discharge. We will again follow the hospitalization of Mr. Jensen to see how discharge orders are written. A summary of what is included in discharge orders is listed below, and a discussion of each element is presented next.

- Disposition (where the patient will go after discharged from the hospital)
- Activity with specific instructions
- Diet
- Medications, including pre-hospital medications that should be resumed and any new medications
- Follow up instructions (when and who)
- Notification instructions (signs or symptoms that could signal complications)

Disposition

The first discharge order usually indicates the disposition, or where the patient will go when discharged. The patient may go home or may be transferred to another facility such as an extended care or rehabilitation facility. In the case of Mr. Jensen, he will return home because he does not require specialized care.

Activity Level

The patient's activity level should be specified in the discharge orders. Mr. Jensen has an abdominal incision, so he should not do any heavy lifting or straining in

order to prevent dehiscence of the wound. An order that says, "avoid heavy lifting" is vague, and the patient is usually not in the position to determine how much weight is too heavy. It is best to give a specific weight limit. A fairly low weight is advised for Mr. Jensen; 20 pounds is the maximum he should lift at this time, although some surgeons might limit the weight to 10 pounds. Patients who have had surgery are often instructed not to drive for a certain amount of time after surgery. For patients who have had abdominal surgery, 1 to 2 weeks are usually a minimum restriction; some procedures, especially orthopedic, might require an even longer restriction period.

Mr. Jensen has a surgical incision, so activity orders should include care of the wound or specific instructions related to the wound. The wound can get wet but should not be immersed in water. Therefore, an order should specify that he may shower but should not take a tub bath, sit in a hot tub, or go swimming. Mr. Jensen will need to continue wound care at home. Instead of writing out the specific wound care orders, an order may be written for the nursing staff to instruct on wound care.

Diet

Consider what type of diet the patient should have at home. Ideally, the patient's diet has been advanced during the hospital stay to the same that it was before hospitalization. Mr. Jensen has a history of hypertension and dyslipidemia, so the diet order should reflect the need for a special diet. A reasonable order for Mr. Jensen is a low-fat, low-cholesterol diet.

Medication

Just as you had to write orders for medications while the patient was hospitalized, the discharge orders should indicate what medications the patient will continue after discharge. First, consider what medications the patient was taking before hospitalization. In Mr. Jensen's case, he was taking Lotensin HCT 20/12.5 and Mevacor. Because these medications treat chronic conditions that he still has, they should be continued. An order should be written to continue usual dosages of these medications. Next, consider what medications might be indicated related to the reason for the hospitalization. Mr. Jensen had major abdominal surgery and will need pain medication after discharge. Usually, the same oral analgesic that was given in the hospital will be continued at home because its efficacy has been established, and the patient has been tolerating it without any problems. A prescription should be written for any medications the patient has not taken previously, so you will need to write a prescription for an analgesic (prescription writing is discussed in Chapter 10). Finally, consider whether other medications, prescription or over-the-counter, are needed. Some medications that may be needed include stool softeners, sleep aids, and nonsteroidal anti-inflammatory medications for mild to moderate pain. Be sure to write a prescription for any medications that are not available over the counter.

Follow-Up Care

Follow-up care should also be part of the discharge orders. Specify when and by whom the patient will be seen. Mr. Jensen will see the surgeon, Dr. Sanders, 1 week from the time of discharge for wound evaluation, removal of staples or sutures, and a routine postoperative checkup. Follow-up care should also include special instructions for the patient, such as notifying Dr. Sanders if any symptoms of complications occur. You should specify what should be reported because the patient may not realize the importance of certain symptoms. Consider what postoperative complications might occur and what symptoms might be associated with those complications. Any patient who has had major abdominal surgery will be at risk for developing wound infection, pneumonia, deep vein thrombosis, or pulmonary embolus. Symptoms that correspond to these conditions include fever, redness or increased pain at the incision site, difficulty breathing, and pain in the leg. "Fever" is somewhat subjective (just like "heavy lifting" discussed earlier), so it is best to state a specific temperature that would be of concern. A typical order would read, "notify Dr. Sanders of temperature greater than 100.5°F, redness or increased pain at incision site, cough, difficulty breathing, or pain or swelling of the leg."

Mr. Jensen would also follow up with his primary care provider (PCP), Dr. Vernon Scott, because he has chronic conditions that need continued monitoring and management that the surgeon would not typically provide. The time frame of follow-up will vary depending on the patient's overall health status and whether the chronic conditions are stable or unstable. Because Mr. Jensen's hypertension and dyslipidemia are stable, he should see Dr. Scott in 1 to 2 months. The entire set of discharge orders for Mr. Jensen would be as follows:

1. Discharge to home
2. No lifting greater than 10 pounds; no driving, exercising, or strenuous activity until released by Dr. Sanders
3. May shower but no tub bath, hot tub use, or swimming until released by Dr. Sanders
4. Instruct on routine wound care
5. Low-fat, low-cholesterol diet
6. Continue Lotensin HCT 20/12.5 and Mevacor at home
7. Ibuprofen 800 mg PO q6h with food prn mild to moderate pain
8. Oxycodone 1 or 2 tablets PO q4h prn moderate to severe pain
9. Colace 100 mg PO twice daily for 1 week to prevent constipation
10. F/U with Dr. Sanders in 1 week.
11. Notify Dr. Sanders if T >100.5°F, redness or increased pain at incision site, cough, difficulty breathing, or pain in legs.
12. Follow-up with Dr. Scott in 1 month for routine care.

MEDICOLEGAL ALERT !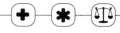

Failure to provide adequate follow-up instructions is one of the leading causes of litigation against healthcare providers. The provider has the responsibility to anticipate what complications the patient might develop and to educate the patient on the signs and symptoms that could indicate such a complication. Patients cannot be expected to know what signs or symptoms need to be reported. Your follow-up instructions and the documentation of such instructions should be as specific as possible. It is a good idea to verify that the patient has understood the follow-up instructions by asking the patient to repeat back to you what he or she has heard about the follow-up instructions. When you do this, you should document that the patient appeared to understand follow-up instructions. It is also recommended that you provide written follow-up instructions as well because the patient is not likely to remember everything you said verbally. You should also include family members or others who may be caring for the patient after discharge and document who, besides the patient, received follow-up instructions.

Discharge Summary

The discharge summary is a synopsis of the patient's entire hospitalization and is required for any hospital stay longer than 24 hours. Often, members of the health-care team, insurance carriers or other third-party payers, and quality assurance personnel request a copy of the discharge summary. The discharge summary must be completed before the hospital can submit for payment. For these reasons, the discharge summary should be completed in a timely manner. Regulations for participating in federal reimbursement programs, for example, require that hospital records be completed within 30 days following the patient's discharge. The discharge summary is usually dictated, and transcribed copies are placed in the chart and sent to the admitting physician and other consulting providers as indicated.

One sample format is provided here, and we will again refer to Mr. Jensen as we discuss the discharge summary. The format used for discharge summaries will vary from institution to institution.

The headings shown below (and in Table 9-1) indicate what information should be part of the discharge summary.

- Date of admission
- Date of discharge
- Admitting diagnosis (or diagnoses)
- Discharge diagnosis (or diagnoses)
- Attending physician
- Primary provider and consulting physician(s) (if any)
- Procedures (if any)
- Brief history, pertinent physical examination findings, and pertinent laboratory values (at time of admission)
- Hospital course
- Condition at discharge
- Disposition
- Discharge medications
- Discharge instructions and follow-up instructions
- Problem list

The dates of admission and discharge are easily determined from the chart. The admitting diagnosis can be found in the initial admitting orders. The discharge diagnosis might be the same as or different from the admitting diagnosis or might include several different diagnoses. If you have not been following the patient on a regular basis, you may have to read through the entire chart to identify all the diagnoses.

Table 9-1 Discharge Summary Contents and Brief Description

Item	Description
Date of admission	List date of admission
Date of discharge	List date of discharge
Admitting diagnosis (or diagnoses)	Principal or presumptive reason for admission
Discharge diagnosis (or diagnoses)	Actual or final reason for admission that was evident by the time of discharge
Attending physician	List attending physician
Referring and consulting physician (if any)	List names of those who provided consultations for this patient during the course of hospitalization; if none, omit heading
Procedures (if any)	If none, omit heading
Brief history, pertinent exam findings and pertinent lab values	Events leading up to hospitalization, pertinent PMH, pertinent exam findings at time of admission, and pertinent lab values at time of admission
Hospital course	Narrative of the details of the daily progress of the patient and response to treatment
Condition at discharge	Avoid one-word descriptions, state why patient is able to be discharged
Disposition	Where patient will go at time of discharge (home, extended care facility, etc.)
Discharge medication	List pre-hospital medications as well as any medications added during hospitalization that patient will continue taking after discharge
Discharge instructions and follow-up	Include activity level, signs or symptoms of potential complications that patient should report, and when patient should be seen for follow-up
Problem list	Include discharge diagnosis, any pre-existing conditions or chronic problems, as well as any new problems patient developed while in hospital; indicate if active problem or resolved

The discharge diagnosis should be the primary reason for hospitalization; secondary diagnoses will be listed as well. For Mr. Jensen, elective right hemicolectomy is the discharge diagnosis, with secondary diagnoses of adenocarcinoma of the colon, hypertension, and dyslipidemia.

The attending (or admitting) physician is the provider primarily responsible for the patient during the entire hospitalization. For a surgical admission, this is almost always the surgeon. For a medical admission, this may be the PCP or a hospitalist. When hospitalists manage the patient, a copy of the discharge summary should always be sent to the PCP to keep with the patient's records. This helps provide continuity of care and documents important details of the hospitalization that could affect management of the patient after hospitalization. Any consulting physicians involved in the care of the patient should be listed and should receive a copy of the discharge summary. It is helpful to include the name of consulting physicians and also their specialty. This is particularly helpful when a patient has had a complicated hospital course and was seen by multiple specialists. This helps provide continuity of care and ensures that the PCP has a record of the specialists who have already seen the patient in case consultation is needed in the future.

Any surgical procedures the patient had during the hospitalization should be listed. Some diagnostic or therapeutic procedures should be listed as well, such as a coronary arteriogram, a bronchoscopy, or wound débridement. Minor procedures, such as insertion or removal of a drain, are rarely included here.

The brief history, pertinent physical examination findings, and laboratory data are in the admission history and physical examination (H&P). Do not repeat everything already documented in these sections; instead, highlight any pertinent findings that relate to the reason for the current hospitalization. The goal is to summarize the information already in the medical record. For the history, include enough information to indicate why hospitalization was necessary. In the case of Mr. Jensen, it is appropriate to mention his initial presentation of fatigue, the finding of blood in the stool, and the subsequent diagnosis of adenocarcinoma. Pertinent findings from the past medical history, current medications, and allergies are customarily included in this section of the discharge summary. There were no significant findings from Mr. Jensen's physical examination; thus, it is permissible to state, "The physical exam findings were unremarkable." Pertinent baseline laboratory data should be summarized. For a surgical admission, the preoperative H&H is usually included (even if normal) as well as any abnormal findings from chemistry

studies, such as the carcinoembryonic antigen (CEA) of 17 for Mr. Jensen. His dyslipidemia is a chronic problem, so you could document the total cholesterol and triglyceride values; however, because this chronic condition was not likely to have had an effect on this hospitalization, it is not necessary to include these values. Any abnormality that needed correction before surgery or that would significantly affect the patient's overall hospitalization would be documented in the discharge summary.

Hospital Course

The hospital course is the most important part of the discharge summary. It can also be the most difficult part to document. Up to this point, the information in the discharge summary has been taken directly from other sections of the medical record. The hospital course narrative is a summary of information that is already recorded in daily progress notes, consultants' notes, or procedure notes, but the challenge is learning what to include and what can be omitted. It takes practice in the art and science of medicine and documentation to develop a concise and informative hospital course narrative without being too verbose or leaving out important details. Think of this section as the story of the course of events of the hospitalization. Summarize the daily progress of the patient and the patient's response to treatment as documented in the daily progress notes. A great deal of detail usually is not needed, but include enough information to avoid ambiguity or an incomplete record of the patient's hospital stay. Some providers summarize the events of each hospital day; this format works well when the stay is brief and the patient's recovery is uneventful. This approach is not recommended if the hospitalization is longer than 5 days or if the patient has multiple problems. In those instances, the narrative is sometimes constructed to summarize the details of each problem and the patient's response to treatment for each problem. Some hospitals may require the use of a specified format.

Application Exercise 9.1

Read the hospital course narrative for Mr. Jensen that is provided in Example 9.1.

EXAMPLE 9.1

Mr. Jensen underwent an elective hemicolectomy without complications. Routine postoperative care was initiated. On POD 1, his maximum temperature was 99.1°F; maximum heart rate was 98, and blood pressure range was 102/70 to 136/86. He had adequate pain relief with PCA morphine administration and required only one bolus dose. Mr. Jensen did not have any specific complaints. On exam, no bowel sounds were heard, so he was kept NPO with IV fluids. The wound edges were dry and intact without any warmth to touch or redness. On POD 2, Mr. Jensen's diet was advanced to clear liquids, which he tolerated well. The catheter was removed, and he was able to void without difficulty. He was able to ambulate with assistance and did not have significant pain. Mr. Jensen had elevated blood pressure readings with systolic consistently above 130 and diastolic consistently above 90, so his antihypertensive medication was restarted. He was also started back on Mevacor. His physical exam was unchanged. On POD 3, the diet was advanced to full liquids. The PCA morphine was discontinued, and he was started on oral oxycodone. On POD 4, Mr. Jensen's vital signs were all stable, the wound was healing as expected, and he was tolerating a regular diet. He was able to ambulate without assistance and felt to be ready for discharge.

Based on the example, answer the following questions: When did bowel sounds return? Did Mr. Jensen have effective pain relief from the oral analgesic? Did Mr. Jensen experience any postoperative complications?

Application Exercise 9.1 Answer

We could assume that bowel sounds returned on POD 2 because the diet was advanced from NPO to clear liquids, but this information is not specifically mentioned. There is no documentation of how Mr. Jensen tolerated the oral analgesic, nor is there any specific information about postoperative complications. You might guess that, because none is mentioned, none occurred, but it is always best to provide enough information so that others reading the discharge summary do not have to guess or make assumptions.

The discharge summary should also include a specific assessment of the patient's condition that should indicate why the patient is ready for discharge. Avoid one-word descriptions such as "stable" or "improved." In the case of Mr. Jensen, you could state, "Mr. Jensen is tolerating a regular diet, has adequate pain relief from oral analgesics, and is able to ambulate without assistance and to perform activities of daily living. His postoperative recovery is progressing as expected without complications."

The disposition indicates where the patient goes when leaving the hospital. If the patient is being transferred to another facility, the reason for transfer should be documented. The discharge medications, instructions, and follow-up were discussed in the previous section on writing discharge orders. List the medications, and document any specific instructions in this part of the discharge summary.

Some facilities require that a discharge summary include a list of all the patient's medical problems. This information is particularly helpful to other providers who will be caring for the patient in the future, especially if the patient was managed by a specialist or hospitalist and will receive primary care from a different provider. The problem list includes the discharge diagnosis, any preexisting diagnoses or chronic problems, and any complications or new problems that the patient had during hospitalization. It is also helpful to indicate whether the problem is an ongoing problem or if it has been resolved. The problem list for Mr. Jensen looks like this:

1. Hemicolectomy
2. Adenocarcinoma of the colon
3. Hypertension
4. Dyslipidemia

A discharge summary for Mr. Jensen is shown in Figure 9-1. After reading it, try to answer these questions: When did bowel sounds return? Did Mr. Jensen have effective pain relief from the oral analgesic? Did he experience any postoperative complications? What medications is Mr. Jensen to take at home? When is Mr. Jensen to see Dr. Sanders? A well-written discharge summary will answer most questions a reader might have about the events of the hospitalization.

Patient Leaving Before Discharge

Two events requiring careful documentation are patients leaving the hospital against medical advice (AMA) and elopement. If a patient is advised to remain in the hospital and he or she still chooses to leave, the patient is said to be leaving AMA. The percentage of patients who left the hospital against medical advice increased significantly between 1997 and 2007, according to a brief from the Agency for Healthcare Research and Quality (Statistical Brief # 78, 2009). In 2007, hospitalizations that ended in patients leaving AMA accounted for 368,000 hospital stays (1.2% of the total) compared with only 264,000 discharges in 1997, a 39% increase. Certain characteristics also distinguished the patients leaving AMA. Patients were more likely to be young (average age 46 years) and male. Overall, women are slightly more likely to be hospitalized, but men left AMA 60% more often than women. Three of the five most common diagnoses for patients who left AMA were related to mental health and substance abuse. Nonspecific chest pain and diabetes with complications were the other two top diagnoses.

Discharge Summary for Mr. Jensen

PATIENT: William R. Jensen   MR#: 35-87-26

ADMITTING PHYSICIAN: David K. Sanders, MD

Date of Admission: XX/XX/XXXX   Date of Discharge: XX/XX/XXXX

Admitting Diagnosis:
    1. Adenocarcinoma of right colon
    2. HTN
    3. Dyslipidemia

Discharge Diagnoses:
    1. Right hemicolectomy
    2. Adenocarcinoma of the colon
    3. HTN well controlled
    4. Dyslipidemia, fairly well controlled

PRIMARY CARE PHYSICIAN: Vernon Scott, MD

BRIEF HISTORY OF PRESENT ILLNESS: Mr. Jensen is a 67-year-old Caucasian male who was referred to me after being diagnosed with colon cancer. The patient underwent a diagnostic colonoscopy with biopsies, and pathology report indicated adenocarcinoma. After discussing with Mr. Jensen and his wife the types of treatment available, they both agreed to an elective right hemicolectomy.

PMH: Medical hx includes HTN and dyslipidemia. Surgical history includes repair of right rotator cuff 24 years ago, and left inguinal herniorrhaphy 15 years ago. Current medications include Lotension HCT 20/12.5 once daily and Mevacor 20 mg daily. He also takes a multivitamin daily and fish oil supplements twice daily. Patient is allergic to PENICILLIN, which causes a rash.

PHYSICAL EXAMINATION:
    GENERAL: BP 142/80, P 86 and regular, Temp 97.8 orally. Current weight 174 pounds. WDWN male, A & O x 3.

    HEENT: Unremarkable.

    NECK: Supple, full ROM.

    RESP: Breath sounds without wheezing or crackles. Respiratory excursion symmetrical.

    CV: Heart RRR without murmurs, gallops, or rubs. No JVD or peripheral edema. Distal pulses intact.

    ABD: Soft, nontender. No masses or organomegaly. Bowel sounds physiologic in all four quadrants. No guarding or rebound noted.

    RECTAL/GU: Prostate nontender, not enlarged. Stool guaiac positive. External genitalia exam reveals a circumcised male, both testes descended. No testicular or scrotal masses.

LABORATORY:
    CBC: WBC 5800; Hct 48; Hgb 16. Peripheral smear shows normochromic, normocytic cells, differential WNL. Chemistry panel shows triglycerides of 178; LDL of 208; total cholesterol of 267; CEA of 17; otherwise WNL. Chest x-ray: borderline cardiomegaly, no consolidations of effusions.

    UA: Negative

    PT, PTT: 12.4 and 31.

    ECG: Normal sinus rhythm with rate of 84. No ectopy, no ischemic changes

HOSPITAL COURSE: Elective right hemicolectomy was performed XX/XX/XXXX without complications. Intraoperative findings were consistent with adenocarcinoma with no evidence of metastatic disease. IV of D_5 ½ NS and PCA with morphine for postoperative pain management. On POD #1, patient did not voice any complaints. Blood pressure was 138/88, heart rate 92 max, respirations 20 and shallow. Max temp of 99.1. On exam, good breath sounds in all lung fields, no wheezing or crackles. Heart RRR. Abd soft and nondistended. Incision dry and intact without erythema or drainage. No calf tenderness or swelling. Orders to discontinue catheter. On POD #2, patient remained afebrile, max temp of 98.8, all other vital signs stable, breath sounds clear, heart RRR. Faint bowel sounds were heard throughout. Wound healing well without signs of infection. IV analgesics discontinued, changed to oral Percocet. Restart prehospital meds. Diet advanced to clear liquids. On POD #3, patient reported good pain relief with PO meds and tolerating prehospital meds without difficulty. No nausea or vomiting with liquid diet. Full liquid diet was tolerated well. Patient reports having bowel movement (BM) this morning. Remained afebrile and all vital signs stable. No complaints. Lung and heart exam unchanged. No abdominal tenderness. Wound edges dry without erythema. Patient returned to regular diet. By POD #4, patient still afebrile, VS were WNL, wound healing without complications or signs of infection, tolerating regular diet and meds without difficulty. Patient ready for discharge.

(Continued)

DISCHARGE INSTRUCTIONS: Patient will follow up with Dr. Sanders in one week for suture removal and will follow up with Dr. Scott in 3 weeks for routine care. Continue wound care as instructed. He may shower and get the wound wet, but should not take tub baths or swim. He should be on a low-fat, low-cholesterol diet. Activity level limited to no lifting over 10 pounds, no pulling or straining, until appointment with Dr. Sanders. Patient to notify Dr. Sanders if he develops temp >100.5°F, SOB, swelling in legs, leg pain, or severe abdominal pain, cramping, or rectal bleeding.

MEDICATIONS: Patient will continue Mevacor and Lotensin HCT. Given prescription for Percocet 5 mg, 1–2 po every 4–6 hrs PRN pain. Mr. Jensen was advised not to drive, drink alcohol, or operate any machinery while taking the Percocet. He should also drink lots of water to help avoid constipation, and may take Colace 100 mg (OTC) if needed.

Figure 9-1 Discharge summary for Mr. Jensen.

Patients leave AMA for a variety of reasons. When asked, they most commonly cite family problems or emergencies; personal or financial obligations; feeling bored, fed up, or well enough to leave; or dissatisfaction with their treatment. Although many patients who leave AMA have substance abuse problems, few of them attribute their decision to leave to their addiction. It seems likely that leaving AMA puts patients at increased risk for adverse health outcomes. This concern is supported by several studies that found that patients who leave AMA have significantly higher readmission rates than other patients. Hwang and colleagues (2003) conducted a study of general medical patients who left AMA and found that the readmission rate within the first 15 days after discharge was 21%, compared with 3% in matched controls. The rate of readmission over the subsequent 75-day period was similar in the two groups. No specific factors were found to strongly predict readmission among patients leaving AMA.

When a patient states a desire to leave the hospital before being ready for discharge, the attending physician should be notified immediately. Fully competent patients are legally able to discharge themselves without completing treatment. The attending physician should ascertain that the patient is competent and should discuss with the patient the benefits of continued hospitalization and treatment and the risks associated with leaving and not completing treatment. In most hospitals, this conversation is documented in the medical record, and the patient is asked to sign a form indicating that he or she is aware of the risks and is leaving against medical advice. An example of such a form is shown in Figure 9-2.

Name and relationship to the patient (if applicable) of any witnesses to the conversation should be included in the documentation. Direct quotes of the patient's statements should be used to explain why the patient wants to leave. Do not document your own interpretation of why the patient is leaving or include any judgmental or derogatory remarks about the patient. Every effort should be made to arrange follow-up care for the patient. Document

the discharge instructions and follow-up care just as you would for any other patient.

EXAMPLE 9.2

Below is an example of an AMA note for Mr. Sanford, a 43-year-old man who was admitted because of chest pain.

xx/xx/xxxx, 1548. I was informed by Karen Macayo, RN, nurse manager of telemetry 5B unit, that Mr. Sanford has decided to leave the hospital against medical advice. He states, "I am a single father and I just cannot stay here and leave my kids alone. My sister was taking care of them, but she has to leave." The patient is competent and understands the risks of leaving, including serious cardiac disease, permanent disability, and sudden cardiac death. Mr. Sanford had an opportunity to ask questions about his condition, and I answered them to the best of my ability. He has been informed that he may return for care at any time. Follow-up has been arranged with his PCP in 2 days.
Signature of attending physician

Patient elopement occurs when a patient leaves the hospital without being discharged. Eloping patients are often at risk for serious harm, and there are many cases in which patient elopement has resulted in death. Patients rarely tell the nursing or medical staff they want to leave; they just leave. There is no chance to discuss with the patient the risks of leaving and benefits of remaining in the hospital for treatment. Elopement is different than *wandering*, which refers to when a patient strays beyond the view or control of staff without the intent of leaving (often because of cognitive impairment).

If a patient elopes, document the date and time you were informed of the elopement and who notified you. The documentation should contain only facts and not speculation on why the patient eloped. A discharge summary is still required. In the disposition part of the discharge summary, state that the

---

Release Against Medical Advice   **Memorial Hospital**

Patient Name _____

Medical Record Number: _____

Date _____ Time _____ ☐ AM ☐ PM

I understand that I am leaving the above facility against medical advice. I have been informed of the risks associated with leaving the facility and, knowing these risks, I wish to leave this facility. I assume full responsibility for my own care and welfare.

By signing this form, I release the attending physician, the facility, and its personnel from all liability for any adverse effects, which may result from my leaving against medical advice.

Patient Signature: _____

If the patient is unable to consent by reason of age or some other factor, state the reasons _____

_____

Signature of legally authorized representative _____

Witness _____

Relation to Patient: _____

Attending Physician signature: _____

Figure 9-2 Sample AMA form.

patient eloped. An elopement prevents the patient from receiving specific discharge instructions and follow-up care information, and it is customary to document that you were unable to provide this information to the patient.

EXAMPLE 9.3

Suppose that Mr. Sanford, the patient mentioned in Example 9.2, had eloped rather than telling the staff that he was leaving AMA. A sample elopement note for Mr. Sanford is shown below.

xx/xx/xxxx, 1548. I received a call from Karen Macayo, head nurse of telemetry 5B unit, regarding Mr. Sanford. The nurse who was assigned to care for him on the 3–11 shift was making rounds when she first came on duty and noticed Mr. Sanford was not in his room. His IV had been disconnected, and the tubing was lying on the bed. The IV catheter was still attached, and a small pool of blood was noted on the bedding. The oxygen tubing was found on the bedside table. A hospital gown was found on the bed. The nurse checked the imaging schedule to be sure the patient was not in that department; no imaging studies had been ordered for Mr. Sanford, and a call to the department confirmed that he was not there. Nursing staff stated that Mr. Sanford had not indicated to them that he was planning to leave. Several overhead pages asking Mr. Sanford to return to his room were made without success. Security was notified, and they checked the hospital grounds. Mr. Sanford was not found and is presumed to have eloped.

Signature of attending physician

To reinforce the content of this chapter, please complete the worksheets that follow.

Discharge Orders and Discharge Summary

1. List three components of the discharge orders.

_____

_____

_____

2. List three components that should be addressed when instructing a patient on activity at the time of a hospital discharge.

_____

_____

_____

3. List at least seven components of a discharge summary.

_____

_____

_____

_____

_____

_____

_____

_____

4. List at least three entities that may ask for (or are likely to receive a copy of) the discharge summary.

_____

_____

_____

_____

5. List at least three diagnoses for patients who are most likely to leave a hospital AMA.

_____

_____

_____

_____

6. List at least three elements that should be included in an AMA note.

_____

_____

_____

Discharge Summary for Ronald Hearst

Refer to Figure 9-3 and read the discharge summary for Mr. Ronald Hearst, an 84-year-old man who is being transferred to a psychiatric facility upon discharge from the hospital.

Discharge Summary—Ronald Hearst

PATIENT: Hearst, Ronald W.   MR#: 427-08-733

SEX: Male   DOB: 05/17/XXXX

DATE OF ADMISSION: 03/22/XXXX

DATE OF DISCHARGE: 04/01/XXXX

DISCHARGE DIAGNOSES
    1. Chest pain. No myocardial infarction.
    2. Right hip fracture due to fall in hospital, status post open reduction and internal fixation.
    3. Right fifth metacarpal fracture.
    4. Coronary artery disease with prior stents.
    5. Paroxysmal atrial fibrillation.
    6. Diabetes mellitus, type 2.
    7. Acute renal failure, resolved.
    8. Mild abnormality of liver enzymes, history of chronic hepatitis B.
    9. Malnutrition.
    10. Urinary tract infection, treated.
    11. Encephalopathy with acute illness postoperative delirium in addition to dementia.

ATTENDING PHYSICIAN:
    Reginald Dykstra, MD

Consulting Physicians:
    Connor Everett, DO; Cardiology
    Burton Samuelson, MD; Neurology
    Wayne Billingsly, MD; Orthopedics
    Edward Dobrison, MD; Psychiatry

    For details of the presenting history and physical examination, please refer to the H&P in the chart.

Hospital Course:
    In brief, the patient is an 84-year-old man. He was initially admitted from the emergency room with complaint of chest pain. He had a history of coronary artery disease and prior stents. An MI was ruled out with serial enzymes. He did have some paroxysmal atrial fibrillation, then stayed in sinus rhythm. He was seen during the hospitalization by Dr. Everett from Cardiology. The first night of admission, the patient got up unassisted owing to confusion, fell, and had a fracture of the right hip. He was treated by Dr. Billingsly for orthopedic surgery. He also had some acute renal failure when he came in the hospital probably due to dehydration; this returned to normal. The patient underwent ORIF of the hip. He had no further chest pains. His diabetes was monitored and covered. He was seen by Dr. Samuelson for Neurology and Dr. Dobrison for Psychiatry. He was quite agitated and assaultive at times. They were managing him with medications and recommended an inpatient psychiatry unit. The patient will be transferred to an inpatient pyschiatric facility when a bed is available. His condition is improved and stable at time of transfer. Prognosis is fair.

Medicatons:
    Risperidone 1 mg three times a day; Levaquin 250 mg daily; Lactulose twice daily; thiamine 100 mg a day; nitroglycerin ointment 2%, 1 inch every 6 hours; metoprolol 50 mg orally twice a day; enoxaprin 80 mg subcutaneous daily; and multivitamin once a day. He is on sliding scale insulin. He will be up as directed by physical therapy. He will be on his heart healthy diabetic diet.

Figure 9-3 Discharge summary—Ronald Hearst.

Based on the discharge summary, answer the questions that follow.

1. How long was Mr. Hearst in the hospital?

_____

2. Which discharge diagnoses listed are not addressed in the narrative of the hospital course? (list)

_____

_____

_____

3. Mr. Hearst will be transferred to a psychiatric facility. If you were a provider at the receiving facility, what criticisms would you have of this discharge summary?

_____

_____

_____

_____

_____

_____

4. What findings support that Mr. Hearst is ready for discharge from the hospital?

_____

_____

5. Refer to Figure 9-1, Discharge Summary for Mr. Jensen. Identify at least three elements included in that discharge summary that are not included in Mr. Hearst's discharge summary.

_____

_____

_____

_____

Discharge Summary for Henry Oliver

Refer to Figure 9-4 and read the discharge summary for Mr. Henry Oliver, a 53-year-old man who was hospitalized for orthopedic surgery. Based on the discharge summary, answer the questions that follow.

Discharge Summary for Henry Oliver

PATIENT: Oliver, Henry P.   MR#: 441-07-638

SEX: Male   DOB: 10/25/XXXX

DATE OF ADMISSION: 07/14/XXXX

DATE OF DISCHARGE: 07/18/XXXX

ADMITTING DIAGNOSIS: Quadriceps tendon rupture of the right knee status post prior total knee arthroplasty.

DISCHARGE DIAGNOSIS: Quadriceps tendon rupture of the right knee status post prior total knee arthroplasty.

ATTENDING PHYSICIAN: Richard Lyons, MD

PRIMARY CARE PHYSICAN: Melinda Knowles, DO

HOSPITAL COURSE: The patient was admitted on 07/14/XXXX after he was noted to have an extensor mechanism rupture. He presented to the emergency department initially. Internal Medicine was consulted for medical optimization and clearance. On 07/15/XXXX, he was taken to the operating room, where he underwent a quadricepsplasty of the right leg for apparent augmentation of the quadriceps rupture with allograft augmentation, a lateral release, and an anterior synovectomy. The patient tolerated the procedure well. He was placed in a long-leg bulky Robert Jones dressing. He was admitted to the orthopedic unit and was allowed weight-bearing as tolerated in the splint. He had daily physical therapy. Intraoperative cultures were obtained. Initial Gram stain was negative. Final cultures were negative at 72 hours. On postoperative day #2, the patient's hemoglobin dropped to 9.0, and he was transfused with 2 units packed red blood cells. He was noted to have decreased magnesium and potassium, which were replaced. On postoperative day #3, the patient was able to ambulate 200 feet with physical therapy and was stable for discharge home.

CONDITION ON DISCHARGE: Stable

DIET: Regular

DISCHARGE MEDICATIONS:
1. Colace 100 mg bid
2. Ferrous sulfate 325 mg bid
3. Aspirin 325 mg bid
4. Multivitamin daily
5. Tramadol 50 mg every 6 hours

DISCHARGE INSTRUCTIONS: The patient is discharged home. He will be weight-bearing as tolerated in the splint. He will present next week to be placed in a long-leg cast. He will remain on aspirin therapy for 6 weeks for DVT prophylaxis. All questions were answered and discussed, and the patient is agreeable.

Figure 9-4 Discharge summary—Henry Oliver.

1. What complications developed postoperatively that are not listed as discharge diagnoses?

_____

2. If you were Dr. Knowles, the patient's primary care provider, what information would you like to know that is not included in this discharge summary?

_____

_____

_____

_____

_____

_____

3. What type of culture was obtained and what is the significance of the results reported in the discharge summary?

_____

_____

4. What findings support that Mr. Oliver is ready for discharge from the hospital?

_____

_____

5. What specific information is missing from the discharge instruction section of the summary?

_____

_____

_____

_____

Discharge Summary for Mrs. Gladys McLaughlin

Refer to Figure 7-10 and read the admission H&P for Mrs. McLaughlin. Read the daily progress notes that follow and use the information to write a discharge summary.

HOSPITAL DAY #1, 0920

S: Mrs. McLaughlin states she did not sleep well last night. She attributes this to noise from the hallway. She specifically denies having any chest pain or pressure. She did ambulate 2 or 3 times yesterday with minimal dizziness. She denies any dizziness at the present time. She has not experienced any shortness of breath. She does not have any new complaints.

O: A&O × 3. VS: BP 116/68, P 103, R 16. Neck: no JVD. Heart: rhythm still irregular. 2/6 systolic murmur; unchanged. Lungs: clear to auscultation all fields. Ext: no peripheral edema. IV Cardizem infusing. Serial troponin levels have remained WNL. Serial ECGs show persistence of atrial fibrillation but no ischemic patterns. She received the Lantus dose this morning, 22 units. She has been on sliding-scale insulin also. Max blood glucose of 402 last evening, and she was covered with 10 units of regular insulin. Accu-Chek this morning was 385, and she received 8 units regular insulin. Cardiology consult appreciated; note reviewed and agree with starting patient on metoprolol. Wait another 24 hours to see if patient's rhythm will be restored to NSR.

A: (1) Atrial fibrillation. (2) Chest pain resolved; MI ruled out. (3) Hypertension. (4) uncontrolled diabetes. (5) UTI.

P: Will continue IV Cardizem. Start metoprolol 50 mg PO bid. Will wait on starting back on lisinopril because the beta-blocker will be started. Continue sliding-scale insulin. Consider endocrinology consult if not within acceptable range in another 24 hours. Add Cipro 500 mg PO bid for 7 days.

HOSPITAL DAY #2, 0745

S: Doing well. States no dizziness in the past 24 hours. Specifically denies chest pain.

O: A&O × 3. VS: BP 132/84, P 92, R 18. No JVD. Heart rate slower today and now regular. Remainder of physical exam unchanged. ECG shows NSR with rate of 94. BP up over the past 24 hours at all readings. Blood glucose range of 240–380 over past 24 hours. Still receiving sliding-scale insulin per routine doses. Urine culture was positive for >100,000 colonies E. coli.

A: (1) Atrial fibrillation resolved, now with NSR. (2) Hypertension with persistently elevated readings over past 24 hours. (3) Uncontrolled diabetes. (4) UTI with positive cultures.

P: Discontinue IV Cardizem. Restart lisinopril 5 mg PO daily. Continue with sliding-scale insulin per routine orders. Continue Cipro and all other regular medications.

HOSPITAL DAY #3, 0820

S: Patient says she did not sleep well again last night. Specifically denies any chest pain or pressure or SOB. Attributes not sleeping well to being away from home and in a different environment. She is ambulating with assistance. No further dizziness or lightheadedness. Appetite is improving.

O: A&O × 3. BP 126/84, P 88, R 16. Heart rate regular. Breath sounds clear. No change in exam. Telemetry strips reviewed; patient with mostly sinus rhythm over the past 24 hours. She did have a few runs of atrial fib but remained asymptomatic. Blood glucose range 160–230. She is requiring less sliding-scale insulin coverage. Continues on Cipro for UTI.

A: (1) Atrial fibrillation mostly resolved; doing well on metoprolol. (2) Hypertension; stable. (3) Type 2 diabetes; glucose control improving but not yet at goal. (4) UTI; currently being treated.

P: Continue present management. Social services to consult for discharge planning.

HOSPITAL DAY #4, 0750

S: Patient without any complaints. Has not had any further episodes of dizziness or lightheadedness. Denies SOB. Ambulating without difficulty. Nurse reports that patient slept through the night.

O: A&O × 3. BP 134/80, P 90, R 16. Heart RRR, systolic murmur 2/6. Lungs clear all fields. No peripheral edema. All recorded blood pressures in acceptable range of <130 systolic and <80 diastolic. Blood glucose range 140s to 180s. Has only required 2 interval doses of insulin in the past 24 hours. Social services note seen; patient has daughter who can stay with her for a few days.

A: (1) Atrial fib; converted and maintaining NSR on metoprolol. (2) Hypertension; stable. (3) Type 2 diabetes; better control now that UTI is resolving.

P: Continue metoprolol and present management. If glucose stays within normal range without sliding scale coverage, anticipate discharge tomorrow.

HOSPITAL DAY #5, 0900

S: Patient denies any chest pain or pressure, dizziness, or SOB. Feels like she is ready to go home.

O: A&O × 3. All vital signs have been within normal range for the past 24 hours. Blood glucose max was 144. Patient did not require any sliding-scale doses in past 24 hours. Heart RRR, 2/6 systolic murmur. Lungs clear. Abdomen soft with bowel sounds throughout. No CVA tenderness. No peripheral edema.

A: (1) Atrial fib, controlled on metoprolol. (2) MI ruled out; no further chest pain. (3) Hypertension, stable on lisinopril. (4) Type 2 diabetes, stable on regular dose of Lantus. (5) Resolving UTI.

P: Patient asymptomatic now. Ambulating without difficulty. No recurrence of chest pain or dizziness. Stable for discharge to home. Will continue her on metoprolol 50 mg PO bid. Continue Cipro 500 mg PO bid for 2 more days. Continue Lantus 22 units daily in a.m. Continue all other regular home medications. Patient should not drive for 2 weeks, until she has had time to adjust to all medications. Otherwise, activity as tolerated. Continue on 1800-calorie ADA, heart-healthy diet. Notify Dr. Rosenberg immediately if any episodes of chest pain or pressure, dizziness, or any new symptoms. Otherwise, follow up with Dr. Rosenberg in 1 week. Follow up with cardiologist in 2 weeks. Discharge instructions discussed with patient and daughter. All questions answered. Patient is agreeable to discharge.

Discharge Orders for Mrs. Gladys McLaughlin

Read the daily progress notes for Mrs. McLaughlin shown in Worksheet 9.4. Write corresponding discharge orders based on the information provided.

Abbreviations

These abbreviations were introduced in Chapter 9. Beside each, write the meaning as indicated by the context of the chapter.

AMA _____

BM _____

MI _____

ORIF _____

RN _____

Chapter 10

Prescription Writing and Electronic Prescribing

OBJECTIVES

- Discuss the role of the Drug Enforcement Agency (DEA) in regulating controlled substances.
- Discuss federal and state laws that govern prescribing authority.
- Identify safeguards for prescribers to protect their DEA number and prevent prescription tampering and fraud.
- Define controlled and noncontrolled substances.
- Identify required elements of a prescription.
- Identify dangerous abbreviations that should be avoided.
- Identify common prescription-writing errors.
- Define electronic prescribing (e-prescribing).
- Discuss key federal initiatives that have been part of the impetus for e-prescribing.
- Identify the criteria for qualified e-prescribing.
- Discuss benefits of and barriers to e-prescribing.

According to the National Ambulatory Medical Care Survey, 963.6 million visits were made to office-based health-care providers during 2005. In more than two thirds of these visits, there was "mention of medications," which is defined as medications provided, prescribed, or continued. At 40% of all visits, two or more drugs were recorded. According to the IMS Health Report, 3.9 billion prescriptions were dispensed in the United States in 2009, reflecting a 5.1% increase over 2008. It has been estimated that another 1 billion prescriptions are written each year that are never filled.

The medication use process is particularly susceptible to errors because of the large number of drugs available, a lack of precisely defined best practices, and confusion between drug names, dosage forms, routes of administration, doses, and units of dose measurement. The number of look-alike and sound-alike drug names is a matter of such concern that the Food and Drug Administration (FDA) has instituted a program to better distinguish between them. Additionally, the FDA approves one or two new drugs each week and makes a dozen or so changes in indications for current medications already approved. Physicians, nurse practitioners, and physician assistants cannot possibly keep up with all the relevant information available on all the medications they might prescribe. When you factor in the current practice of handwriting prescriptions by most prescribers and the number of steps between writing a prescription and dispensing a medication, it is easy to see how errors can occur.

Between 1.5% and 4% of prescriptions written are found to contain errors that could result in serious patient risk. These errors are most often a result of illegible handwriting, incoherent abbreviations and dose designations, unclear telephone or verbal orders, or ambiguous orders and fax-related problems. According to one study that looked at the use of Computerized Physician Order Entry (CPOE) in ambulatory settings (Johnston et al., 2004), adverse drug events (ADEs) were identified in 5% to 18% of

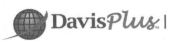 **DavisPlus** | Visit **http://davisplus.fadavis.com** for complete learning activities on actual EMR software at, Keyword: Sullivan

prescriptions written for ambulatory patients. The use of electronic prescribing, or e-prescribing, has been touted as an important practice that will help eliminate nearly 2.1 million ADEs per year in the ambulatory patient population. E-prescribing will be discussed in detail later in this chapter. However, before looking at e-prescribing, it is necessary to understand basic concepts related to prescribing, such as the role of the Drug Enforcement Agency (DEA), state and federal laws that govern prescribing authority, and controlled versus noncontrolled substances. Likewise, a prescriber has to understand the elements that are required in a prescription, regardless of the means by which the prescription is generated.

Federal and State Regulations and Prescribing Authority

The DEA was established in 1973 to serve as the primary federal agency responsible for the enforcement of the Controlled Substances Act (CSA). The CSA sets forth the federal law regarding both illicit and licit (pharmaceutical) controlled substances. With respect to pharmaceutical controlled substances, the DEA's statutory responsibility is twofold: to prevent diversion and abuse of these drugs while ensuring an adequate and uninterrupted supply is available to meet the country's legitimate medical, scientific, and research needs. In carrying out this mission, the DEA works in close cooperation with state and local authorities and other federal agencies.

Under the framework of the CSA, the DEA is responsible for ensuring that all controlled substance transactions take place within the "closed system" of distribution established by Congress. Under this "closed system," all legitimate handlers of controlled substances—manufacturers, distributors, practitioners, pharmacies, and researchers—must be registered with the DEA and maintain strict accounting for all distributions. Under the CSA, the term "practitioner" is defined as a physician, dentist, veterinarian, scientific investigator, pharmacy, hospital, or other person licensed, registered, or otherwise permitted, by the United States or the jurisdiction in which the practitioner practices or performs research, to distribute, dispense, conduct research with respect to, administer, or use in teaching or chemical analysis a controlled substance in the course of professional practice or research.

Every person or entity that handles controlled substances must be registered with the DEA or be exempt by regulation from registration. The DEA registration grants practitioners federal authority to handle controlled substances. The registration is used to track practitioners' controlled substances prescribing practices and to control the unauthorized prescribing of controlled substances. Each qualified practitioner is assigned a unique DEA identifier number. A prescription for a controlled substance that does not have an authorized DEA number on it cannot be filled. The DEA provides a practitioners' manual to assist prescribers in understanding their responsibilities under the CSA and to provide guidance in complying with federal regulations. The manual may be found at the DEA's website at www.DEAdiversion.usdoj.gov. Any DEA-registered practitioner may only engage in those activities that are authorized under state law for the jurisdiction in which the practice is located. When federal law or regulations differ from state law or regulations, the practitioner is required to abide by the more stringent aspects of both the federal and state requirements. In many cases, state law is more stringent than federal law, and must be complied with in addition to federal law. If a state requires a separate controlled substance license, it should be obtained first and should be included in the federal application. Practitioners should be certain they understand their state as well as DEA controlled substance regulations. The DEA regulations prohibit a physician from delegating the use of his or her signature and DEA registration to another person. Therefore, if a mid-level provider is delegated the authority to prescribe controlled substances, the provider must also be registered with the DEA. Appendix F and Appendix G provide a summary of physician assistant and nurse practitioner prescribing authority by state, respectively.

On April 1, 2008, all written prescriptions for outpatient drugs prescribed to a Medicaid beneficiary were required to be on paper with at least one tamper-resistant feature as outlined by the Centers for Medicare and Medicaid Services (CMS). CMS outlined three baseline characteristics of tamper-resistant prescription pads, although each state defined which features it would require to meet those characteristics. To be considered tamper resistant, a prescription pad must have at least one of the following three characteristics:

- One or more industry-recognized features designed to prevent unauthorized copying of a completed or blank prescription form
- One or more industry-recognized features designed to prevent the erasure or modification of information written on the prescription by the prescriber
- One or more industry-recognized features designed to prevent the use of counterfeit prescription forms

By October 1, 2008 these same prescriptions had to be on paper that met all three baseline characteristics of tamper-resistant pads.

Safeguards for Prescribers

In enforcing the CSA, it is the DEA's responsibility to ensure drugs are not diverted for illicit purposes. Unfortunately, the United States is now experiencing an alarming prescription drug abuse problem. More than 6 million Americans are abusing prescription drugs—that is more than the number of Americans abusing cocaine, heroin, hallucinogens, and inhalants, combined. Researchers from the Centers for Disease Control and Prevention (CDC) report that opioid prescription painkillers now cause more drug overdose deaths than cocaine and heroin combined. All prescribers have an obligation to protect their DEA number and minimize the risk of prescription forgery and tampering. In addition to the federally required security controls, practitioners can use additional measures to ensure security:

- Keep all prescription blanks in a safe place where they cannot be stolen; minimize the number of prescription pads in use.
- Write out the actual amount prescribed in addition to giving a number to discourage alterations of the prescription order.
- Use prescription blanks only for writing a prescription order and not for notes.
- Never sign prescription blanks in advance.
- Assist the pharmacists when they telephone to verify information about a prescription order; a corresponding responsibility rests with the pharmacist who dispenses the prescription to ensure the accuracy of the prescription.
- Contact the nearest DEA field office to obtain or furnish information regarding suspicious prescription activities.
- Use tamper-resistant prescription pads.
- Do not include your DEA number on preprinted prescription pads. Instead, leave a blank line and write it in only when required for a controlled substance.
- Keep an inventory of the number of prescription pads you have on hand, making it easier to identify whether pads are missing.
- Do not use your DEA number as an identifier. Some pharmacies, suppliers of durable medical equipment, and insurance companies ask for the DEA number as a provider identifier. Some journals use it to obtain access to online articles. Using your DEA number for identification increases the risk of misuse and the possibility of forged prescriptions.
- Do not display your DEA certificate. File it in a locked cabinet.
- Limit the number of people who have access to your DEA number. Instruct office staff to refer all requests for your DEA number directly to you.

Controlled and Noncontrolled Substances

The drugs and other substances that are considered controlled substances under the CSA are divided into five schedules. A complete list of the schedules is updated and published annually in the DEA regulations, Title 21 of the Code of Federal Regulations, Sections 1308.11 through 1308.15. Substances are placed in their respective schedules based on whether they have a currently accepted medical use in treatment in the United States and on their relative abuse potential and likelihood of causing dependence when abused.

All drugs listed in Schedule I have no currently accepted medical use and therefore may not be prescribed, administered, or dispensed for medical use. In contrast, drugs listed in Schedules II through V all have some accepted medical use and therefore may be prescribed, administered, or dispensed. Table 10-1 presents the categories of controlled substances as defined by the CSA, and Appendix D provides examples of the drugs in each schedule.

Elements of a Prescription

Certain elements should be included in every prescription, whether it is for a noncontrolled or a controlled substance. The basic elements include the following:

- Date the prescription was written
- Prescriber identification
- Patient identification

Table 10-1	Drug Enforcement Agency Classification of Controlled Substances*
Schedule	**Comments**
I	High potential for abuse. No accepted medical use.
II	High potential for abuse. Use may lead to severe physical or psychological dependence.
III	Some potential for abuse. Use may lead to low to moderate physical dependence or psychological dependence.
IV	Low potential for abuse. Use may lead to limited physical or psychological dependence.
V	Subject to state and local regulations. Abuse potential is low.

*As in the Controlled Substances Act of 1970. Drugs are categorized according to their potential for abuse: the greater the potential, the more severe the limitations on their prescription.

- The inscription
- The subscription
- Signa
- Indication
- Refill information
- Generic substitution
- Warnings
- Container information
- Prescriber's signature

A summary of these elements is shown in Table 10-2.

Writing Prescriptions for Noncontrolled Medications

Prescriber identification. In many cases, this is preprinted on a standard prescription form. This includes the name and title of the prescriber and the address and telephone number of the practice or institution. When the prescriber is a nonphysician, some states require that the supervising physician's name be printed on the prescription form as well.

Patient identification. This includes the patient's name, address, age or date of birth, and sometimes, weight. It is recommended, and in some states it is required, that you use the patient's legal name instead of a nickname. If you are unsure of the patient's legal name, ask to see a driver's license or an insurance card if available. This helps avoid confusion and correctly identifies the patient. The date of birth is more commonly requested than the patient's age because it allows more specific identification. When a prescription is written for a pediatric patient, you should include the patient's weight so that the pharmacist can verify the medication has been dosed appropriately.

Inscription. This includes name and strength of the medication. Generic or trade names may be used. Avoid abbreviating names of medications to help reduce the possibility of error. There are exceptions for well-known medications; for instance, trimethoprim-sulfamethoxazole is commonly abbreviated TMP/SMX. The strength is the amount per dosing unit, such as a 50 mg tablet or 250 mg per 5 mL. Some medications come in many different strengths and forms (i.e., tablets and liquids). If you are unsure which strengths and forms are available, you should consult a prescribing guide, pharmacology text, or medication reference book. The strength is not the same as the total amount to be taken by the patient over the course of the prescription.

Subscription. This provides information to the pharmacist on dosage form and number of units or doses to dispense. Instructions about the dosage form may be tablets, capsules, or suspension, for example. If a liquid or semiliquid is to be dispensed, provide the quantity, such as how many milliliters of suspension or how many grams in a tube. The amount dispensed should be the amount needed to complete a course of treatment. For example, if a patient is to take a tablet twice a day for 10 days, the subscription, or amount to dispense, would be 20 tablets. You will often see #20 or Disp: 20 tabs; either is acceptable. Many patients use a mail-order pharmacy service provided by their health insurance plan administrator. Such mail-order pharmacies may have specific requirements on

Table 10-2 Summary of Elements of a Prescription	
Item	**Description**
Date of Prescription	
Prescriber's Information	Name and title, office or institution name, address, and phone number; blank line for DEA number
Patient's Information	Legal name, age or date of birth, address, weight if necessary
Inscription	Name of drug and strength
Subscription	Information for pharmacist regarding dosage form and number of doses to dispense
Signa	Instructions to patients including route of administration, how often to take, special instructions, or indication for medication
Refill information	Number of refills or length of time prescription may be filled
Generic substitution	Indicate if a generic form is permissible or if medication is to be dispensed as written
Warnings	What adverse effects may be caused by the medication, such as drowsiness, feeling shaky, etc.
Container information	Use of childproof containers is required unless specifically indicated to use non-childproof container
Provider's signature and title	

how the quantity should be written and refill information, so it is recommended that you ask the patient whether they use a mail-order service before writing the prescription.

Signa or sig. This provides instructions to the patient on how to take the medication and should be as specific as possible. It should include the route; any special instructions, such as to take on an empty stomach or with food; and how often to take. When the medication is prescribed on a prn basis, the reason for taking the medication should be included. Avoid writing vague or ambiguous instructions, such as take as directed or apply in usual manner. Numerous studies have documented that patients usually do not remember all the information they are given during the course of a provider–patient encounter; therefore, it is necessary to provide instructions that are as detailed and accurate as possible to reduce the chance that the medication may be taken inappropriately.

Indication. Including the indication for the prescription is mandatory in some states. Even when states do not require an indication, the ISMP recommends including it for two reasons. First, many drugs have names that look and sound alike. Second, illegible writing may cause confusion or misinterpretation. Including the indication for the prescribed medication provides another safety check for the prescriber, the pharmacist, and the patient.

Refill information. This should be included on the prescription form and can be written as the number of times a prescription may be refilled or a period during which the prescription may be refilled. Most states impose a 1-year maximal refill period. Patients taking medications for chronic conditions should be assessed at least annually, so it is not prudent to write medication refills for more than a 1-year period. If the patient has prescription coverage as a benefit of an insurance plan, it is a good idea to consult the formulary for that insurance company to see whether the medication you want to prescribe is covered and whether there are regulations about how many can be dispensed in a certain period. Many companies will cover only a 1-month supply of medication at a time. It is usually of monetary benefit to the patient to prescribe a medication that is covered by the insurance plan, but that is not the only factor considered when deciding which medication to prescribe.

Dispense as written. Most prescription forms will allow you to indicate whether the medication should be dispensed as written (DAW) or whether substitution of a generic form of the medication is permitted (Fig. 10-1). Generic medications usually offer considerable cost savings to the patient, and with few exceptions, it is preferable to allow substitution.

Warnings. The prescription should specify what, if any, warning labels should be attached to the medication package or vial. In most instances, the pharmacist filling the prescription will automatically affix the appropriate warnings listed in the prescribing information, but the prescriber should include this information on the form. This provides another safety check between the prescriber and the pharmacist. In many states, the law requires that pharmacists dispense medications in child-proof containers. If the patient taking the medication is likely to have difficulty opening such a container (such as a patient with arthritic hands), indicate that a non–child-proof container should be used.

Signature. The provider's signature authenticates the prescription. On a prescription form, the signature should include the name and the title of the prescriber. Signatures can be unique and may identify people, much like fingerprints, but above all they should be legible. Figure 10-2 shows a completed prescription with all the elements labeled.

Although frequently used when writing the instructions, there is controversy about whether abbreviations should be used at all. A list of commonly used abbreviations is shown in Table 10-3. Some providers and pharmacists think that writing out instructions, rather than using abbreviations, reduces the chance of a medication error. The National Coordinating Council for Medication Error Reporting and Prevention has identified several abbreviations that are particularly dangerous because they have been consistently misunderstood. These abbreviations are shown in Table 10-4. The Council recommends that these should never be used in prescription writing. Refer to Appendix D for the Institute for Safe Medication Practices (ISMP) list of Error-Prone Abbreviations, Symbols, and Dose Designations that should be avoided when writing prescriptions.

Writing Prescriptions for Controlled Medications

Two main differences between noncontrolled and controlled medications are the quantity initially

Primary Care and Pediatric Associates

2400 Main St.   Glendale, AZ 85308

Phone: 623-572-3000   Fax: 623-572-3400

David M. Wright, DO   Debbie D. Sullivan, PA-C

DEA # _____   DEA # _____

Name: _____   Age: _____

Address: _____   Date: _____

Refill _____ times   Childproof Container: ☐ yes   ☐ no

_____   _____

Dispense as written   **Substitution Permitted**

Figure 10-1 Prescription form with signature lines.

dispensed and refills. State laws regulate the quantity of controlled medications that can be prescribed during a certain period. When indicating the quantity, write out the number instead of writing it numerically ("ten" instead of "10"), or do both. An example is shown in Figure 10-3. This helps prevent modification of the prescription. State laws also regulate the number of refills, if any, allowed for controlled substances. It is your responsibility as a provider to know these regulations.

MEDICOLEGAL ALERT ! ___ (+) (✳) (⚖)

According to some studies, up to 25% of ambulatory patients experience adverse medication events. Up to 6% of these adverse events could have been reduced or prevented altogether. Many preventable events involve prescribing a medication to which the patient has a known allergy. Before writing any new prescription for a patient, always ask about allergies to any medications, and prescribe accordingly. Sometimes, when asked about medication allergies, patients may describe what sounds like side effects of a medication rather than describing a true allergic reaction. If you have any doubt whether a patient is truly allergic to a medication, always err on the side of caution and do not prescribe it if there is even a remote chance the patient had an allergic reaction in the past. You should always consider what medications the patient is already taking and determine the likelihood of drug interactions. Sometimes, the benefit of prescribing a specific medication may outweigh the possible risk for a drug

Primary Care and Pediatric Associates

2400 Main St.	Glendale, AZ 85308
Phone: 623-572-3000	Fax: 623-572-3400
David M. Wright, DO	Debbie D. Sullivan, PA-C

1

DEA # _____   DEA # _____

2

Name: ___*Jane Smith*_____   Age: ____*24*_____

Address: ___*11527 N. 83rd Ave. Peoria*_____   Date: ____*XX/XX/XXXX*_____

3 ☐

4 ☐

5 ☐

Augmentin 500 mg tablets

Dispense: 20

Sig: Take one by mouth twice daily for 10 days for infection

Refill ___*0*___ times   Childproof Container: ☐ yes   ☒ no

_____   *Debbie Sullivan, PA-C*_____

Dispense as written	**Substitution Permitted**

1. Prescriber's Information
2. Patient's Information
3. Inscription
4. Subscription
5. Signa or Sig

Figure 10-2 Prescription form showing elements.

interaction or side effect; document in such a way that reflects that you are aware of possible side effects or drug interactions but that you believe the medication still to be the most appropriate treatment for the patient's condition.

Common Errors in Prescription Writing

Almost 70% of provider–patient encounters for acute problems result in the writing of one or more prescriptions. Serious errors can occur, both in writing the prescription and in dispensing the medication. Several studies have identified errors commonly made in the process. These studies have shown that as many as one third of all outpatient prescriptions contain errors. Specific errors fall into these general categories:

- *Illegibility* of any part of the prescription
- *Omissions:* leaving off drug name, strength, or quantity to dispense; minor omissions include not putting patient's name, date, directions for use, or prescriber's name

Table 10-3 — Common Abbreviations Used in Prescription Writing

Latin	Abbreviation	Meaning
ante cibum	ac	before meals
bis in die	bid	twice a day
gutta	gtt	drop
hora somni	hs	at bedtime
oculus dexter	od	right eye
oculus sinister	os	left eye
per os	PO	by mouth
post cibum	pc	after meals
pro re nata	prn	as needed
quaque 3 hora	q3h	every 3 hours
quaque die	qd	every day

- *Dose or direction error:* exceeding recommended dose or substantial departure from recommended dose; not including indication for prn medications
- *Legal requirements not met:* not including DEA number on a controlled substance prescription, dispensing quantity above that allowed by state regulation, not spelling out the quantity of a controlled substance, including refills when not allowed by law
- *Unclear quantity prescribed:* quantity does not match directions, specifying non-trade-size topical preparations or liquid antibiotics
- *Incomplete directions:* not identifying route, quantity to be taken at each dose, frequency of dosing
- *Leading and trailing zeros:* not putting a leading zero before a decimal expression of less than 1, including a trailing zero after a decimal

Electronic Prescribing

In Chapter 1, we discussed several factors influencing the implementation of an electronic medical record (EMR) system as a means of delivering safe, high-quality, efficient, and cost-effective health care. Similarly, electronic prescribing, or "e-prescribing," has been targeted as a key factor in preventing medical errors and reducing ADEs. E-prescribing has been defined as the computer-based electronic generation, transmission, and filling of a prescription, taking the place of paper and faxed prescriptions. A more formal definition is provided in the Medicare Part D prescription drug program:

> *E-prescribing means the transmission, using electronic media, of prescription or prescription-related information between a prescriber, dispenser, pharmacy benefit manager, or health plan, either directly or through an intermediary, including an e-prescribing network. E-prescribing includes, but is not limited to, two-way transmissions between the point of care and the dispenser.*

Federal Initiatives for Electronic Prescribing

Since early 2000, many federal and state organizations have called for the adoption of a national electronic-prescribing system. Several key federal regulations include provisions or mandates related to e-prescribing. Passage of the Medicare Modernization Act of 2003 (MMA) resulted in a significant

Table 10-4 — Dangerous Abbreviations to Avoid

Abbreviation	Intended Meaning	Common Error
U	unit	Mistaken for a 0 or a 4, resulting in overdose; also mistaken for cc when poorly written
μg	micrograms	Mistaken for mg, resulting in overdose
Q.D.	Latin abbreviation for *every day*	The period after the Q has sometimes been mistaken for an l, and the drug has been given qid (four times daily) rather than daily
Q.O.D.	Latin abbreviation for *every other day*	Misinterpreted as Q.D. (daily) or Q.I.D. (four times daily); if the O is poorly written, it looks like a period or an l
SC or SQ	subcutaneous	Mistaken as SL (sublingual) when poorly written
TIW	three times a week	Misinterpreted as *three times a day* or *twice a week*
HS	half strength	Misinterpreted as the Latin abbreviation HS (*hour of sleep*)
cc	cubic centimeter	Mistaken as U (unit) when poorly written
AU, AS, AD	Latin abbreviation for *both ears, left ear, right ear*	Misinterpreted as the Latin abbreviation OU (*both eyes*), OS (*left eye*), OD (*right eye*)

Adapted from National Coordinating Council for Medication Error Reporting and Prevention. Council Recommendations to Enhance Accuracy of Prescription Writing. Available at: http://www.nccmerp.org/council/council1996-09-04.html. Retrieved February 8, 2010.

Primary Care and Pediatric Associates

2400 Main St.   Glendale, AZ 85308

Phone: 623-572-3000   Fax: 623-572-3400

David M. Wright, DO   Debbie D. Sullivan, PA-C

DEA # _____   DEA # __MS1234567_____

Name: __Brenda Cartwright_____   Age: __39_____

Address: __4444 W. Dupont St. Phoenix_____   Date: __8/26/XXXX_____

Hydrocodone Tablets 5/500 mg

Disp: 10 (ten)

Sig: Take one tablet by mouth every 4 hrs as needed for pain.

Refill __0__ times   Childproof Container: ☒ yes   ☐ no

_____   *Debbie Sullivan, PAC*

Dispense as written   **Substitution permitted**

Figure 10-3 Controlled substance quantities.

increase in attention and focus on e-prescribing. One component of the MMA was Medicare Part D, which introduced an entitlement benefit for prescription drug coverage for Medicare beneficiaries. Under the Part D program, the MMA mandates that plans accept electronic prescriptions; it authorizes the Department of Health and Human Services to mandate transactive standards; and it provides economic incentives to prescribers for the adoption of e-prescribing. A report released by the Institute of Medicine in July 2006, *Preventing Medication Errors*, received widespread publicity and helped build awareness of e-prescribing's role in enhancing patient safety. In the same year, CMS enacted three foundation standards

that apply to all electronic prescribing done under Part D of the MMA. The foundation standards cover three broad areas: (1) transactions between prescribers and dispensers for new prescriptions, refill requests, prescription changes and/or cancellations, and related messaging and administrative transactions; (2) eligibility and benefits queries and responses between prescribers and Part D sponsors; and (3) eligibility queries between dispensers and Part D sponsors. MMA also required CMS to implement pilot projects to test additional standards related to formulary and benefit information, prior authorization, medication history, and fill status notification. These are all important components of an electronic prescribing system, especially one that could be implemented nationally. In 2007, electronic prescribing became legal in all 50 states. Congress passed the Medicare Improvements for Patients and Providers Act in 2008. The Act provided for a 2% annual bonus for providers who started e-prescribing in 2009. The incentive will decrease to 1% in 2011 and to 0.5% 2 years later (2013), the last year of the bonus. Penalties will apply for those who have not implemented e-prescribing capabilities; 1% in 2012, 1.5% in 2013, and 2% in 2014 and each subsequent year.

Qualified Electronic Prescribing

Similar to the "meaningful use" standard imposed on EMR adopters, criteria have also been developed for "qualified e-prescribing." To qualify, a system must be capable of all of the following:

• Generating a complete active medication list incorporating electronic data received from applicable pharmacy drug plans if available
• Selecting medications, printing prescriptions, electronically transmitting prescriptions, and conducting all safety checks
• Providing information related to the availability of lower-cost, therapeutically appropriate alternatives (if any)
• Providing information on formulary or tiered formulary medications, patient eligibility, and authorization requirements received electronically from the patient's drug plan

Benefits and Barriers to E-Prescribing

Much of the perceived benefits of e-prescribing are related to decreasing medication errors and the incidence of ADEs. It is important to understand not only how e-prescribing affects patient safety but also how it affects prescribers and their office staff, pharmacists, payers, and employers. E-prescribing provides point-of-care access to patient eligibility and formulary coverage, which helps prescribers determine the most clinically appropriate and cost-effective medication for patients. It allows for immediate access to plan formulary requirements such as prior authorization, quantity restrictions, noncovered drugs, and drug tiers. It provides a real-time view of a patient's medication history to all providers; because all providers see the same information, it

alerts prescribers to potential drug–allergy and drug–drug interactions and decreases the chance of different prescribers giving the same medication. Access to a Clinical Decision Support System (CDSS) helps prescribers make informed decisions about which medication is most effective.

E-prescribing brings automation of the entire prescribing process. New prescriptions go directly to the pharmacy's computer, and renewal requests come back to the prescriber's e-prescribing and EMR application for authorization. This creates a closed system that prevents prescription tampering and fraud. It also eliminates handwritten prescriptions and errors related to illegibility and transcribing and data entry. It decreases the amount of time spent on telephone calls from dispensers to prescribers for queries related to illegibility, noncovered drugs, and prior authorization requirements. This allows prescribers to spend more time providing patient care and results in cost savings to pharmacies and payers. E-prescribing may also increase patient compliance because of cost-effectiveness, convenience, and a decrease in the total time it takes from generation of a prescription to dispensing of a medication.

Many of the potential barriers associated with electronic prescribing are the same as those for using an EMR system. Cost can be an issue to both prescribers and pharmacies. The pharmacy's software vendor charges transaction fees, and there may be a one-time start-up fee and monthly charges. A free stand-alone e-prescribing system is available through the National ePrescribing Patient Safety Initiative, so prescribers may not have to purchase a system; however, they may be charged monthly access fees for certain services. Although Medicare offers a financial incentive for those who meet certain criteria, the burden is on the prescriber to bill appropriately to realize these incentives. Billing codes (the G codes) have been introduced that must be used for billing related to e-prescribing. Given the time and expense of training office staff on these billing procedures, they may result in very little net gain for the prescriber, so the incentive may not be worth the trouble.

Several barriers are related specifically to the absence of standards, certification issues, and technology. There is no standard for drug terminology or prior authorization. There is no standard for the signa, or the instructions to patients on how to take the medication. Some systems allow for free-text, whereas others use a drop-down menu, which may actually increase errors in this part of the prescription. Like EMR systems, e-prescribing systems will have to meet certification criteria. At the time of publication of this text, it is unclear whether e-prescribing certification will be separate from EMR certification.

Federal standards for certification have not yet been defined, and certifying organizations have not yet been identified. Although certain e-prescribing vendors award a "certification," it is not clear whether such certification will meet federal requirements. Other barriers identified include software functionality problems, input errors by prescribers, inaccuracies in formulary information, and system incompatibilities that exist between prescriber software and pharmacy dispensing software.

One barrier was the inability to prescribe controlled substances electronically; however, the DEA recently revised a regulation that gave prescribers the option of writing prescriptions for controlled substances electronically. The Electronic Prescriptions for Controlled Substances rule became effective June 1, 2010. These regulations provide the option of writing prescriptions for controlled substances electronically but do not mandate it. They also permit pharmacies to receive, dispense, and archive these electronic prescriptions. Practitioners who wish to prescribe controlled substances using electronic prescriptions must obtain a third-party audit or certification to certify that each electronic prescription and pharmacy application to be used to sign, transmit, or process controlled substances prescriptions is in compliance with DEA regulations pertaining to electronic prescriptions for controlled substances. More information on the ruling may be obtained at the DEA website: http://www.deadiversion.usdoj.gov/ecomm/e_rx/index.html.

Although e-prescribing has decreased some common prescribing errors, it has actually increased other types of errors. Donyai and colleagues (2007) conducted a hospital-based study that looked at e-prescribing and prescribing quality. They reported an increase in errors related to selection of the incorrect product dose or frequency from a drop-down menu and the inappropriate use or selection of default doses. Another type of error specifically related to e-prescribing with CDSS—called *alert fatigue*—has been identified. A study by Isaac and associates (2009) looked at the e-prescribing records of nearly 2900 community physicians and other prescribers over a 9-month period.

About 1 in 15 prescription orders, or 6.6%, produced an alert for a drug interaction or a drug allergy. Most of the 233,537 alerts (98.6%) were for a potential interaction with a drug the patient was already taking. Researchers found that clinicians overrode more than 90% of the drug interaction alerts and 77% of the drug allergy alerts.

E-prescribing has been proposed as an important tool for improving the safety and efficiency of medication use. So far, the promise of e-prescribing has been realized largely in inpatient settings. The bulk of prescribing, however, occurs in outpatient care, and most of these practice settings still use paper-based prescribing. For the potential of e-prescribing to be achieved, it must be adopted in community-based settings. According to the *National Progress Report on E-Prescribing* by SureScripts (2009), there was an increase in the volume of e-prescribing messages, requests for prescription benefit information, and number of prescription histories delivered to prescribers in 2009 compared with 2008. The number of prescriptions routed electronically grew from 68 million in 2008 to 191 million in 2009. Stand-alone e-prescribing software was deployed more than EMR software (57% and 23%, respectively). The number of prescribers routing prescriptions electronically grew from 74,000 at the end of 2008 to more than 156,000 by the end of 2009. This represents about 25% of all office-based prescribers and is twice the number of office-based prescribers in 2008. Although many clinicians may eventually move to fully integrated EMR systems that include e-prescribing components, at the present time the cost and complexity of acquiring and implementing such systems is prohibitive for many practices, especially smaller physician offices. Even though e-prescribing use is on the upswing nationally, prescribers, dispensers, and state and federal entities must continue to work together to remove barriers to e-prescribing so that the projected cost savings and reductions in medical errors can be realized.

To reinforce the content of this chapter, please complete the worksheets that follow.

Worksheet 10.1

1. State two purposes of DEA registration.

_____

_____

2. If federal prescribing law differs from state law, which must the prescriber follow?

_____

3. List at least two characteristics of tamper-proof prescription pads.

_____

_____

4. List at least five precautions that prescribers should take to control and protect their DEA registration.

_____

_____

_____

_____

_____

5. Match the following terms and definitions.

A. signa	_____ name and strength of the medication
B. inscription	_____ reason the patient is to take the medication
C. subscription	_____ instructions to patient on how to take the medication
D. indication	_____ medical use and abuse potential
E. schedule	_____ information on dosage form and units to dispense

6. List at least five common errors made in prescription writing.

_____

_____

_____

_____

_____

_____

7. List the four elements required to meet the standards for qualified e-prescribing.

_____

_____

_____

_____

8. List at least three benefits to e-prescribing.

_____

_____

_____

_____

9. List at least three barriers to e-prescribing.

_____

_____

_____

_____

10. List at least two types of errors that are unique to e-prescribing.

_____

_____

_____

Worksheet 10.2

Refer to Figure 9-4, discharge summary for Henry Oliver. Review the list of his discharge medications and then complete the following.

1. Look up each of his medications. Indicate which ones are available over the counter and which require a prescription.

_____

_____

_____

_____

2. Look up ferrous sulfate. List at least three different brand names for the drug, the different preparations available, and the strengths available. Write a prescription for a 1-month supply of ferrous sulfate for the dose listed in Mr. Oliver's discharge medications.

_____

_____

_____

_____

3. Look up tramadol. List a brand name for tramadol and the name for tramadol with acetaminophen. List the strengths available in each brand. Write a prescription for a 1-week supply of plain tramadol in the strength listed in Mr. Oliver's discharge medications.

_____

_____

_____

_____

Refer to Worksheet 9.4 and review the discharge medications for Mrs. McLaughlin.

1. Look up all the medications listed and indicate which ones are controlled substances and what schedule.

_____

_____

_____

_____

2. Write a prescription for a 1-month supply of metoprolol.

_____

_____

3. Write a prescription for a 10-day course of Cipro based on twice-daily dosing.

_____

_____

4. Look up Xanax and write all the strengths that are available.

_____

_____

5. Write a prescription for Xanax for 1 week, using the dose indicated in Mrs. McLaughlin's discharge summary and indicating that a generic drug may be substituted for the brand name.

_____

_____

6. Write a prescription for the Lantus based on a dose of 22 units each day and indicate that only name brand medication should be dispensed.

_____

_____

7. Patients sometimes use a mail-order pharmacy to fill prescriptions for medications taken daily. The mail-order pharmacies usually require a 90-day supply to be dispensed at one time, and enough refills to provide medication for 1 year. Write a prescription for the lisinopril based on these requirements.

_____

_____

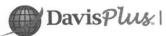 **DavisPlus** | Visit **http://davisplus.fadavis.com** for complete learning activities on actual EMR software at, Keyword: Sullivan

Worksheet 10.4

Refer to Figure 9-1 and review the discharge medications for Mr. Jensen and complete the following as instructed.

1. Look up Lotensin HCT. List the two medications contained in the formulation and the strengths that are available.

_____

_____

2. Write a prescription for a 1-month supply of Lotensin HCT.

_____

_____

3. Look up Mevacor and list the strengths that are available and the generic name for the medication.

_____

_____

4. Write a prescription for a 1-month supply of Mevacor, indicating that a generic drug may be substituted for the brand name.

_____

_____

5. Look up Percocet and identify its schedule. List the generic name of the medication and the strengths that are available. Consult Appendix F and determine the maximum number that may be dispensed by a Physician Assistant practicing in West Virginia and write an appropriate prescription. Consult Appendix G and determine the maximum number that may be dispensed by a Nurse Practitioner practicing in Michigan and write an appropriate prescription.

_____

_____

_____

_____

Abbreviations

These abbreviations were used in this chapter. Beside each, write the meaning pertaining to the context of this chapter.

CSA _____

DAW _____

DEA _____

FDA _____

MMA _____

TMP/SMX _____

Adult Preventive
Care Timeline

Appendix A

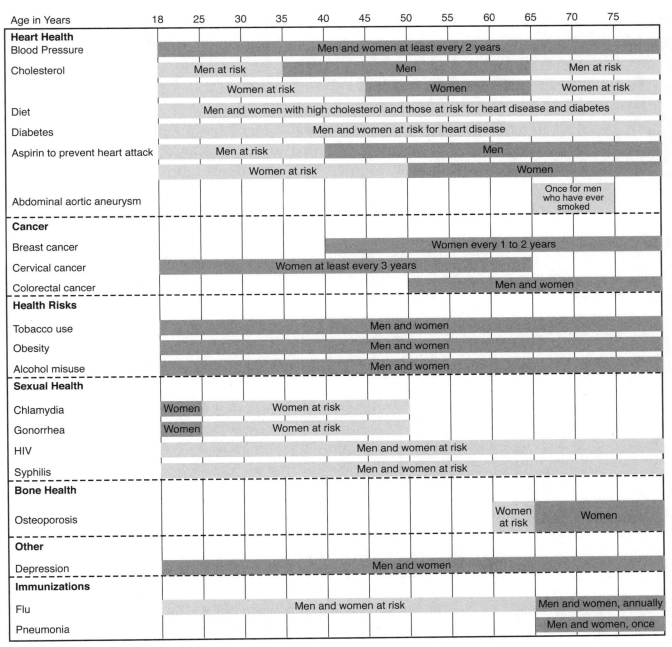

225

A Guide to Sexual History Taking

A Guide to Sexual History Taking

The importance of taking a sexual history

A sexual history is important for all patients to provide information that identifies those at risk for sexually transmitted disease, including HIV, to guide risk-reduction counseling, and to identify what anatomic sites are suitable for STD screening. This basic sexual history tool can be used by clinicians as a guide to determine the patient's risk for STDs. This history can be taken by the clinician as part of the history and physical, or done by the patient as a self-administered questionnaire. This template may not be culturally appropriate for some patients, and it can be adjusted as needed.

Getting started and the 5 Ps

A. *Getting started: introductory statements and questions*

1. ***Teens.*** Care needs to be taken when introducing sensitive topics such as sexuality with teenagers. It is important to interview the teen alone and reinforce confidentiality. For teens, the sexual history can be incorporated into a broader risk assessment that addresses issues related to home, school, drug use, smoking, etc. Discussions should be appropriate for the teen's developmental level.

"Now I am going to take a few minutes to ask you some sensitive questions that are important for me to help you be healthy. Anything we discuss will be completely confidential. I won't discuss this with anyone, not even your parents, without your permission."

"Some of my patients your age have started having sex. Have you had sex?" or

"What are you doing to protect yourself from AIDS, HIV, or other STDs?"

If you identify that the teen is sexually active, you will want to continue with a more complete sexual history...

2. ***Adults.*** *"Now I am going to take a few minutes to ask you some direct questions about your sexual health. These questions are very personal, but it is important for me to know so I can help you be healthy. I ask these questions to all of my patients regardless of age or marital status and they are just as important as other questions about your physical and mental health. Like the rest of this visit, this information is strictly confidential."*

B. *The 5 Ps: Partners, sexual Practices, Past STDs, Pregnancy history and plans, and Protection from STDs*

1. ***Partners.*** For sexual risk, it is important to determine the number and gender of a patient's sexual partners. One should make no assumptions of partner gender in the initial history-taking. If multiple partners, explore for more specific risk factors, such as patterns of condom use and partner's risk factors (i.e., other partners, injection drug use, history of STDs). If one partner, ask about length of the relationship and partner's risk, such as other partners and injection drug use.

- **"Do you have sex with men, women, or both?"**
- **"In the past 2 months, how many people have you had sex with?"**
- **"In the past 12 months, how many partners have you had?"**

If the patient has sex with both men and women, repeat these questions for each specific gender.

2. ***Sexual Practices.*** In addition to determining the gender and number of partners, it is also important to ask about sexual practices and condom use. Asking about sex practices will guide risk-reduction strategies and identify anatomical sites from which to collect specimens for STD testing.

"I am going to be more explicit about the kind of sex you may have been having over the last year so I understand your risks for STDs."

- **"Do you have vaginal sex, meaning penis in vagina sex?"** If answer is yes,
- **"Do you use condoms: never, sometimes, most of the time, or always for this kind of sex?"**
- **"Do you have anal sex, meaning penis in rectum/anus sex?"** If answer is yes,
- **"Do you use condoms: never, sometimes, most of the time, or always for this kind of sex?"**
- **"Do you have oral sex, meaning mouth on penis/vagina?"** If condom use is inconsistent,
- **"In what situations, or with whom, do you not use condoms?"**

3. ***Past history of STDs.*** A history of prior gonorrhea or chlamydia infections increases a person's risk for repeat infection. Recent past STDs indicate higher risk behavior.

- **"What STDs have you had in the past, if any?"**
- **"Have you ever had an STD, such as chlamydia, gonorrhea, herpes, or warts?"** If answer is yes,
- **"Do you know what the infection was and when it was?"**
- **"Have any of your partners had an STD?"** If answer is yes,
- **"Do you know what the infection was and when it was?"**

(Continued)

4. *Pregnancy plans.* Based on partner information already obtained, you may determine that the patient is at risk for becoming pregnant or causing a pregnancy. If so, determine first whether pregnancy is desired.

- **"What are your current plans or desires regarding pregnancy?"** *(Women)*
- **"Are you concerned about getting pregnant or getting your partner pregnant?"**
- **"Are you trying to get pregnant?"** *(Women)*
- **"Are you and a partner trying to get pregnant?"** *(Men)* If answer is no,
- **"What are you doing to prevent a pregnancy?"**

5. *Protection from STDs*

- **"What do you do to protect yourself from sexually transmitted diseases and HIV?"**

With this open-ended question, you allow different avenues of discussion: condom use, monogamy, patient self-perception of risk, and perception of partner's risk. If you have determined that the patient has had one partner in the past 12 months and that partner has had no other partners, infrequent or no condom use may not warrant risk-reduction counseling. Regardless of the patient's risk behavior, if the patient is a woman and is 25 or younger, routine screening for chlamydia is recommended annually.

C. *Additional questions to identify HIV and hepatitis risk.* Immunization history for hepatitis A and B can be noted at this point, as well as past HIV testing. Hepatitis A immunization is recommended for men who have sex with men (MSM) and intravenous drug users (IDU).

- **"Have you or any of your partners ever injected drugs?"**
- **"Have you or any of your partners ever had sex with prostitutes?"**
- **"Have you ever gotten hepatitis B vaccine (all 3 doses)?"**
- **"Have you ever gotten hepatitis A vaccine (2 doses)?" (only MSM, IDU)**
- **"Have you ever been tested for HIV, the virus that causes AIDS?"**

D. **Finishing up. By the end of this section of the interview, the patient may have come up with information or questions that she/he was not ready to discuss earlier.**

- **"Is there anything else about your sexual practices that I need to know about to ensure you good health care?"**
- **"Do you have any questions?"**

At this point, review and reinforce positive, protective behaviors. After reinforcing positive behavior, it is appropriate to address specific concerns regarding higher-risk practices. Your expression of concern can then lead to risk-reduction counseling or a counseling referral.

(Reprinted with permission from the California STD/HIV Prevention Training Center.)

Suggestions for Dictating Medical Records

- Organize your thoughts and your materials before you begin to dictate. This will help decrease the amount of time you spend going through the chart hunting for specific information.
- Speak slowly and clearly. Try to reduce background noise as much as possible.
- Get in the habit of doing a "sound check" at the beginning of a dictation session. Record a few words, then play back the recording to check for clarity of your speech, volume, background noise, and other factors that will influence the quality of your dictation.
- Always spell out the patient's name, even if it is a very common name, such as Mary. It is also a good idea to spell out the names of physicians and other health-care providers involved in the patient's care. It is good practice to spell out the names of medications, especially ones that are not used frequently and new medications.
- If you need to look through the chart for information, use the pause feature on the dictation system. Transcriptionists do not want to listen to you thumbing through pages of a chart. It puts unnecessary gaps in the dictation and can be very distracting.
- When you are dictating, do everything possible to avoid having a conversation at the same time. If someone walks up and asks you a question about Mrs. Smith while you are dictating a record on Mrs. Jones, the answer you provide may inadvertently become part of the medical record for Mrs. Jones. Transcriptionists are responsible for typing out information that is heard on the tape; they are not responsible for editing tapes as they transcribe.
- Remember to protect the patient's confidentiality as much as possible. Be aware of who is within hearing range when you are dictating. If others are in the immediate area, especially other patients or family members of patients, and there is a chance that they may overhear your dictation, move to a more private area to dictate to avoid violating confidentiality.

ISMP's List of Error-Prone Abbreviations, Symbols, and Dose Designations

Description	Intended Meaning	Misinterpretation	Correction
Abbreviations			
µg	Microgram	Mistaken as "mg"	Use "mcg"
AD, AS, AU	Right ear, left ear, each ear	Mistaken as OD, OS, OU (right eye, left eye, each eye)	Use "right ear," "left ear," or "each ear"
OD, OS, OU	Right eye, left eye, each eye	Mistaken as AD, AS, AU (right ear, left ear, each ear)	Use "right eye," "left eye," or "each eye"
BT	Bedtime	Mistaken as "BID" (twice daily)	Use "bedtime"
cc	Cubic centimeters	Mistaken as "u" (units)	Use "mL"
D/C	Discharge or discontinue	Premature discontinuation of medications if D/C (intended to mean "discharge") has been misinterpreted as "discontinue" when followed by a list of discharge medications	Use "discharge" and "discontinue"
IJ	Injection	Mistaken as "IV" or "intrajugular"	Use "injection"
IN	Intranasal	Mistaken as "IM" or "IV"	Use "intranasal" or "NAS"
HS	Half-strength	Mistaken as bedtime	Use "half-strength" or "bedtime"
hs	At bedtime, hours of sleep	Mistaken as half-strength	
IU**	International unit	Mistaken as IV (intravenous) or 10 (ten)	Use "units"
o.d. or OD	Once daily	Mistaken as "right eye" (OD—oculus dexter), leading to oral liquid medications administered in the eye	Use "daily"
OJ	Orange juice	Mistaken as OD or OS (right or left eye); drugs meant to be diluted in orange juice may be given in the eye	Use "orange juice"
Per os	By mouth, orally	The "os" can be mistaken as "left eye" (OS—oculus sinister)	Use "PO," "by mouth," or "orally"
q.d. or QD**	Every day	Mistaken as q.i.d., especially if the period after the "q" or the tail of the "q" is misunderstood as an "i"	Use "daily"
qhs	Nightly at bedtime	Mistaken as "qhr" or every hour	Use "nightly"
qn	Nightly or at bedtime	Mistaken as "qh" (every hour)	Use "nightly" or "at bedtime"
q.o.d. or QOD**	Every other day	Mistaken as "q.d." (daily) or "q.i.d." (four times daily) if the "o" is poorly written	Use "every other day"
q1d	Daily	Mistaken as q.i.d. (four times daily)	Use "daily"
q6PM, etc.	Every evening at 6 PM	Mistaken as every 6 hours	Use "6 PM nightly" or "6 PM daily"
SC, SQ, sub q	Subcutaneous	SC mistaken as SL (sublingual); SQ mistaken as "5 every"; the "q" in "sub q" has been mistaken as "every" (e.g., a heparin dose ordered "sub q 2 hours before surgery" misunderstood as every 2 hours before surgery)	Use "subcut" or "subcutaneously"
ss	Sliding scale (insulin) or ½ (apothecary)	Mistaken as "55"	Spell out "sliding scale;" use "one-half" or "½"
SSRI	Sliding scale regular insulin	Mistaken as selective-serotonin reuptake inhibitor	Spell out "sliding scale (insulin)"
SSI	Sliding scale insulin	Mistaken as Strong Solution of Iodine (Lugol's)	
i/d	One daily	Mistaken as "tid"	Use "1 daily"

Description	Intended Meaning	Misinterpretation	Correction
Abbreviations (continued)			
TIW or tiw **BIW or biw**	TIW: 3 times a week BIW: 2 times a week	TIW mistaken as "3 times a day" or "twice in a week" BIW mistaken as "2 times a day"	Use "3 times weekly" Use "2 times weekly"
U or u**	Unit	Mistaken as the number 0 or 4, causing a 10-fold overdose or greater (e.g.,4U seen as "40" or 4u seen as "44"); mistaken as "cc" so dose given in volume instead of units (e.g., 4u seen as 4cc)	Use "unit"
UD	As directed ("ut dictum")	Mistaken as unit dose (e.g., diltiazem 125 mg IV infusion "UD" misinterpreted as meaning to give the entire infusion as a unit [bolus] dose)	Use "as directed"
Dose Designations and Other Information			
Trailing zero after decimal point (e.g., 1.0 mg)**	1 mg	Mistaken as 10 mg if the decimal point is not seen	Do not use trailing zero for doses expressed in whole numbers
"Naked" leading zero before a decimal point (e.g., .5 mg)**	0.5 mg	Mistaken as 5 mg if the decimal point is not seen	Use zero before a decimal point when the dose is less than a whole unit
Drug name and dose run together (especially problematic for drug names that end in "l" such as Inderal40 mg; Tegretol300 mg)	Inderal 40 mg Tegretol 300 mg	Mistaken as Inderal 140 mg Mistaken as Tegretol 1300 mg	Place adequate space between the drug name, dose, and unit of measure
Numerical dose and unit of measure run together (e.g.,10mg, 100mL)	10 mg 100 mL	The "m" is sometimes mistaken as a zero or two zeros, risking a 10- to 100-fold overdose	Place adequate space between the dose and unit of measure
Abbreviations such as mg. or mL. with a period following the abbreviation	mg mL	The period is unnecessary and could be mistaken as the number 1 if written poorly	Use mg, mL, etc. without a terminal period
Large doses without properly placed commas (e.g., 100000 units; 1000000 units)	100,000 units 1,000,000 units	100000 has been mistaken as 10,000 or 1,000,000; 1000000 has been mistaken as 100,000	Use commas for dosing units at or above 1,000, or use words such as 100 "thousand" or 1 "million" to improve readability
Drug Name Abbreviations			
ARA A	vidarabine	Mistaken as cytarabine (ARA C)	Use complete drug name
AZT	zidovudine (Retrovir)	Mistaken as azathioprine or aztreonam	Use complete drug name
CPZ	Compazine (prochlorperazine)	Mistaken as chlorpromazine	Use complete drug name
DPT	Demerol-Phenergan-Thorazine	Mistaken as diphtheria-pertussis-tetanus (vaccine)	Use complete drug name
DTO	Diluted tincture of opium, or deodorized tincture of opium (Paregoric)	Mistaken as tincture of opium	Use complete drug name
HCl	hydrochloric acid or hydrochloride	Mistaken as potassium chloride (The "H" is misinterpreted as "K")	Use complete drug name unless expressed as a salt of a drug
HCT	hydrocortisone	Mistaken as hydrochlorothiazide	Use complete drug name
HCTZ	hydrochlorothiazide	Mistaken as hydrocortisone (seen as HCT250 mg)	Use complete drug name
MgSO4**	magnesium sulfate	Mistaken as morphine sulfate	Use complete drug name
MS, MSO4**	morphine sulfate	Mistaken as magnesium sulfate	Use complete drug name

Description	Intended Meaning	Misinterpretation	Correction
Drug Name Abbrevations (continued)			
MTX	methotrexate	Mistaken as mitoxantrone	Use complete drug name
PCA	procainamide	Mistaken as patient controlled analgesic	Use complete drug name
PTU	propylthiouracil	Mistaken as mercaptopurine	Use complete drug name
T3	Tylenol with codeine No. 3	Mistaken as liothyronine	Use complete drug name
TAC	triamcinolone	Mistaken as tetracaine, Adrenalin, cocaine	Use complete drug name
TNK	TNKase	Mistaken as "TPA"	Use complete drug name
ZnS04	zinc sulfate	Mistaken as morphine sulfate	Use complete drug name
Stemmed Drug Names			
"Nitro" drip	nitroglycerin infusion	Mistaken as sodium nitroprusside infusion	Use complete drug name
"Norflox"	norfloxacin	Mistaken as Norflex	Use complete drug name
"IV Vanc"	intravenous vancomycin	Mistaken as Invanz	Use complete drug name
Symbols			
℥ ♏	Dram Minim	Symbol for dram mistaken as "3" Symbol for minim mistaken as "mL"	Use the metric system
x3d	For three days	Mistaken as "3 doses"	Use "for three days"
> and <	Greater than and less than	Mistaken as opposite of intended; mistakenly use incorrect symbol; "<10" mistaken as "40"	Use "greater than" or "less than"
/ (slash mark)	Separates two doses or indicates "per"	Mistaken as the number 1 (e.g., "25 units and 110" units)	Use "per" rather than a slash mark to separate doses
@	At	Mistaken as "2"	Use "at"
&	And	Mistaken as "2"	Use "and"
+	Plus or and	Mistaken as "4"	Use "and"
°	Hour	Mistaken as a zero (e.g., q2° seen as q 20)	Use "hr," "h," or "hour"

** These abbreviations are included on TJC's "minimum list" of dangerous abbreviations, acronyms, and symbols that must be included on an organization's "Do Not Use" list, effective January 1, 2004. Visit www.jointcommission.org for more information about this TJC requirement. © ISMP 2007.

Worksheet Answer Key

Chapter 1

Worksheet 1.1 Answers

General and Medicolegal Principles

1. In addition to other health-care providers, list 5 different types or groups of people who could read medical records you create.
   Any of the following: (1) attorneys, (2) researchers, (3) consulting providers, (4) patient, (5) peer reviewers, (6) insurance companies, (7) state or federal payers

2. List at least 5 general principles of documentation that are based on CMS guidelines.
   Any of the following: (1) record should be complete and legible; (2) for each encounter, document reason, relevant history, exam findings and diagnostic test results, assessment, and plan for care; (3) date and legible identity of person documenting; (4) rationale for ordering test or services; (5) past and present diagnoses; (6) health risk factor identification; (7) patient's progress and response to treatment; (8) identify CPT codes and ICD-9 codes.

3. Describe how to make a correction in a medical record.
   Draw a single line through the entry, label it as an error, initial and date it.

4. Beside each of the following, indicate whether the statement is acceptable (A) or unacceptable (U) according to generally accepted documentation guidelines.
   __A__ Use of either the 1995 or 1997 CMS guidelines
   __A__ Making a late entry in a chart or medical record
   __U__ Using correction fluid or tape to obliterate an entry in a record
   __U__ Making an entry in a record before seeing a patient
   __A__ Amending an entry in a medical record
   __U__ Stamping a record "signed but not read"

Medical Billing and Coding

1. Indicate whether the following statements are true (T) or false (F).
   __T__ CPT codes reflect the level of evaluation and management services provided.
   __F__ The three key elements of determining the level of service are history, review of systems, and physical examination.
   __T__ Time spent counseling the patient and the nature of the presenting problem are two factors that affect the level of service provided.
   __T__ ICD-9 codes indicate the reason for patient services.
   __T__ ICD-9 codes are used to track mortality and morbidity statistics internationally.
   __F__ ICD-10 code sets have more than 155,000 codes but do not have the capacity to accommodate new diagnoses and procedures.
   __T__ "V" codes are used for reasons other than illness or disease.
   __T__ The medical record must include documentation that supports the assessment.
   __F__ Assignment of appropriate CPT and ICD-9 codes that support the level of E/M services provided is only dependent on adequate documentation of the history and physical examination.
   __F__ An ICD-9 code should be as broad and encompassing as possible.
   __T__ There is no code for "rule out."
   __T__ The complexity of medical decision making takes into account the number of treatment options.

2. ICD-9 codes are used to identify which of the following? (underline all that apply)
   HPI   **Diagnosis**   Treatment
   Physical   Treating facility   **Symptoms**
   exam findings
   Surgical history   **Complaints**   Tests ordered
   Reason for   Level of service   **Conditions**
   office visit

3. Translate the following lay terms into medical terminology.

flu	influenza
rash	exanthem
navel	umbilicus
heartburn	gastroesophageal reflux disease
stroke	cerebrovascular accident
kidney stone	renal calculus
flat feet	pes planus
vitamin B$_{12}$ deficiency	pernicious anemia
sugar diabetes	diabetes mellitus
tiredness	fatigue
stomach	abdomen
tennis elbow	lateral epicondylitis

heel	calcaneus
heart attack	myocardial infarction
pink eye	conjunctivitis
emphysema	chronic obstructive pulmonary disease
light intolerance	photophobia
tubal pregnancy	ectopic pregnancy
ear drum	tympanic membrane
blood thinner	anticoagulant

Electronic Medical Records

1. List at least five functions that an EMR system should be able to perform.
   Any of the following: (1) store health information and data; (2) result management for diagnostic tests; (3) order management; (4) decision support; (5) electronic communication and connectivity; (6) patient support; (7) administrative processes; (8) reporting.
2. Identify at least five perceived benefits of an EMR system.
   Any of the following: (1) immediate access to key information such as allergies, lab results; (2) alert to duplicate orders; (3) alert to drug interactions; (4) reduce duplication; (5) enhance legibility; (6) reduce fragmentation; (7) improve the speed with which orders are executed; (8) alert to screenings and preventive measures needed; (9) improve continuity of care; (10) reduce frequency of adverse events; (11) increase timeliness of diagnoses and treatment; (12) provide decision-making support to increase compliance with best clinical practices.
3. Identify at least five potential barriers to implementing an EMR system.
   Any of the following: (1) cost of implementation; (2) reduced workflow and productivity during implementation; (3) unreliable technology; (4) lack of interoperability; (5) safety and security of systems; (6) debate over who owns data; (7) technical matters such as accessibility, vendor support, down time.
4. List at least two criteria required to meet "meaningful" use standards.
   Any of the following: (1) certified system; (2) electronic prescribing; (3) quality reporting; (4) capable of exchanging data with other systems

HIPAA

1. Indicate whether each statement about the Health Insurance Portability and Accountability Act is true (T) or false (F).
   T___ Establishes standards for the electronic transfers of health data
   F___ Provides health care for everyone
   F___ Limits exclusion of preexisting medical conditions to 24 months
   T___ Gives patients more access to their medical records
   T___ Protects medical records from improper uses and disclosures
   F___ Federal HIPAA regulations preempt state laws.
   T___ The Privacy Rule only applies to covered entities that transmit medical information electronically.
   T___ Protected Health Information is data that could be used to identify an individual.
   T___ Covered entities include doctors, clinics, dentists, nursing homes, chiropractors, psychologists, pharmacies, and insurance companies.
   T___ A covered entity may disclose PHI without patient authorization for purposes of treatment, payment, or its health-care operations.
   F___ PHI cannot be transmitted between covered entities by e-mail.
   F___ Patients are entitled to a listing of everyone with whom their health-care provider has shared their PHI.
   T___ PHI may be disclosed to someone involved in the patient's health care without written authorization.
   T___ The Privacy Rule allows certain minors access to specified health care,
   T___ A Notice of Privacy Practice explains how patients' PHI is used and disclosed by the covered entity.
   F___ An employee cannot be terminated for violating the Privacy Rule.
   T___ An individual may not sue the insurance company over an HIPAA violation.
   T___ Criminal penalties for HIPAA violations can result in fines and imprisonment.
   F___ The confidentiality, integrity, and availability of PHI only need to be protected when the PHI is transmitted, not when it is stored.
   T___ Employees are required to attend periodic security awareness and training.
   T___ The Security Rule requires covered entities to install and regularly update antivirus, anti-spyware, and firewall software.
   T___ Physical and technical safeguards must be in place to prevent PHI from being transmitted over the Internet.
   T___ A process to develop contracts with business associates that will ensure they will safeguard PHI is required by HIPAA.
   F___ HIPAA may not audit a practice for compliance without notice.

2. From the list below, underline each that would be considered a covered entity according to HIPAA.

<u>chiropractors</u> social worker <u>psychologists</u>
<u>nurse</u> medical <u>nursing homes</u>
<u>practitioners</u> assistants
<u>doctors</u> <u>HMOs</u> lawyers
office <u>PPOs</u> <u>Veterans</u>
managers <u>Administration</u>
  <u>hospitals</u>
<u>Medicare</u> <u>Medicaid</u> employers
<u>hospitals</u>

3. Identify at least two conditions that are considered *sensitive* PHI.
Any of the following: (1) HIV status; (2) mental health conditions; (3) substance abuse.

4. Patients have the right to review and obtain copies of their medical records except in certain circumstances. List two.
Any of the following: (1) psychotherapy notes; (2) information compiled for a lawsuit; and (3) information that, in the opinion of the health-care provider, may cause harm to the individual or another.

5. Indicate by a yes (Y) or no (N) whether disclosure of PHI to the specific entity would require patient authorization.
N___ Specialist/consultant
N___ Patient's health plan
Y___ Life insurance company
N___ Hospital accounting department
Y___ Patient's employer
Y___ Pharmaceutical companies
N___ Reporting a gunshot wound to police
N___ Reporting names of patients with a communicable disease to a county health department
N___ Reporting suspected child abuse to a child protection agency
N___ Medical billing and coding department
Y___ Friends and family not involved in a patient's health care

Worksheet 1.2 Answers

Abbreviations

AMA	American Medical Association
AMI	acute myocardial infarction
ARRA	American Recovery and Reinvestment Act
CE	covered entity
CMS	Centers for Medicare and Medicaid Services
CP	chest pain; cerebral palsy
CPR	computer-based patient record
CPT	*Current Procedural Terminology*
DM	diabetes mellitus

EHR	electronic health record
E/M	evaluation and management
EMR	electronic medical record
EPR	electronic patient record
HHS	Health and Human Services
HIMSS	Healthcare Information and Management Systems Society
HIPAA	Health Insurance Portability and Accountability Act
HITECH	Health Information Technology for Economic and Clinical Health Act
HIV	human immunodeficiency virus
HMO	health maintenance organization
ICD-9	International Classification of Diseases, 9th Revision
ICD-10	International Classification of Diseases, 10th Revision
PHI	protected health information
URI	upper respiratory infection

Chapter 2

Worksheet 2.1 Answers

1. Does this document meet the CMS guidelines for documentation of a comprehensive history and physical? Why or why not?
No. All elements of the HPI are not documented. The family history does not document any medical conditions of first-degree relatives. The ROS only addresses four systems; therefore, it is incomplete.

2. Critically analyze the H&P and list any errors. The chief complaint is not in the patient's own words. There are contradictory statements in the document; for example, Drixoral and Robitussin are listed as medications, but there is a statement, "patient does not take any medications." Pain is listed in the HPI, but not explored, so it is unclear where the patient is having pain. Seasonal allergies should be listed in past medication history and not as an allergy. There is no documentation of the type of reaction the patient has when she takes penicillin. There is objective information (vital signs) in the ROS, which is for subjective data. More information should be documented in the psychosocial history. The documentation of the ROS does not follow the recommended order and does not address all of the 14 systems that CMS identifies. Dizziness is listed in the respiratory system. The HEENT examination is not thorough. There is no documentation of examination of the musculoskeletal system or GU/GYN, which is indicated for a new patient. Is

"tenderness to palpation in both upper quadrants" a significant finding? There is no exploration of GI history to correlate with this finding.

3. Did any questions come to mind that you are unable to answer after reading the H&P? Some questions arise because of the lack of documenting a complete ROS. Is the patient still menstruating? If so, when was the date of the last menstrual period? Does she use any contraception? Does the patient take Drixoral and Robitussin all the time, or has she taken them only since her symptoms began? Does the patient use tobacco? Has she used alcohol or illicit drugs in the past?

4. Are the diagnoses listed in the assessment section reasonably supported by the history? There is not enough information documented to support a definitive diagnosis of pneumonia. It is reasonable to include the patient's history of tonsillectomy. There could be other symptoms, conditions, or risk factors not identified because of the lack of a thorough PMH, family history, psychosocial history, and ROS.

5. Did you identify other differential diagnoses or conditions that could be included in the assessment? If so, list.
Bronchitis, upper respiratory infection, gastroesophageal reflux disease, costochondritis, pleuritis, allergic rhinitis.

6. Is the plan reasonable based on the assessments listed? Why or why not?
There is nothing in the assessment to support the need for CBC, CMP. Although it is reasonable to do this because the patient is new to the practice and her last physical was 2 years ago, the plan should be linked to an assessment. It is not clear when the patient should return for follow-up. No patient education has been documented.

Worksheet 2.2 Answers

1. Does this document meet the CMS guidelines for documentation of a comprehensive history and physical examination? Why or why not?
Yes. It documents all the elements cited by the guidelines.

2. Critically analyze the H&P and list any errors. Identify any strengths.
Gynecological history would typically document whether deliveries were vaginal or by cesarean section; this is not documented. Readers are unable to determine whether the

abortion was spontaneous or induced based on the documentation. No specific health information is documented for Ms. Gordon's parents. Although the statement "no history of familial diseases" is documented, it is not clear which familial diseases were inquired about. Strengths: well organized, and subjective and objective information listed appropriately. Thorough ROS and examination. The history of the migraine headaches is well documented. Able to follow the NP's reasoning for each assessment. Although the patient did not present with a specific complaint, the NP analyzed the data presented and recognized that the patient displays several symptoms of a thyroid disorder. The plan is well organized and thorough.

3. Did any questions come to mind that you are unable to answer after reading the H&P?
Is there any family history of thyroid disease?

4. Are the conditions listed in the assessment section reasonably supported by the history? Why or why not?
Yes; the NP shows her analysis of the data by listing the weight loss, anxiety, and increased reflexes as findings associated with Graves' disease. She also makes an assessment of the migraine headaches.

5. Did you identify other differential diagnoses or conditions that could be included in the assessment? If so, list.
None identified.

6. List the ICD-9 code for each assessment shown.
Weight loss: _____783.21_____
Graves' disease: _____242.0_____
Migraine headache: __346.0 or 346.2__
Anxiety: _____300.0_____

7. Would it be appropriate to include the ICD-9 code for Graves' disease when billing for this visit? Why or why not?
No. It is a valid differential diagnosis, but has not been definitively diagnosed. The results of the laboratory studies are needed before reaching a definitive diagnosis.

8. Is the plan reasonable based on the assessments listed? Why or why not?
Yes. The NP has documented her reasoning and the need to rule out thyroid disease, so it is reasonable to order the TSH, T_3, and T_4. CBC and CMP are also appropriate in the work-up of a patient who presents with weight loss. Because the Imitrex is effectively managing the patient's migraine headaches, there is no need to change the medication. The appropriate information

on how to use the medication is documented. Follow-up instructions are included. It is reasonable to conduct the well-woman examination at another appointment.

Worksheet 2.3 Answers

Abbreviations

AV	arteriovenous
BMI	body mass index
BP	blood pressure
CAD	coronary artery disease
CBC	complete blood count
CC	chief complaint
CMP	comprehensive metabolic panel
CN	cranial nerves
COPD	chronic obstructive pulmonary disease
CV	cardiovascular
CVA	costovertebral angle
DOB	date of birth
DOE	dyspnea on exertion
DTR	deep tendon reflex
ECG, EKG	electrocardiogram
ENT	ears, nose, throat
EOMs	extraocular movements
G3, P2, AB1	gravida 3, parity 2, abortion, 1
GI	gastrointestinal
GU	genitourinary
GYN	gynecologic, gynecology
H&P	history and physical examination
HA	headache
Hct	hematocrit
HEENT	head, eyes, ears, nose, throat
Hgb	hemoglobin
HHS	Health and Human Services
HIV	human immunodeficiency virus
HPI	history of present illness
Ht	height
HTN	hypertension
LDL	low-density lipoprotein
MSK	musculoskeletal
OLD CHARTS	onset, location, duration, character, alleviating/aggravating, radiation, temporal pattern, symptoms associated
OTC	over the counter
P	pulse
PEARL	pupils equal and reactive to light
PMH	past medical history
PQRST	palliative or provocative factors, quality of pain, region affected, severity of pain, timing
PRN	as needed

PSA	prostate-specific antigen
Pt	patient
R, RR	respirations, respiratory rate
R/O	rule out
ROM	range of motion
ROS	review of systems
RRR	regular rate and rhythm
SH	social history
S/P	status post
SH	social history
SOAP	subjective, objective, assessment, plan
SOB	shortness of breath
T	temperature
TB	tuberculosis
TMs	tympanic membranes
TSH	thyroid-stimulating hormone
T_3	triiodothyronine
T_4	thyroxine
UA	urinalysis
UTD	up to date
WBC	white blood cell
WNL	within normal limits
Wt	weight

Chapter 3

Worksheet 3.1 Answers

1. List the five components of the adult preventive care examination.
   Risk factor identification, age- and gender-specific screening, laboratory and diagnostic screening tests, patient education and counseling, assessment of immunization status

2. List at least five risk factors that should be screened for in the personal history.
   Any of the following: exercise, nutrition, BMI, tobacco use, alcohol use, other substance use, sex-related risk factors, IPV, safety measures, occupational exposures, oral health, blood or blood product transfusion

3. List at least three diseases that are associated with tobacco use.
   Any of the following: heart disease, cancer, COPD, stroke

4. List the four questions that make up the CAGE questionnaire.
   Have you ever felt the need to cut down on drinking?
   Have people annoyed you by criticizing your drinking?
   Have you ever felt guilty about drinking?
   Have you ever taken a drink first thing in the morning to steady your nerves or get rid of a hangover?

5. List one advantage of the AUDIT screening tool compared with the CAGE questionnaire. AUDIT has greater sensitivity than CAGE in populations with a lower prevalence of alcoholism.

6. List at least five substances that are screened for with the NIDA Modified ASSIST. Any of the following: tobacco products, alcoholic beverages, cannabis, cocaine, stimulants, methamphetamine, inhalants, sedatives, hallucinogens, opioids, other.

7. List the five Ps of the sexual history. Partners, practices, protection from STD, past history of STD, prevention of pregnancy

8. List three questions that are used to screen for IPV.
Within the past year, have you been hit, slapped, kicked, or otherwise physically hurt by someone?
Are you in a relationship with a person who threatens or physically hurts you?
Has anyone forced to you participate in sexual activities that made you feel uncomfortable?

9. List at least four facts that should be documented when a patient discloses IPV.
Any of the following: victim's description of abuse, name of alleged perpetrator and relationship to the victim, detailed description of all physical injuries, any information or referral provided to the victim, detailed description of the victim's demeanor, photographs of injuries

10. List at least three potential complications associated with blood transfusion.
Any of the following: transmission of disease, hemolytic reaction, febrile nonhemolytic reaction, iron overload, bacterial infection from contamination

11. List at least four conditions that have a genetic predisposition that should be screened for when taking a patient's family medical history.
Any of the following: diabetes, cardiovascular disease, hypertension, hyperlipidemia, cancer, asthma, osteoporosis

12. List at least five activities of daily living.
Any of the following: bathing, dressing, toileting, transferring, continence, feeding

13. List at least five independent activities of daily living.
Any of the following: food preparation, housekeeping, laundering, handling one's own finances, handling one's own medications, using the telephone, shopping, or transportation

14. List at least five factors that may contribute to falls in elderly patients.

Any of the following: inadequate lighting, pets in the home, clutter or throw rugs, medications, loss of flexibility, decrease in vision, chronic health conditions

15. Inez Lewis is a 68-year-old woman who presents for her annual WWE. She has a personal history of hypertension and a family history of glaucoma. List at least five screening examinations that could be ordered for Ms. Lewis.
Any of the following: measure blood pressure, colonoscopy, eye exam, mammogram, fecal occult blood testing, Pap smear, bone densitometry, assess risk for falling, ADLs, IADLs, immunization screening

16. Gene Ankar is a 52-year-old man who presents for his annual well-man examination. List two specific physical examination components and at least three screening tests that could be ordered for this patient, based on USPSTF recommendations.
Any of the following: prostate exam, hernia exam, testicular exam, PSA, colonoscopy, fecal occult blood testing, immunization screening, substance abuse screening, measure blood pressure, measure cholesterol and lipid levels

Worksheet 3.2 Answers

1. What additional information should have been included Ms. Erwin's sexual history?
Any of the following: gender of sexual partners, how often her partners use condoms, what type of STD she was treated for and when, if any partners have had an STD, what she does to protect herself from STD/HIV, future plans for pregnancy

2. What counseling or education would you provide to Ms. Erwin during this visit?
Any of the following: recommend condom use to protect from STD/HIV, the number of sexual partners increases her risk for contracting STD/HIV, find out if any partners have had an STD, could educate her on hepatitis transmission, discuss screening for STDs, educate her that some STDs can result in infertility

3. What physical examination should be done during this visit?
Standard physical examination, plus clinical breast exam and pelvic and bimanual exams

4. List at least three screening examinations or tests (including those recommended by the USPSTF) that could be done during this visit.

Any of the following: Pap smear to screen for cervical cancer; testing for gonorrhea, chlamydia and possible HIV/syphilis; measure blood pressure; screen for tobacco, alcohol, and substance use/abuse; screen for depression

Worksheet 3.3 Answers

Geriatric Screening

1. Based on the information above, how would you interpret Mr. Hammel's Mini Cog results?
   Abnormal clock and only one item recall is considered positive for cognitive impairment.
2. What additional screening examinations could be conducted as part of the evaluation of Mr. Hammel's weight loss?
   Any of the following: MUST, MNA-SF, ADLs
3. Based on the USPSTF Adult Preventive Care Timeline, what other screening tests could be done at this visit?
   Any of the following: measure blood pressure and cholesterol, colorectal cancer screening, depression screening, immunizations
4. Based on his age, Mr. Hammel could be screened for other risk factors; name at least four.
   Any of the following: risk for falls, gait and balance, depression, IADLs, sensory deficits such as vision changes and hearing changes.

Worksheet 3.4 Answers

Family History Screening

1. Identify the red flags from this patient's family history.
   Two first-degree relatives with the same condition (colon cancer)
   A family member with two related conditions (father with HTN, high cholesterol)
2. What conditions with a known genetic familial tendency should Mr. Shipley be screened for at this time?
   Coronary artery disease, colon cancer
3. Based on recommendations from the USPSTF, what additional screening should Mr. Shipley have at this time?
   Any of the following: blood pressure and cholesterol (would be done to monitor chronic conditions because he is already known to have these); diet; tobacco use; obesity; alcohol misuse; depression; fecal occult blood testing; colonoscopy (because he is at high risk, unless one has been done); ECG (because of personal and family risk factors for CAD)

4. What patient counseling or education should be provided to Mr. Shipley and documented in his medical record?
   Any of the following: education about a low cholesterol diet; importance of monitoring blood pressure and cholesterol levels and keeping both in a desired range because of his personal and family history of CAD; increased personal risk for colon cancer because of family history and measures that can be taken to reduce his risk; importance of screening for colon cancer; importance of avoiding tobacco use because of his personal and family history of CAD.

Worksheet 3.5 Answers

Adult Immunizations

1. What vaccines are indicated for a 40-year-old man who has sex with men who had his last tetanus immunization 6 years ago?
   Any of the following: varicella, hepatitis A, hepatitis B, seasonal influenza
2. Which three vaccines are contraindicated in pregnant women?
   Varicella, zoster, MMR
3. What vaccines are recommended for a 21-year-old woman who plans to start nursing school in 6 months who received one HPV vaccine at age 12?
   Any of the following: tetanus/diphtheria/pertussis (Tdap), HPV, varicella, zoster, MMR, influenza, hepatitis A, hepatitis B, meningococcus
4. What vaccines are recommended for a 63-year-old woman who volunteers at a public library and has diabetes?
   Any of the following: varicella, zoster, MMR, seasonal influenza, pneumococcus, meningococcus
5. A 34-year-old man undergoes splenectomy following an accident in which he sustained blunt abdominal trauma. Which vaccines are indicated for this patient? Which vaccine is contraindicated in this patient?
   Any of the following are indicated: Tdap, varicella, zoster, MMR, influenza, pneumococcus, hepatitis A, hepatitis B
   Contraindicated: meningococcus

Worksheet 3.6 Answers

ADL	activities of daily living
AHRQ	Agency for Healthcare Research and Quality
AUDIT	Alcohol Use Disorders Identification Test

BMD	bone mineral density
BPH	benign prostatic hyperplasia
CAD	coronary artery disease
CDC	Centers for Disease Control and Prevention
CDT	clock-drawing test
CTS	carpal tunnel syndrome
DAST-10	Drug Abuse Screening Test—10 Item
FBS	fasting blood sugar
FOBT	fecal occult blood test
GDS	Geriatric Depression Scale
HDDA	Hearing-Dependent Daily Activities
HDL	high-density lipoprotein
HPV	human papillomavirus
HTLV-1	human T-lymphotrophic virus, type 1
HTLV-2	human T-lymphotrophic virus, type 2
IADL	independent activities of daily living
IPV	intimate partner violence
MNA-SF	Mini-Nutrition Assessment— Short Form
MUST	Malnutrition Universal Screening Test
NIDA	National Institute of Drug Abuse
Modified ASSIST	Modified Alcohol, Smoking and Substance Involvement Screening Tool
OSHA	Occupational Safety and Health Administration
PID	pelvic inflammatory disease
PPD	packs per day
STD	sexually transmitted disease
STI	sexually transmitted infection
USPSTF	United States Preventive Services Task Force
VDRL	Venereal Disease Research Laboratory
WWE	well-woman examination

Chapter 4

Worksheet 4.1 Answers

1. List five components of pediatric health maintenance visits.
   Growth and development screening; laboratory screening tests; assessment of immunization status; anticipatory guidance; risk factor identification.
2. List three growth parameters that should be measured and documented from birth to 24 months of age.
   Height, weight, head circumference
3. At what age is BMI screening introduced?
   2 years
4. Name three widely used resources available from the CDC.

Growth charts; immunization schedules; BMI charts

5. List at least three tools that are used to screen children for achievement of developmental milestones.
   Any of the following: Denver Developmental Screening Test, 2nd edition; PEDS; PEDS-DM; ASQ-3; Bayley Scales of Infant Development
6. List at least four of the six most commonly included laboratory tests that are part of mandatory newborn screening.
   Any of the following: phenylketonuria, medium-chain acyl-CoA dehydrogenase deficiency, congenital hypothyroidism, neonatal hyperbilirubinemia, biotinidase deficiency, sickle cell anemia
7. For each of the ages listed, list at least three topics that should be discussed with parents/caregivers as part of anticipatory guidance.
   6 months:
   Any of the following: injury prevention; cup, finger foods; no bottles in bed; pool and tub safety; teething; poisons; nutrition; sleep position
   2–3 years:
   Any of the following: appetite; brushing teeth; toilet training; reading to the child; independence/dependence; car, home, and pool safety; preschool; control of TV viewing
   10–14 years:
   Any of the following: safety issues; nutrition; dental hygiene; peer pressure; smoking, alcohol and drugs; puberty; safe sex, contraception, STD prevention; communication
8. List at least four conditions (maternal or paternal) that should be explored as part of the genetic and teratology history.
   Any of the following: thalassemia; neural tube defects; congenital heart disease; Tay-Sachs, Canavan, Niemann-Pick disease; sickle cell disease or trait; muscular dystrophy; cystic fibrosis; Huntington's chorea; mental retardation; autism; hemophilia; RH sensitized; Down syndrome; other inherited genetic or chromosomal disorder
9. List at least four infections that could cause fetal malformation or birth defects that should be explored as part of the maternal evaluation.
   Any of the following: mumps, measles, rubella, rubeola, varicella zoster, hepatitis B, HIV, HPV, syphilis, gonorrhea, chlamydia, toxoplasmosis, cytomegalovirus, group B streptococcus
10. What does the FISTS mnemonic stand for?
    Fights, injuries, sexual violence, threats, self-defense strategies

11. List the four recognized types of child abuse.
   Neglect, physical, emotional, and sexual
12. List at least two screening tools that can be used to screen for child abuse or maltreatment. Any of the following: Childhood Trauma Questionnaire; Youth at Risk Screening; Childhood Maltreatment Interview Schedule—Short Form
13. List at least four topics that should be explored when taking the history of a child who presents for a preparticipation sports examination. Any of the following: personal and family history of cardiovascular disease, congenital or acquired heart disease, hypertension, cardiac murmurs, shortness of breath, syncope or near-syncope with exercise, hypertrophic cardiomyopathy, Marfan syndrome, unexplained sudden death in family members younger than 50, cocaine or anabolic steroid use
14. What three systems should be emphasized when examining a child who presents for a preparticipation sports examination? Cardiovascular, respiratory, and musculoskeletal

Worksheet 4.2 Answers

Weight-for-age percentiles: Girls, birth to 36 months

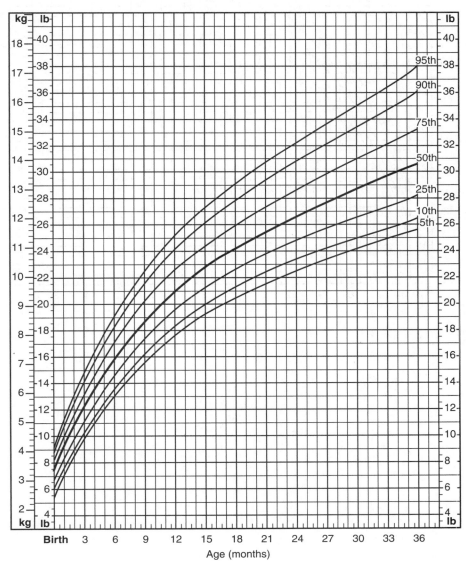

Length-for-age percentiles: Girls, birth to 36 months

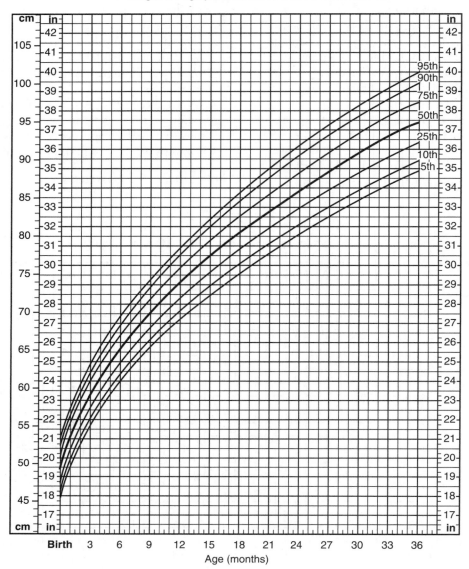

Head circumference-for-age percentiles: Girls, birth to 36 months

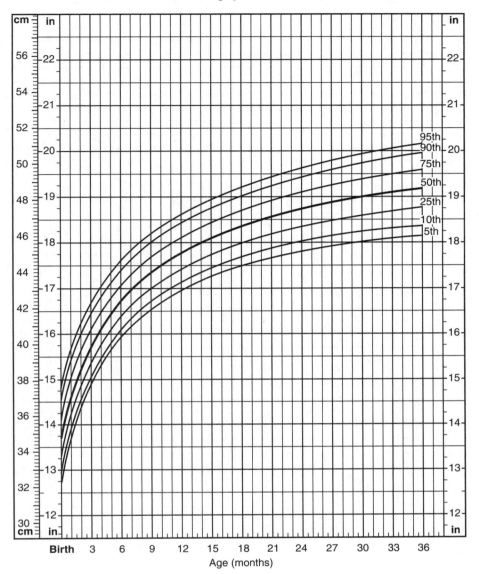

95th
90th
75th
50th
25th
10th
5th

Age (months)

Weight-for-age percentiles: Boys, birth to 36 months

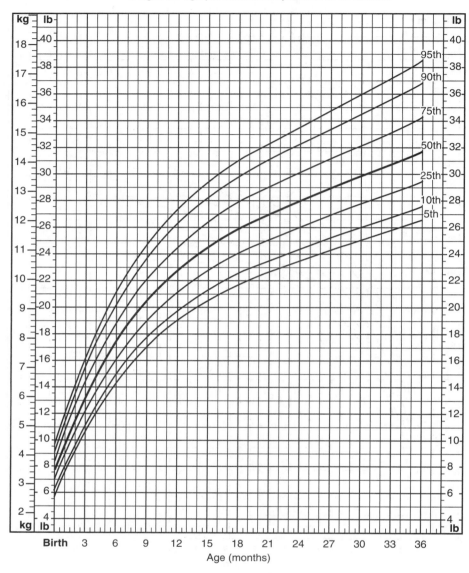

Length-for-age percentiles: Boys, birth to 36 months

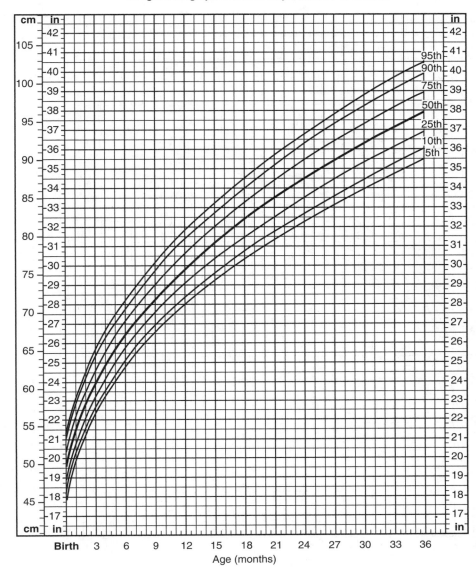

Head circumference-for-age percentiles: Boys, birth to 36 months

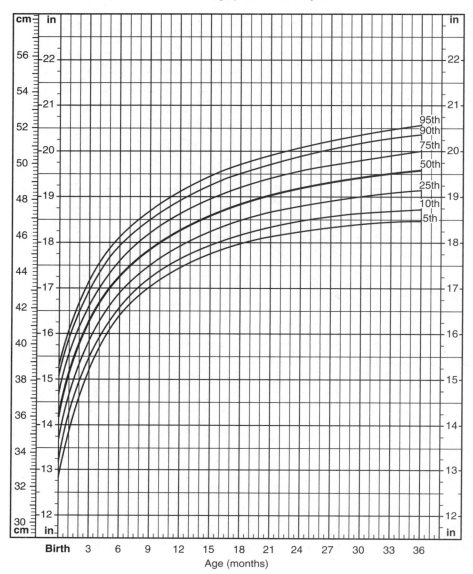

95th
90th
75th
50th
25th
10th
5th

Age (months)

Birth 3 6 9 12 15 18 21 24 27 30 33 36

Worksheet 4.3 Answers

HEEADSSS Write-Up

1. Based on the information in this write-up, list any risk factors that you identified for Allison. Any of the following risks: pregnancy, sexually transmitted diseases, head injury from not wearing a helmet when bike riding, second-hand smoke exposure

2. Critically analyze the content of this write-up. Identify other topics or additional information that should have been included in this write-up. Any of the following: more information on home situation, such as if she has her own room, ages of siblings, relationship with them; explore relationship with stepmother/stepbrother, any fights or violence, etc.; ask if she has moved recently or if she has ever lived away from home; explore interests/favorite classes in school; determine whether there is a reason for lower grades last quarter; if she has changed schools lately; eating history needs to be fully explored; what she does in free time with family/friends; determine whether Allison or any of her friends use alcohol and follow up as needed; explore Allison's ideas of "safe sex"; ask if Allison has difficulty sleeping; any thoughts of harming self or others; has she ever ridden with a drunk driver; explore for any sexual abuse/rape

3. Do you feel additional screening is needed at this time? Why or why not? If yes, what screening should be done?
   Any of the following: screen for intimate partner violence, sexually transmitted diseases, pregnancy, respiratory or ENT problems that could be associated with second-hand smoke exposure

4. What anticipatory guidance should be provided to Allison's mother at this visit?
   Any of the following: safety issues, dental hygiene; smoking, alcohol, and drugs; safe sex, contraception, STD prevention; communication; dating; peer pressure; motor vehicle safety; sports safety; staying in school

Worksheet 4.4 Answers

Abbreviations

AAP	American Academy of Pediatrics
ASQ-3	Ages and Stages Questionnaires, 3rd edition
CAPTA	Child Abuse Prevention and Treatment Act
CMIS-SF	Child Maltreatment Interview Schedule—Short Form
CTQ	Childhood Trauma Questionnaire
DDST-II	Denver Developmental Screening Test II
DTP	diphtheria, tetanus, pertussis
EPSDT	Early Periodic Screening, Diagnosis, and Treatment
FISTS	Fighting, Injuries, Sexual violence, Threats, Self-Defense
GAPS	Guidelines for Adolescent Preventive Services
HEEADSSS	Home, education/employment, eating, activities, drugs, sexuality, suicide/depression, safety
HIB-c	*Haemophilus influenzae* type B vaccine, conjugate
HRSA	Health Resource Services Administration
MCAD	Medium-chain acyl-CoA dehydrogenase deficiency
MCHB	Maternal and Child Health Bureau
MMR	measles, mumps, rubella
NHANES	National Health and Nutrition Examination Survey
OCP	oral contraceptive pill
PEDS	Parents' Evaluation of Developmental Status
PEDS-DM	Parents' Evaluation of Developmental Status—Developmental Milestones
PKU	Phenylketonuria
Td	tetanus, diphtheria

Chapter 5

Worksheet 5.1 Answers

Part A

A 45-year-old woman presents with a chief complaint of right hand pain. List the seven cardinal aspects of the history of present illness that should be documented in the subjective information.

Onset
Location
Duration of pain
Character of pain
Alleviating and aggravating factors
Radiation
Temporal pattern
Symptoms associated
List several pertinent aspects of the PMH that should be documented.
Medications, allergies, hand dominance, any surgery involving the hand, medical conditions that could cause pain, such as arthritis
What information about the patient's social history would be important to document?
Occupation/work history to determine whether job activities are a contributing factor

Part B

Onset, severity, aggravating factor, pertinent positive associated symptom, pertinent negative associated symptom

Part C

The patient is allergic to penicillin; the patient has no chronic medical conditions; the patient takes Zantac daily; could also include the patient works as a mechanic

Part D

History obtained from spouse
Medications
Review of systems

Onset of chief complaint
Could also include x-ray report (it could also be in objective)

Part E

1. __5__ The abdomen is soft and nondistended.
2. __2__ The oropharynx shows some erythema of the posterior pharyngeal wall but no exudates.
3. __4__ Auscultation of the lungs does not reveal any abnormal breath sounds.
4. __3__ The neck is supple with full range of motion, and there are no signs of meningeal irritation.
5. __1__ The skin is warm to touch and without cyanosis.

Worksheet 5.2 Answers

Medical Terminology

Next to each lay term, write an acceptable medical term and the ICD-9 code for each.

	Lay term	Medical term	ICD-9
1.	miscarriage	spontaneous abortion	634
2.	mole	neoplasm, nevus	448.1
3.	nearsightedness	myopia	367.1
4.	stiff neck	torticollis	723.5
5.	athlete's foot	tinea pedis	110.4
6.	hives	urticaria	708.8
7.	measles	rubeola	055
8.	tingling	paresthesias	782.0
9.	loss of appetite	anorexia	783.0
10.	shingles	varicella zoster	052.9
11.	canker sore	aphthous ulcer	528.2
12.	stye	hordeolum	373.11

Worksheet 5.3 Answers

Assessment and Plan

S: This 6-year-old child presents with a sore throat times 3 days. His mother states that he has had a fever of 101.5 orally, seems to have difficulty swallowing, and complains of a headache. His appetite is decreased. He has a runny nose with clear discharge. Denies cough, abdominal pain, vomiting, or diarrhea. There are no known exposures to communicable diseases. Tylenol helps the fever and sore throat "a little." PMH is negative. Meds: none. NKDA. The child is generally healthy. He is up to date on his immunizations.

O: T 100.8 (oral), P 98, R 20, BP 100/64
General: WDWN Caucasian male in NAD.
Skin: no rash
HEENT: Canals and TMs are unremarkable. Nasal mucosa is slightly congested with pink turbinates and clear discharge. Pharynx shows 3+ injected tonsils with scant exudates.

NECK: Supple. Tender, moderately enlarged tonsillar lymph nodes.
HEART: Rate 98 and regular without murmur.
LUNGS: Clear to auscultation. No adventitious sounds. Nonlabored breathing.
Abdomen: Soft, nondistended. Mildly tender throughout without guarding, rebound, or change in facial expression. No organomegaly or masses. Bowel sounds are normoactive.

1. What is your assessment of the patient described in the preceding example?
   Sore throat, R/O streptococcus pharyngitis
   Upper respiratory infection
   Viral syndrome
2. What tests, if any, would you order? How might the results affect your DX?
   Rapid strep test, if positive, would give definitive diagnosis of strep rather than symptom of sore throat
3. Write a Plan for this patient using all of the components discussed.

Rapid strep test now; if positive, prescribe amoxicillin.

Gargle with warm salt water 3 to 4 times a day. Use OTC throat sprays or lozenges as needed for comfort. Drink a lot of fluids to maintain hydration.

Follow up in 2 days if not improved, sooner if any vomiting and can't keep down medications or any difficulty breathing.

Worksheet 5.4 Answers

Plan Components

Which of the following would be documented in the plan? Underline all that apply.

physical examination findings
information from medical records
patient education
CBC results
R/O ankle fracture
laboratory and x-ray orders
vital signs
recommended OTC medications
follow-up instructions
review of systems
referrals

Number the following sentences in the suggested order they should appear in the plan.

4	Discussed the DDX with patient.
6	Follow-up in 2 weeks.
1	CT of chest if symptoms not resolved within 2 weeks.
2	Refer to respiratory for pulmonary function testing.
7	Go to the ED if shortness of breath worsens despite albuterol
5	Handout on monitoring peak expiratory flow readings given and explained.
3	Albuterol inhaler 1–2 puffs every 4–6 hours prn wheezing.

Worksheet 5.5 Answers

Sandra Harris Case

1. Analyze the subjective portion of the note. List additional information that should be included in the documentation.
   No documentation of any aggravating or alleviating factors. Need to document more associated signs and symptoms, such as abdominal pain, fever, chills, body aches, urinary symptoms. No documentation of any medication allergies. Patient is in age group in which she is probably still menstruating—need to know if she is and if

so, date of LMP. Should document whether any PMH that might contribute to symptoms. Need to document surgical history, especially if the patient has had abdominal surgery.

2. Analyze the objective portion of the note. List additional information that should be included in the documentation.
   Should document assessment of hydration status, such as skin turgor and appearance of mucous membranes. Reasonable to include ENT examination because DDX is broad. Need more documentation of abdominal examination, such as whether abdomen is soft, rigid, distended, or nondistended, and any tenderness to palpation.

3. Is the assessment supported by the subjective and objective information? Why or why not?
   No. The HX as documented does not support food poisoning. There is no documentation of any HX that supports GERD, such as indigestion; nausea and vomiting is not a typical presentation of GERD, so it is unlikely.

4. Did you consider other differential diagnoses than the ones documented? If so, list.
   Yes: viral gastritis/gastroenteritis, small bowel obstruction, lactose ingestion

5. What condition/symptom/diagnosis would be most appropriate to document for this visit? Can you find an ICD-9 code for it?
   Nausea and vomiting, 787.0; or gastritis, 535.0

6. Does the plan correspond to the assessment? Why or why not?
   No; IV fluid bolus and ibuprofen might be reasonable, but this is not the only therapeutic management that could be done and would not treat hepatitis A or GERD. CBC and BMP are not needed to diagnose food poisoning; there is no definitive test for food poisoning.

7. Did you consider other interventions that could be included in the plan? If so, list.
   Give the patient an antiemetic agent, preferably by intravenous route or rectally. UA should be done and possibly a pregnancy test depending on the date of the patient's last menstrual period and her gynecologic history. If patient has had abdominal surgery in the past, consider obtaining flat and upright abdominal radiographs.

Worksheet 5.6 Answers

SOAP Analysis

1. Analyze the subjective portion of the note. List additional information that should be included in the documentation.
   Considering the setting of emergency department, no additional subjective information is

needed. The HPI and the PMH are sufficiently focused to the chief complaint and setting, and the documentation is thorough.

2. Analyze the objective portion of the note. List additional information that should be included in the documentation.
No additional information needed. The general assessment reassures readers that the patient is not in any acute distress. Given the chief complaint and the setting, the examination is appropriately focused.

3. Is the assessment supported by the subjective and objective information? Why or why not?
Yes. Even though there is no objective swelling or difficulty breathing at the time the patient is seen in the ED, the subjective content sufficiently documented the patient's symptoms, his self-treatment, and the resolution of his symptoms.

4. Did you consider other differential diagnoses than the ones documented? If so, list.
Allergic reaction to medication or other substance; drug interaction

5. What condition/symptom/diagnosis would be most appropriate to document for this visit? Can you find an ICD-9 code for it?
Adverse effect of medication, 995.20
Allergy, unspecified, 995.3
Urticaria, 708

6. Does the plan correspond to the assessment? Why or why not?
Yes. Plan addresses the assessment by stopping the medication, informing the patient to follow up with PCP for medication management and what action to take if symptoms recur.

7. Did you consider other interventions that could be included in the plan? If so, list.
No; plan is appropriate

Worksheet 5.7 Answers
SOAP Note Analysis: Cassandra Fields

1. Analyze the subjective portion of the note. List additional information that should be included in the documentation.
None identified.

2. Analyze the objective portion of the note. List additional information that should be included in the documentation.
None identified.

3. Is the assessment supported by the subjective and objective information? Why or why not?
Yes; it is appropriate to list the presenting symptom followed by differential diagnoses that are being considered and require further work-up.

4. Did you consider other differential diagnoses than the ones documented? If so, list.
No.

5. What condition/symptom/diagnosis would be most appropriate to document for this visit? Can you find an ICD-9 code for it?
LLQ pain, 789.4
Constipation, 564.0

6. Does the plan correspond to the assessment? Why or why not?
Plan is extremely detailed and documents patient education that was provided regarding her condition; patient's desire to be treated as an outpatient because of caring for her husband; details of medical management, possible complications, and when to return for routine follow-up; and symptoms that prompt immediate call to provider.

7. Did you consider other interventions that could be included in the plan? If so, list.
None identified.

Worksheet 5.8 Answers
SOAP Note From Narrative
This is one possible SOAP note for Ms. Jacobs' visit.

SUBJECTIVE: Ms. Jacobs is a 57-year-old woman who presents with complaints of urine incontinence for the past 6 months. Initially, she had mostly stress incontinence with sneezing or coughing. In the past week, the problem is worse. She reports urgency, frequency, and nocturia. She also notes a strong odor to the urine. She has tried decreasing fluid intake and has quit drinking coffee, but this has not impacted her symptoms. PMH: no active or chronic diseases. Surgical history includes sinus surgery at age 28 and right carpal tunnel release at age 46. Medications: calcium supplement and multivitamin daily. She states an allergy to PCN, which causes a rash and swelling of the lips. OB history: G5 P5, all vaginal deliveries. Menopause since age 49. FH: Both parents deceased. Father died at age 61 from MI. Mother had diabetes; died from complications of colon cancer. Three siblings; one with HTN, one with diabetes. SH: married, monogamous relationship with spouse. Denies tobacco use. Alcohol intake limited to wine 2–3 times a month. Denies any illicit drug use. Typically drinks 2–3 cups of coffee and 3–4 glasses of tea daily, but has decreased fluid intake for the past week in hopes of alleviating urinary frequency. Exercise consists of daily walks, but she has not been able to do that for the past week as she is concerned about urinary incontinence when out walking.

ROS: General: denies fever, chills, weight loss or weight gain. HEENT: denies any problems. CV: denies chest pain, palpitations. RESP: denies cough, SOB, DOE. GI: denies abdominal pain. No change in bowel habits. GYN: reports some vaginal dryness, requiring use of lubricant for sexual activity. Denies hot flashes, mood swing. GU: denies burning or pain with urination. Other symptoms as reported in HPI. Denies hematuria. ENDO: denies polydipsia, polyphagia. No fluctuation in weight. No heat or cold intolerance.

OBJECTIVE EXAM:

General: WDWN female appearing stated age, in no distress. A&O, cooperative.

Vital signs: BP 124/72 P 86 RR 18 T 99.1 Wt: 174 lbs Ht: 5'8"

HEENT: head normocephalic, atraumatic. PEARL. TMs intact bilaterally.

NECK: supple, full ROM. No thyromegaly. No cervical adenopathy.

HEART: RRR, no gallops or murmurs.

LUNGS: CTA all fields.

ABD: soft, nondistended. Bowel sounds present all 4 quadrants. No organomegaly or masses. No tenderness to palpation. No flank tenderness.

PELVIC: atrophic changes noted of the external genitalia, but no erythema, lesions or masses. Vaginal mucosa pale, loss of ruga consistent with age-related changes. Cervix parous, pale, without discharge. Rectovaginal wall intact. Positive dribbling of urine with cough and bearing down.

RECTAL: no perirectal lesions or fissures. External rectal sphincter tone intact; rectal vault with soft brown stool; no masses.

LABS: urine dip test in office shows urine to be dark amber, clear. Specific gravity of 1.022; pH is 6.5. Negative for nitrites, leukocyte esterase, protein, blood, glucose, urobilinogen and bilirubin.

ASSESSMENT:

1) urinary incontinence, no signs of infection
2) post-menopausal
3) atrophic vaginitis

PLAN:

1) will send urine for culture
2) check post-void residual
3) discussed types of incontinence and provided pt with handout on incontinence
4) instructed pt on pelvic floor exercises and handout given
5) will have patient keep 24 hour urine diary for 3 days out of each week for the next 4 weeks
6) start topical Estrace Vaginal Cream 42.5 g nightly at bedtime
7) pt to return in 4 weeks for follow-up evaluation

Worksheet 5.9 Answers

Abbreviations

A&O	alert and oriented
BID	twice a day
BMP	basic metabolic panel
cm	centimeter
CT	computed tomography
CVA	cerebrovascular accident
DDX	differential diagnosis
DM	diabetes mellitus
ED	emergency department
FH	family history
GERD	gastroesophageal reflux disease
HgbA1c, HbA1c	hemoglobin A1c or glycosylated hemoglobin
HCTZ	hydrochlorothiazide
HR	heart rate
HX, Hx	history
IV	intravenous
JVD	jugular venous distention
LLQ	left lower quadrant
MCH	mean corpuscular hemoglobin
MCHC	mean corpuscular hemoglobin concentration
MCV	mean corpuscular volume
mg	milligram
MRI	magnetic resonance imaging
NAD	no acute distress
NKDA	no known drug allergies
NSR	normal sinus rhythm
N/V	nausea and vomiting
OB/GYN	obstetrics and gynecology
PCP	primary care provider
PPD	packs per day
PRN	as required
RBC	red blood cell
RDW	red blood cell distribution width
RICE	rest, ice, compression, elevation
RLQ	right lower quadrant
UTI	urinary tract infection
WDWN	well developed, well nourished

Chapter 6

Worksheet 6.1 Answers

1. In addition to a SOAP note, identify at least four types of documentation that could be kept in a patient's medical record.

Any of the following: demographic information, billing information, problem list, medication list, flow sheet, noncompliance note, results of laboratory or other diagnostic studies, communication from other providers, medical records from other providers, advance directives, documentation of telephone calls and e-mails

2. Explain the rationale for using a medication list.
   Any of the following: The medication list provides a way to get a lot of information quickly. It allows the provider to see all the medications a patient is taking, the dose, how long on the medication, and the reason for it. It also allows the provider to see allergies, OTC products, supplements, etc. It provides a place to list the pharmacy, phone number and location, and insurance information that may be needed when writing prescriptions.

3. Figure 6-5 shows a flow sheet used to track information for a patient who is on anticoagulation therapy. Identify at least three other conditions for which a flow sheet might be used and the information that could be included.
   Any of the following: diabetes, to track blood glucose and $HgbA1_C$ levels; anemia, to track Hgb and Hct levels or treatment, such as vitamin B_{12} injections; dyslipidemia, to record levels of cholesterol, HDL, LDL, triglycerides; birth control, to record dates of injections; hypertension, to record blood pressure readings; COPD, to record results of pulmonary function tests, etc.

4. Identify the two basic kinds of advance directives.
   Living will and durable power of attorney.

5. Describe the purpose of a living will.
   A living will expresses the patient's preference for medical care in such matters as cardiopulmonary resuscitation, artificial nutrition and hydration, mechanical ventilation, etc.

6. Describe the purpose of a durable power of attorney.
   A durable power of attorney appoints someone to make decisions about health care in the event that the patient is unable to make his or her own decision.

7. Caring Connections is a program of the National Hospice and Palliative Care Organization. Visit their website at www.caringinfo.org and find your state's requirements for a living will and power of attorney.

8. Identify at least four components of a telephone call that should be documented and placed in the patient's medical record.
   Any of the following: date, time, identity of caller, relationship to patient if not the patient, complaint or signs and symptoms, advice given, recommendations for care, disposition, follow-up care

9. Identify three advantages to using e-mail to communicate with patients.
   Any of the following: eliminates phone tag, may result in fewer interruptions to the provider, can be done at a time convenient for the patient and the provider, establishes written record of what was said or not said, potential cost savings

10. Identify three disadvantages to using e-mail to communicate with patients.
    Any of the following: requires encrypted e-mail system; can be intercepted, altered, or delivered to the wrong person; may not reach the intended person; lack of reimbursement; poorly written or misinterpreted e-mails may cause legal problems; potential abuse of e-mail by patients; patients expect immediate response; may transmit computer viruses

11. Visit the websites of the American Medical Association (AMA) and the American Medical Informatics Association (AMIA). Identify at least four guidelines for providers who choose to communicate with patients by e-mail.
    Any of the following: establish turn-around time for messages; do not use e-mail for urgent matters; inform patient about privacy issues; patients should know who besides addressee processes messages during addressee's usual business hours and during addressee's vacation or illness; print all messages, with replies and confirmation of receipt, and place in the patient's chart; inform patients that e-mail communications will be kept in the medical record; establish types of transactions (prescription refill, appointment scheduling, etc.) and sensitivity of subject matter (HIV, mental health, etc.) permitted over e-mail; instruct patients to put the category of transaction in the subject line of the message for filtering—prescription, appointment, medical advice, billing question; request that patients put their name and patient identification number in the body of the message; configure automatic reply to acknowledge receipt of messages; send a new message to inform patient of completion of request; request that patients use auto-reply feature to acknowledge reading clinician's

message; develop archival and retrieval mechanisms; maintain a mailing list of patients, but do not send group mailings in which recipients are visible to each other; use blind copy feature in software; avoid anger, sarcasm, harsh criticism, and libelous references to third parties in messages; append a standard block of text to the end of e-mail messages to patients that contains the physician's full name, contact information, and reminders about security and the importance of alternative forms of communication for emergencies; explain to patients that their messages should be concise; when e-mail messages become too lengthy or the correspondence is prolonged, notify patients to come in to discuss or call them; remind patients when they do not adhere to the guidelines; for patients who repeatedly do not adhere to the guidelines, it is acceptable to terminate the e-mail relationship

12. Identify three benefits that providers, hospitals, or health systems can realize with social networking.
Any of the following: market services they provide; communicate with colleagues; quickly disseminate research findings; attract new patients; share practice management tips; build consensus on issues; increase presence in the community; stay abreast of medical news

13. List three concerns related to providers having pages on social networking sites.
Any of the following: blurring of professional and private lives; violating boundaries of patient–provider relationship; use of information by residency programs, potential employers, etc. to make decisions; no control over the information posted; permanence of information on the Internet; no anonymity; breach of patient confidentiality

14. Identify at least three recommendations to providers who choose to have a presence on a social networking site.
Any of the following: maintain separate sites for professional and personal use; establish guidelines for postings and who is granted access to the site; post a disclaimer stating that the provider is not giving medical advice

Worksheet 6.2 Answers

Jennifer Erwin

Health History / Problem List

Name: Jennifer Erwin	S.S.# ____-____-_____	Male____	Adv. Directives Yes __ No __
DOB:	Tel.# ____-____-_____	Fem ___G __ P __ Ab __	Organ Donor Yes __ No__
PROBLEM LIST		ALLERGIES:	
1.		Hospitalizations:	Surgeries:
2.		Date:	Reason:	Date:	Reason:
3.			
4.			
5.			
6.			
7.			
8.			
9.			
10.			

Social History	Family History	CANCER: colon ____ breast ____ other ____
S ____ M ____ D ____ W ____	Father:	HTN: CAD: CVA:
Smoking: ETOH:	Mother:	DM:
Caffeine: Exercise:	Siblings:	Osteoporosis:
Occup:	Children:	Other:

Breast	Date						
	Result						
Pap/Pelvic Exam	Date						
	Result						
Mammogram	Date						
	Result						
Prostate/Testicular	Date						
	Result						
PSA	Date						
	Result						
Colonoscopy/Sigmoid	Date						
	Result						
FOBT Cards	Date						
	Result						
CBC	Date						
	Result						
CMP	Date						
	Result						
TSH	Date						
	Result						
Total Cholesterol	Date						
	Result						
HDL	Date						
	Result						
LDL	Date						
	Result						
Triglycerides	Date						
	Result						
CXR	Date						
	Result						
ECG	Date						
	Result						
DEXA	Date						
	Result						

Worksheet 6.3 Answers
Ms. Monica Jacobs

Health History / Problem List

Name: Jacobs, Monica	S.S.# ____-____-_____	Male ____	Adv. Directives Yes __ No __
DOB:	Tel.# ____-____-_____	Fem _X_ G _5_ P _5_ Ab __	Organ Donor Yes __ No__

PROBLEM LIST | ALLERGIES: penicillin

PROBLEM LIST	Hospitalizations:	Surgeries:

1. urinary incontinence		
2.	Date:	Reason:	Date/Age:	Reason:
3.			28	sinus surgery - chronic inf.
4.			46	R carpal tunnel release
5.				
6.				
7.				
8.				
9.				
10.				

Social History	Family History	CANCER: colon _X_ breast ____ other ____
S ____ M _X_ D ____ W ____	Father:	HTN: X CAD: X CVA:
Smoking: ETOH:	Mother:	DM: mother, type 2 and sister
Caffeine: Exercise:	Siblings:	Osteoporosis:
Occup:	Children:	Other:

Breast	Date / Result							
Pap/Pelvic Exam	Date / Result							
Mammogram	Date / Result							
Prostate/Testicular	Date / Result							
PSA	Date / Result							
Colonoscopy/Sigmoid	Date / Result							
FOBT Cards	Date / Result							
CBC	Date / Result							
CMP	Date / Result							
TSH	Date / Result							
Total Cholesterol	Date / Result							
HDL	Date / Result							
LDL	Date / Result							
Triglycerides	Date / Result							
CXR	Date / Result							
ECG	Date / Result							
DEXA	Date / Result							

Worksheet 6.4 Answers

Recording Telephone Calls

This is one example of how this call could be documented.

Peoria Pediatrics Telephone Log Form

Date: _6 / 22 / xx_   Time __1610__

Caller/Relationship: __Cindy Florinda, mother__

Patient: __Tyler Florinda__   Age: __15 months__

Reason for call: __fever and rash__

HPI / PMH: __Fever onset last night, rash today. Decreased appetite. No N/V/D, + runny nose. No cough. Last wet diaper 4 hours ago. No ill contacts. Rash nonpruritic. Decreased appetite but taking fluids OK. Fever down with Advil. Had MMR vaccine about 10 days ago.__

Medications: __Advil 200 mg PRN, no regular meds.__

Allergies: __NKDA__

Diagnosis: __Vaccine side effect.__

Recommendations/Rx: __Continue Advil; observe.__

Disposition: __home__

Follow-up: __Notify if fever > 48 hr, no wet diaper > 6 hours, or lethargy.__

Pharmacy: _____ Phone: _____

Billing:

Worksheet 6.5 Answers

Abbreviations

ACE, ACEI	angiotensin-converting enzyme, angiotensin-converting enzyme inhibitor
AHIMA	American Health Information Management Association
AMIA	American Medical Informatics Association
AP	anteroposterior
CTA	clear to auscultation
INR	International Normalized Ratio
MMR	measles, mumps, rubella
N/V/D	nausea, vomiting, diarrhea
POA	power of attorney
PT	prothrombin time
SSN	social security number

Chapter 7

Worksheet 7.1 Answers

1. Is this a medical or surgical admission?
   Medical
2. The medication listed for this patient is aspirin. Based on the documented PMH, what is the indication for this medication?
   Nothing documented in PMH or HPI to indcate why he is taking aspirin, so the indication for it is unknown.

3. What additional information should be documented about the medication?

How many milligrams per dose, dosing frequency, route, and indication

4. Do you feel that the information documented in the social history is sufficient? Why or why not?

No; it does not address some of the important information that should be documented, such as his support system, living arrangements, education, language, etc. Does not document quantity and frequency of alcohol intake.

5. List the systems explored in the ROS and the total number of systems reviewed.

Genitourinary, cardiovascular, respiratory, abdominal, hematologic, neurologic, eyes, for seven systems

6. Does the ROS meet CMS guidelines for documentation? Why or why not?

Yes. Although CMS identifies 14 systems, the guidelines do not specifically say how many systems have to be reviewed. The number of systems reviewed may affect the level of E/M and billing.

7. Do you think the H&P contains enough information to justify hospital admission? Why or why not?

Yes, there are enough problems identified that the patient would need hospitalization. It would be difficult to justify a need for hospitalization based only on HPI, but the document as a whole demonstrates that the patient has multiple problems that need to be managed.

8. Read the assessment section and then the laboratory data section. Identify any additional information that you think should be recorded in the laboratory data section.

Results of urinalysis should be documented, especially because his chief complaint is related to the genitourinary system.

9. After reading and critically analyzing the H&P, identify strengths and weaknesses of the document.

Weaknesses: More information in HPI, addressing all the cardinal elements. Including dates of the surgeries might be helpful, especially if the TURP had been done recently and might affect the patient's overall management. Need more information about the aspirin, as noted previously. More psychosocial history. Document UA results in laboratory data. One assessment documented is the result of a diagnostic test; this could be relevant, but the documentation does not establish the relevancy.

Strengths: The assessment and plan are well-documented, and the enumerated lists make it easy to identify the problems and follow the plan of care.

Worksheet 7.2 Answers

This is one possible order set for Mr. Hunter.

Admit to Dr. Samuel Mason to medical floor
Diagnosis: (1) Urosepsis
             (2) Acute renal failure
             (3) Hx of TURP
Stable condition
Up ad lib, encourage ambulation
Vital signs every 8 hours while awake
Allergies: NKDA
Regular diet
NS at 200 cc/hr
Daily intake and output
ASA 81 mg daily by mouth for CVD prophylaxis
Metronidazole 500 mg IV every 6 hours; start after blood and urine cultures obtained
Acetaminophen 500 mg tabs one or two every 4 hours prn temp >101.5° or for headache
Esomeprazole 40 mg PO daily
Urine culture, Gram stain and sensitivity
Blood cultures times 2 at 30-minute interval
PSA
CBC, BUN, creatinine daily times 3 days
Urology consultation with Dr. David Parrack
Notify Dr. Mason of temp >102° or patient unable to void for >6 hours

Worksheet 7.3 Answers

This is one possible admit note for Mr. Hunter.

> Date: xx/xx/xx
> Time: 1502

Admit note: Mr. Hunter is a 76-year-old man who has had urinary frequency and urgency for 1 week. He developed a fever 2 days ago and has developed nausea but no vomiting. History significant for TURP approximately 8 months ago by Dr. David Parrack. Patient's current medication is ASA only for CVD prophylaxis. NKDA. Temp is 100.3°, other vital signs stable. UA shows hematuria, bacteriuria. CBC with WBC of 12.9. Creatinine 1.4; BUN 25. Urine and blood cultures pending. Will admit and begin antibiotic therapy, GI prophylaxis with Nexium. Consult Dr. Parrack to see this patient in a.m. Admission H&P done and dictated XX/XX/XX at 1437. Samuel Mason, MD.

Worksheet 7.4 Answers

1. Is this a medical or surgical admission?

Medical

2. Review the PMH and identify strengths and weaknesses as documented.

Strengths: HPI is okay. PMH easy to follow with the numbered list, as is medication list. Examination is appropriately focused to problem responsible for admission.

Weaknesses: There is no indication of the present status of the conditions listed in PMH. No reaction to the medications to which patient is allergic. Route not indicated for several of the medications. Social history not well documented. Not sure which systems were reviewed in ROS.

3. The author states, "10-point review of systems is negative." Identify any information you find in other parts of the document that could be counted as ROS. List the systems reviewed and the total number of systems reviewed. Cardiovascular, neurological, eyes, respiratory, musculoskeletal, gastrointestinal; six systems identified.

4. Based on the discussion of documenting the psychosocial history in Chapter 2, what elements could be added to the social history to make it more complete?

If the patient has a support system; what are her current living arrangements; if she may need help at time of discharge; if she has any religious or dietary practices that she wishes to observe while in the hospital; who she wants involved in medical decision making, if anyone. Frequency and quantity of alcohol intake are not documented.

5. The assessment and plan in this admission H&P is a slightly different format compared with other H&Ps you have seen in this chapter. Do you feel the assessment and plan sections, as documented, sufficiently reflect a reason for hospitalization for this patient? Does it meet CMS guidelines for documentation? Why or why not? Yes, new onset of atrial fibrillation with symptoms is a reason for hospitalization. Probably does meet CMS guidelines for documentation, although it would be helpful to have a specific comment on the status of all the patient's comorbid conditions.

Worksheet 7.5 Answers

This is one possible order set for Mrs. McLaughlin.

Date: xx/xx/xx
Time: 1132
Admit to Dr. JoAnn Brooks to telemetry floor
Diagnoses:
(1) New-onset atrial fibrillation with fast ventricular response
(2) Type 2 diabetes, uncontrolled
(3) Peripheral neuropathy
(4) Hypertension

(5) Hx of mitral regurgitation
Condition: stable
Activity: up with assistance
Continue cardiac monitor
Oxygen at 2 L/min via nasal cannula
Consult Dr. Victor Kaplan, cardiology
Vital signs every 4 hours
ALLERGIES: PENICILLIN, SULFA
2000-calorie ADA diet
Accu-Chek before meals and at bedtime
Saline lock
Diltiazem bolus of 20 mg IV then continuous infusion at 10 mg/hr
Metoprolol 50 mg PO bid for rate control
Enoxaparin 40 mg subcutaneously (subQ) once daily
Xanax 0.25 mg PO twice daily for anxiety
Lantus insulin 22 units in the morning subcutaneously
Regular insulin per sliding scale as follows:

Blood Glucose:	Units of Insulin
151–200	3
201–250	5
251–300	7
301–350	10
351–400	12
>400	notify physician

Hold lisinopril at present
Troponin and ECGs at 1700 and 2200
Notify if heart rate <60 or >150 beats/min

JoAnn Brooks, MD

Worksheet 7.6 Answer

This is one possible admit note for Mrs. Gladys McLaughlin.

xx/xx/xx
1145

This is a 74-year-old woman with a Hx of type 2 diabetes, peripheral neuropathy, HTN, mitral regurgitation, and osteoporosis who presented to her PCP Dr. Rosenberg today with complaint of lightheadedness. Onset of symptoms yesterday that have persisted. ECG at Dr. Rosenberg's office earlier today showed new-onset atrial fibrillation. She denies associated chest pain or pressure, syncope, SOB or DOE, slurred speech, or difficulty moving extremities. Presently her blood pressure is 109/67, pulse is 110 and irregular, respirations are 16, temperature is 97.8°. Heart irregular, slightly tachycardic, 2/6 systolic murmur. No JVD. Lungs are clear. Repeat ECG with atrial fibrillation and fast ventricular response around 150 with right bundle branch block. Initial troponin negative. Will admit to telemetry, consult with Dr. Kaplan. Start rate control with IV diltiazem and oral metoprolol. Start enoxaparin. Hold

ACE for now. Glucose today was 481. Will continue Lantus 22 units subcutaneously and start Regular insulin by sliding scale. Continue with R/O MI per usual protocol. Admit H&P done and dictated at 1157.

JoAnn Brooks, MD

Worksheet 7.7 Answers

Abbreviations

ADA	American Diabetes Association
AD CAVA DIMPLS	admit, diagnosis, condition, activities, vital signs, allergies, diet, interventions, medications, procedures, labs, special instructions
ADE	adverse drug event
AP	anteroposterior
BR	bed rest
BRP	bathroom privileges
BUN	blood, urea, nitrogen
CDSS	clinical decision support system
CEA	carcinoembryonic antigen
CPOE	computerized physician (or provider) order entry
D5NS	5% dextrose in normal saline
H&H	hematocrit and hemoglobin
ICS	incentive spirometry
ISMP	Institute for Safe Medical Practice
LDL	low-density lipoprotein
NCEP	National Cholesteral Education Program
NPO	nothing per os, or nothing by mouth
NS	normal saline
OCR	Office of Civil Rights
OOB	out of bed
PACU	postanesthesia care unit
PCA	patient-controlled analgesia
PT	physical therapy
RLL	right lower lobe
SDS	same day surgery
S/P	status post, or after
SR	slow release
SVN	single volume nebulizer
TID	three times daily
TURP	transurethral resection of the prostate

Chapter 8

Worksheet 8.1 Answers

1. List several questions that should be answered daily for postoperative patients.
   Any of the following: Is the patient the same, better, or worse? Is the patient getting adequate pain relief? Has bowel function returned? Can the activity level be advanced? Can the diet be advanced? Can any sutures, staples, tubes, or drains be removed? Is the patient having any fever, cough, shortness of breath, or difficulty breathing?
2. A postoperative patient has been on a full liquid diet for the past 24 hours. He now has full bowel sounds and says he is hungry. Write an order for a change in diet.
   Advance diet to regular diet as tolerated.
3. List seven components of a procedure note.
   name of procedure; indication for procedure; consent; anesthesia; details of the procedure; findings; complications
4. List at least five components of an operative note.
   Any of the following: date of procedure; name of procedure; indication; surgeon; surgical assistant; anesthesia; preoperative diagnosis; postoperative diagnosis; EBL; drains, if any; type of specimens obtained, if any; complications; disposition
5. List at least five components of a delivery note.
   Any of the following: type of delivery; estimated gestational age of the fetus; viability of fetus; sex of fetus; Apgar scores at 1 and 5 minutes; weight of fetus; delivery of placenta; if any lacerations or episiotomy; EBL; condition of mother immediately after delivery
6. List the five Ws that could be sources of postoperative fever.
   Wind, wound, water, walk, wonder drugs

Worksheet 8.2 Answers

Here is one possible operative note for Mrs. Stevens.

Date of procedure: xx/xx/xxxx
Name of procedure: right carpal tunnel release
Indication: right hand chronic with intractable pain, numbness, and tingling
Surgeon: Ralph Benedict, DO
Surgical Assistant: Susan Carmichael, PA-C
Anesthesia: distal wrist block; Wendy Falconetti, CRNA
Preoperative diagnosis: carpal tunnel syndrome, right hand
Postoperative diagnosis: carpal tunnel syndrome, right hand, severe
EBL: <40 cc
Complications: none
Disposition: awake, alert, and to recovery in stable condition

Susan Carmichael, PA-C

Worksheet 8.3 Answers

1. What additional information about consent should be documented in the procedure note?

The risks of the procedure, benefits of the procedure, potential complications, and the name and relationship of the person giving consent

2. After critically analyzing the note and comparing it with the one presented in the chapter, what additional information should be documented in the note?

   Any of the following: the type of local anesthetic solution used; type of solution used to prep the skin; date and time the procedure was done; description of the fluid that was obtained

   Digging deeper: Information about paracentesis was not specifically presented in this chapter; however, you are encouraged to read about this procedure and answer the following questions.

3. List at least two laboratory values that are typically evaluated and documented before a paracentesis is performed.

   Any of the following: PT/PTT, INR, platelet count

4. List at least three tests that are typically ordered to evaluate ascitic fluid.

   Any of the following: protein, albumin, specific gravity, glucose, bilirubin, amylase, lipase, triglyceride, LDH; cell count and differential

Worksheet 8.4 Answers

1. List at least three problems, symptoms, or complaints documented in the H&P that should be followed up when rounding on Mr. Hunter the day after his admission and documented in the subjective portion of the daily visit note. State your rationale for including each one.

   Any of the following:
   - Is he still having urgency or frequency; because this was a complaint on admission
   - Is he still having nausea; because this was a complaint on admission
   - Has he vomited; could be part of his illness and/or medication side effect
   - Does he feel about the same, better, or worse; to get the patient's perspective on how he feels and compare with your own assessment
   - Ask if any new problems or complaints; to identify whether Mr. Hunter has developed problems other than those present at time of admission

2. List at least three findings that should be documented in the objective portion of the daily visit note and state your rationale for including each one.

   Any of the following:
   - Temperature; because he was febrile at the time of admission
   - General assessment; because this should be documented in every daily visit note

- Heart examination; because this should be documented in every daily visit note
- Lung examination; because this should be documented in every daily visit note
- Result of PSA, if available; because this was ordered, and time of admission and results of all laboratory tests ordered should be followed up and documented
- Review of urology consult if available; to determine whether any change in management is recommended by the specialist

3. List at least three problems, symptoms, or complaints documented in the H&P that should be followed up when rounding on Mrs. McLaughlin the day after her admission and documented in the subjective portion of the daily visit note. State your rationale for including each one.

   Any of the following:
   - Any lightheadedness; because this symptom was present at time of admission
   - Any chest pain; because she was admitted to continue work-up to rule out MI
   - If she feels the same, better, or worse; to get the patient's perspective on how she feels and compare with your own assessment
   - If she has had any difficulty breathing; because this symptom could be associated with having an MI or an arrhythmia
   - If she has any new problems or complaints; to monitor for new problems that could indicate side effects of treatment or change in condition

4. List at least three findings that should be documented in the objective portion of the daily visit note and state your rationale for including each one.

   Any of the following:
   - General assessment; because this should be documented as part of every daily visit note
   - Heart rate and rhythm; to assess response to treatment for her arrhythmia
   - Results of cardiac enzymes, ECG, or any other diagnostic tests; to determine whether there are any changes from baseline because she is being observed to rule out MI
   - BP range or most recent reading; because she has a history of hypertension and her antihypertensive medication is being held at this time
   - Blood glucose range or most recent reading; because she has uncontrolled diabetes mellitus
   - Heart examination; because she is admitted for a cardiac problem, and it should be documented in every daily visit note
   - Lung examination; because it should be documented in every daily visit note

Worksheet 8.5 Answers

CRNA	certified registered nurse anesthetist
EBL	estimated blood loss
I&O	intake and output
IM	intramuscular
NSVD	normal spontaneous vaginal delivery
POD	postoperative day
SMA	superior mesenteric artery
SR	sustained release

Chapter 9

Worksheet 9.1 Answers

Discharge Orders and Discharge Summary

1. List three components of the discharge orders.
   Any of the following: disposition; activity with specific instructions; diet; medications; follow-up instructions; notification instructions

2. List three components that should be addressed when instructing a patient on activity at the time of a hospital discharge.
   Specific restrictions on driving, lifting
   How long restrictions are in place
   Wound care instructions

3. List at least seven components of a discharge summary.
   Any of the following: date of admission; date of discharge; attending physician; consulting physician(s); admitting diagnoses; discharge diagnoses; brief history; physical examination findings; laboratory results; medications; hospital course; follow-up instructions; notification instructions

4. List at least three entities that may ask for (or are likely to receive a copy of) the discharge summary.
   Any of the following: primary care provider; consulting physician; facility to which the patient is being transferred; insurance or payer

5. List at least three diagnoses for patients who are most likely to leave a hospital AMA.
   Chest pain, substance abuse problems, mental health diagnoses

6. List at least three elements that should be included in an AMA note.
   Any of the following: document the benefits and risks associated with leaving; name and relationship of any witnesses to the conversations; quotes by the patient of why he or she is leaving; follow-up care and other discharge instructions

Worksheet 9.2 Answers

Discharge Summary for Ronald Hearst

1. How long was Mr. Hearst in the hospital?
   11 days

2. Which discharge diagnoses listed are not addressed in the narrative of the hospital course? (list)
   Right fifth metacarpal fracture, abnormality of liver enzymes, hepatitis B, malnutrition, urinary tract infection

3. Mr. Hearst will be transferred to a psychiatric facility. If you were a provider at the receiving facility, what criticisms would you have of this discharge summary?
   Any of the following: The narrative of the hospital course is extremely limited considering the patient was in the hospital for 11 days; does not include any H&P information, only refers to H&P; no baseline laboratory values for comparison; no information on how long patient was in PAT or how that was treated; no information on treatment of fifth metacarpal fracture; acute renal failure is mentioned, but no corresponding laboratory values related to kidney function are provided; do not know patient's kidney function at time of discharge; no mention of when urinary infection developed or how it was treated; no specific information on diabetes or the status of it during the hospitalization; no information on encephalopathy; lacking details of the patient's psychiatric/behavioral problems (when developed, how treated, specific details of agitation; how patient was managed); no specific information on patient's condition to show that he is ready for discharge.

4. What findings support that Mr. Hearst is ready for discharge from the hospital?
   Only information provided is that patient is improved and stable; lacks specific criteria assessed to determine his readiness for transfer

5. Refer to Figure 9-3, Discharge Summary for Mr. Jensen. Identify at least three elements included in that discharge summary that are not included in Mr. Hearst's discharge summary.
   Any of the following: brief history of present illness; past medical history; physical examination findings; vital signs; laboratory results

Worksheet 9.3 Answers

Discharge Summary for Henry Oliver

1. What complications developed postoperatively that are not listed as discharge diagnoses?
   Anemia requiring transfusion; hypomagnesemia; hypokalemia

2. If you were Dr. Knowles, the patient's primary care provider, what information would you like to know that is not included in this discharge summary?
   Any of the following: HPI/PMH; events leading up to need for surgery; baseline physical examination; preoperative work-up (e.g., radiographs,

CT, MRI); what was cultured; what was patient's H&H on postoperative day 2 before and after the transfusion; magnesium level; potassium level; treatment for the electrolyte imbalance; how long patient will be in a long leg cast; when should patient have the cast applied; what limitations does the patient have while the cast is on; when is the patient to follow up with PCP or orthopedist.

3. What type of culture was obtained and what is the significance of the results reported in the discharge summary?
   The culture source is not identified; final cultures were negative, but without knowing the source, it is difficult to determine the significance of these results.

4. What findings support that Mr. Oliver is ready for discharge from the hospital?
   He is able to ambulate 200 feet with physical therapy, and he is stable.

5. What specific information is missing from the discharge instruction section of the summary?
   Any of the following: what limitations patient has while wearing splint; how much weight should he place on affected leg; exactly when he should be seen to have cast placed; when to follow up with PCP; when to follow up to have cast removed.

Worksheet 9.4 Answers

Discharge Summary for Mrs. Gladys McLaughlin

This is one possible discharge summary for Mrs. McLaughlin. This is certainly not the only way the discharge summary could be written.

Date of Admission: xx/xx/20xx
Date of Discharge: xx/xx/20xx
Admitting Diagnosis:
1. Atrial fibrillation
2. Hypertension
3. Type 2 diabetes mellitus, uncontrolled
4. Osteoporosis
5. Mitral regurgitation
6. Peripheral neuropathy due to diabetes
7. Kyphosis
Discharge Diagnosis:
1. Atrial fibrillation; converted to NSR; stable
2. Hypertension; stable
3. Type 2 diabetes mellitus, improved control
4. Osteoporosis; stable
5. Mitral regurgitation; stable
6. Peripheral neuropathy due to diabetes; stable
7. Kyphosis
8. Urinary tract infection; resolving
Attending Physician: JoAnn Brooks, MD
Primary Care Physician: Charles Rosenberg, MD

Consulting Physician: Dr. Trent Kendall, cardiologist

Brief History: This is a 74-year-old woman who presented to Dr. Rosenberg for a routine physical. At the time, she did have some complaints of dizziness. An ECG in his office showed atrial fibrillation. She did not have any chest pain or pressure or other cardiac symptoms, but because this was a new onset, she was admitted to rule out myocardial infarction and get control of her rate. Her PMH is significant for HTN, type 2 diabetes, peripheral neuropathy, GERD, mitral regurgitation, and osteoporosis. Regular home medications include the following:

Lantus 22 units in the morning subcutaneously
Lisinopril 5 mg daily
Omeprazole 40 mg daily
Celebrex 200 mg daily
Xanax 0.25 mg twice daily
Aspirin 81 mg daily
Boniva 150 mg monthly
Mirtazapine 30 mg daily at bedtime

The patient is **ALLERGIC TO PENICILLIN AND SULFA** drugs. She cannot recall any specific reaction to penicillin. She states that she breaks out in a rash from sulfa medications. On admission, her physical examination was positive for irregular heart rate and a 2/6 systolic murmur. Her blood pressure was 109/67. She has marked kyphosis. The examination was otherwise unremarkable. Pertinent laboratory results include an ECG showing atrial fibrillation with a fast ventricular response and a right bundle branch block. Her initial troponin level was normal. Her glucose was elevated at 481. Urinalysis was positive for WBCs and was sent for culture.

Hospital Course: The patient was admitted to rule out MI and to get control of her diabetes and heart rate. She was continued on her regular home medications except for the lisinopril, which was held because her pressure was a little low, and she was having dizziness. She was started on a Cardizem drip. Serial ECGs and cardiac enzymes were obtained. There were no ischemic changes on any of the ECGs. All cardiac enzymes were negative. She was seen in consultation by Dr. Kendall, who agreed that the patient did not have an MI. He added metoprolol for rate control. The heart rhythm converted from atrial fibrillation to normal sinus rhythm after 48 hours. The Cardizem was discontinued, and the patient did well on metoprolol with appropriate rate control. Her blood pressure increased on the second hospital day, and she was started back on lisinopril. Her blood glucose levels continued to be elevated. She was on her usual dose of Lantus insulin of 22 units and also had sliding scale coverage with regular insulin. She was also found to have a UTI confirmed by positive culture. She was started on Cipro 500 mg bid for the UTI. Over the course of the next 3 days, her blood glucose levels normalized. She remained asymptomatic without dysuria or frequency. She did not develop any new problems during the hospital stay. She was able to ambulate without difficulty.

Condition at Discharge: No more dizziness and no episodes of chest pain or pressure; atrial fibrillation converted to NSR, so the patient was stable from a cardiac standpoint. Her glucose levels came down with the Lantus and sliding-scale coverage. Her glucose was stable over the past 24 hours without any sliding-scale coverage. Her hypertension was well controlled on the lisinopril. She was thought to be ready for discharge.

Disposition: home with daughter
Discharge medications:
1. Metoprolol 50 mg PO bid; prescription written
2. Cipro 500 mg PO bid × 2 days; prescription written
3. Lisinopril 5 mg PO daily in a.m.
4. Omeprazole 40 mg PO daily
5. Celebrex 200 mg PO daily
6. Xanax 0.25 mg PO daily
7. Lantus 22 units subQ daily in a.m.
8. Aspirin 81 mg PO daily
9. Boniva 150 mg once monthly
10. Mirtazapine 30 mg PO daily at bedtime

Discharge Instructions: Follow up with Dr. Rosenberg in 1 week and Dr. Kendall (cardiologist) in 2 weeks. No driving for 2 weeks; otherwise, activity as tolerated. Resume 1800-calorie ADA, heart-healthy diet. Notify Dr. Rosenberg of any episodes of chest pain or pressure, dizziness, or any new symptoms.

Worksheet 9.5 Answers
Discharge Orders for Mrs. Gladys McLaughlin

Here is one possible set of discharge orders for Mrs. McLaughlin.

1. Discharge patient home in care of daughter.
2. No driving for 2 weeks; otherwise, activity as tolerated
3. 1800-calorie ADA, heart-healthy diet
4. Metoprolol 50 mg PO bid; prescription written
5. Cipro 500 mg PO bid × 2 days; prescription written
6. Lisinopril 5 mg PO daily in a.m.
7. Omeprazole 40 mg PO daily
8. Celebrex 200 mg PO daily
9. Xanax 0.25 mg PO daily
10. Lantus 22 units subQ daily in a.m.
11. Aspirin 81 mg PO daily
12. Boniva 150 mg once monthly
13. Mirtazapine 30 mg PO daily at bedtime
14. Follow up with Dr. Rosenberg in 1 week
15. Follow up with Dr. Kendall, cardiologist, in 2 weeks
16. Notify Dr. Rosenberg immediately of any chest pain or pressure, dizziness, or any new symptoms

Worksheet 9.6 Answers
Abbreviations

AMA	against medical advice
BM	bowel movement
MI	myocardial infarction
ORIF	open reduction, internal fixation
RN	registered nurse

Chapter 10

Worksheet 10.1 Answers

1. State two purposes of DEA registration.
   Prevent diversion and abuse of controlled substances; ensure adequate supply of medications for valid reasons.
2. If federal prescribing law differs from state law, which must the prescriber follow?
   Whichever is the most stringent.
3. List at least two characteristics of tamper-proof prescription pads.
   Any of the following: features that prevent unauthorized copying; features that prevent the erasure or modification of information written on the prescription; features that prevent use of counterfeit prescription forms
4. List at least five precautions that prescribers should take to control and protect their DEA registration.
   Any of the following: keep prescription blanks in a safe place where they cannot be stolen; do not use prescription pads for writing notes; use tamper-resistant pads; do not print the DEA number on pads, but write it in only when needed; do not use DEA number as an identifier; control the number of people who have access to DEA number; do not display DEA certificate.
5. Match the following terms and definitions.

   A. signa   __B__ name and strength of the medication

   B. inscription   __D__ reason the patient is to take the medication

   C. subscription __A__ instructions to patient on how to take the medication

D. indication   __E__   medical use and abuse potential

E. schedule   __C__   information on dosage form and units to dispense

6. List at least five common errors made in prescription writing.

Any of the following: illegibility; omissions, such as leaving off drug strength or quantity to dispense; exceeding recommended dose; not including the indication for prn medication; not meeting legal requirements, such as including DEA number or dispensing quantity above that allowed by law; quantity does not match directions; incomplete directions; omitting a leading zero or including a trailing zero.

7. List the four elements required to meet the standards for qualified e-prescribing.

Generating a complete active medication list; selecting medications, printing prescriptions, electronically transmitting prescriptions, and conducting all safety checks; providing information related to the availability of lower cost, therapeutically approved alternative medications; providing information on formulary or tiered formulary medications, patient eligibility, and authorization requirements received electronically from the patient's drug plan

8. List at least three benefits to e-prescribing.

Any of the following: legibility; preventing drug–drug interaction errors; providing alerts to allergies or drug interactions or drug–disease interactions; preventing transcribing errors; decreasing the amount of time pharmacy staff spends on phone calls to clarify prescriptions; cost-effectiveness; may increase patient compliance

9. List at least three barriers to e-prescribing.

Any of the following: cost of implementing an electronic system; interruption in workflow; fees charged by software vendors; monthly fees for certain services; burden to bill to receive Medicare incentives in on the prescriber; DEA prohibits electronic transmission of controlled substances; pharmacies must maintain dual prescription filling system; absence of standards; certification issues; technological barriers

10. List at least two types of errors that are unique to e-prescribing.

Any of the following: selection error from drop-down menus; inappropriate use or selection of default doses; alert fatigue

Worksheet 10.2 Answers

1. Look up each of his medications. Indicate which ones are available over the counter and which require a prescription.

Over the counter: Colace, aspirin, multivitamin
Prescription: Ferrous sulfate, tramadol

2. Look up ferrous sulfate. List at least three different brand names for the drug, the different preparations available, and the strengths available. Write a prescription for a 1-month supply of ferrous sulfate for the dose listed in Mr. Oliver's discharge medications.

Any of the following name brands: Feosol, Feostat, Fergon, Feratab, Hemocyte, Hytinic, Ircon, Mol-Iron.

Preparations available: comes in regular, coated, and extended-release tablets; regular and extended-release capsules, and oral liquid
Strengths available:
Ferrous sulfate: *capsule:* 250 mg, 324 mg; *capsule, extended release:* 250 mg; *elixir:* 220 mg/5 mL; *enteric-coated tablet:* 325 mg; *liquid:* 25 mg/mL, 75 mg/0.6 mL, 300 mg/5 mL; *solution:* 300 mg/5 mL; *syrup:* 90 mg/5 mL; *tablet:* 195 mg, 300 mg, 324 mg, 325 mg; *tablet, extended release:* 250 mg, 525 mg
Ferrous sulfate, dried: *capsule, extended release:* 150 mg, 159 mg; *enteric-coated tablet:* 200 mg; *tablet:* 200 mg; *tablet, extended release:* 152 mg, 159 mg, 160 mg

3. Look up tramadol. List a brand name for tramadol and the name for tramadol with acetaminophen. List the strengths available in each brand. Write a prescription for a 1-week supply of plain tramadol in the strength listed in Mr. Oliver's discharge medications.

Tramadol alone is sold as Ultram or Ryzolt; Ultracet is tramadol plus acetaminophen. Ultram is available in a 50-mg tablet. and Ultram ER (extended release) is available in 100-mg, 200-mg, and 300-mg tablets. Ryzolt is available in the same doses as Ultram ER. Ultracet is 37.5 mg of tramadol and 325 mg of acetaminophen.

Worksheet 10.3 Answers

Refer to Worksheet 9.4 and review the discharge medications for Mrs. McLaughlin.

1. Look up all the medications listed and indicate which ones are controlled substances and what schedule.
Xanax is a category IV scheduled drug.

2. Write a prescription for a one-month supply of metoprolol.

3. Write a prescription for a ten-day course of Cipro based on twice daily dosing.

General Hospital
14000 Hospital Blvd.
Phoenix, AZ 85305

Name: _Gladys McLaughlin_____ Age: _74_

Address: _____

RX:

Metoprolol 50 mg tabs

Disp: 60 tabs

Sig: one po twice daily

Refills: (NR) 1 2 3 4 5

_Debbie Sullivan, PA C_____
Signature   DAW
                                 if circled

General Hospital
14000 Hospital Blvd.
Phoenix, AZ 85305

Name: _Gladys McLaughlin_____ Age: _74_

Address: _____

RX:

Cipro 500 mg tabs

Disp: 20 tabs

Sig: one po BID x 10 days

Refills: (NR) 1 2 3 4 5

_Debbie Sullivan, PA C_____
Signature   DAW
                                 if circled

4. Look up Xanax and write all the strengths that are available.
Xanax is available in 0.25 mg, 0.5 mg, 1 mg, and 2 mg tablets.

5. Write a prescription for Xanax for one week, using the dose indicated in Mrs. McLaughlin's discharge summary and indicating that a generic drug may be substituted for the brand name.

6. Write a prescription for the Lantus based on a dose of 22 units each day and indicate that

name brand only medication should be dispensed.

7. Patients sometimes use a mail-order pharmacy to fill prescriptions for medications taken daily. The mail-order pharmacies usually require a 90-day supply to be dispensed at one time, and enough refills to provide medication for one year. Write a prescription for the lisinopril based on these requirements.

```
General Hospital
14000 Hospital Blvd.
Phoenix, AZ 85305

Name: _Gladys McLaughlin_____ Age: _74_

Address: _____

RX:

            Lisinopril 5 mg tabs

               Disp: 90 tabs

            Sig:  one po daily for HTN


Refills:   NR   1   2  (3)  4   5

Debbie Sullivan, PA-C
Signature                              DAW
                                       if circled
```

```
General Hospital
14000 Hospital Blvd.
Phoenix, AZ 85305

Name: _____ Age: _____

Address: _____

RX:




Refills:   NR   1   2   3   4   5

_____
Signature                              DAW
                                       if circled
```

Worksheet 10.4 Answers

1. Look up Lotensin HCT. List the two medications contained in the formulation and the strengths that are available.
   Benazepril and hydrochlorothiazide; available in 5/6.25; 10/12.5; 20/12.5; and 20/25
2. Write a prescription for a 1-month supply of Lotensin HCT.

3. Look up Mevacor and list the strengths that are available and the generic name for the medication.
   Lovastatin; available as 10 mg, 20 mg, and 40 mg
4. Write a prescription for a 1-month supply of Mevacor, indicating that a generic drug may be substituted for the brand name.

```
General Hospital
14000 Hospital Blvd.
Phoenix, AZ 85305

Name: _William Jensen_____ Age: _67_

Address: _____

RX:

        Lotensin HCT 20/12.5 mg

              Disp: 30 tabs

        Sig:  take one tablet by mouth daily for HTN


Refills:  (NR)  1   2   3   4   5

Debbie Sullivan, PA-C
Signature                              DAW
                                       if circled
```

```
General Hospital
14000 Hospital Blvd.
Phoenix, AZ 85305

Name: _William Jensen_____ Age: _67_

Address: _____

RX:

          Mevacor 20 mg tabs

             Disp: 30 tabs

          Sig:  one po daily for dyslipidemia


Refills:  (NR)  1   2   3   4   5

Debbie Sullivan, PA-C
Signature                              DAW
                                       if circled
```

5. Look up Percocet and identify its schedule. List the generic name of the medication and the strengths that are available. Consult Appendix F and determine the maximal number that may be dispensed by a Physician Assistant practicing in West Virginia and write an appropriate prescription. Consult Appendix G and determine the maximal number that may be dispensed by a Nurse Practitioner practicing in Michigan and write an appropriate prescription.

Percocet is a class II narcotic. Generic name is oxycodone plus acetaminophen. It is available in 2.5/325 mg; 5/325 mg; 7.5/500 mg; 10/325 mg and 10/650 mg

Worksheet 10.5 Answers

Abbreviations

CSA	Controlled Substances Act
DAW	dispense as written
DEA	Drug Enforcement Agency
FDA	Food and Drug Administration
MMA	Medicare Modernization Act
TMP/SMX	trimethoprim-sulfamethoxazole

PA in West Virginia - 72 hr. limit

General Hospital
14000 Hospital Blvd.
Phoenix, AZ 85305

Name: *William Jensen*   Age: _67_

Address: _____

RX:

       Percocet 5/325 mg

          Disp: 18 (eighteen)

        Sig: one po every 4 hrs PRN pain

Refills: (NR) 1 2 3 4 5

Debbie Sullivan, PA-C
Signature   DAW
DEA MS 1234567   if circled

NP in Michigan - 1 week limit

General Hospital
14000 Hospital Blvd.
Phoenix, AZ 85305

Name: *William Jensen*   Age: _67_

Address: _____

RX:

       Percocet 5/325 mg

          Disp: 42 (forty-two) tabs

        Sig: one po every 4 hrs PRN pain

Refills: (NR) 1 2 3 4 5

Debbie Sullivan, NP
Signature   DAW
DEA: MS0123456   if circled

Physician Assistant Prescribing Summary by State

Jurisdiction	Restrictions	Controlled Substances
Alabama		Sch. III-V[1]
Alaska		Sch. II-V
Arizona		Sch. II-III limited to 14-day supply with board prescribing certification (72-hr. without); Sch. IV-V not more than 5 times in 6-month period per patient
Arkansas		Sch. III-V
California		Sch. II-V[2]
Colorado		Sch. II-V
Connecticut		Sch. II-V
Delaware		Sch. II-V
District of Columbia		Sch. II-V
Florida	Formulary of prohibited drugs	
Georgia	Formulary	Sch. III-V
Guam		Sch. III-V
Hawaii		Sch. III-V
Idaho		Sch. II-V
Illinois		Sch. III-V[3]
Indiana		Sch. III-V
Iowa		Sch. II-V; Sch. II (except depressants)
Kansas		Sch. II-V
Kentucky		None
Louisiana		Sch. III-V
Maine		Sch. III-V (Medical Board may approve Sch. II for individual PAs practicing with MD supervision. No such provision for Osteopathic board.)
Maryland		Schedule II-V
Massachusetts		Schedule II-V
Michigan		Sch. III-V; Sch. II (7-day supply) as discharge meds
Minnesota	Formulary	Sch. II-V
Mississippi		Sch. II-V
Missouri		Sch. III-V
Montana		Sch. II-V (Sch. II limited to 34-day supply)
Nebraska		Sch. II-V
Nevada		Sch. II-V
New Hampshire		Sch. II-V
New Jersey		Sch. II-V (certain conditions apply)
New Mexico	Formulary	Sch. II-V
New York		Sch. II-V
North Carolina		Sch. II-V (Sch. II-III limited to 30-day supply)
North Dakota		Sch. II-V
Ohio		Sch. III-V
Oklahoma	Formulary	Sch. III-V (limited to 30-day supply)
Oregon		Sch. II-V
Pennsylvania	Formulary	Sch. II-V (Sch. II limited to 72 hours for initial therapy; 30 days for ongoing therapy)
Rhode Island		Sch. II-V
South Carolina		Sch. III-V

Continued

Jurisdiction	Restrictions	Controlled Substances
South Dakota		Sch. II-V (Sch. II limited to 30-day supply)
Tennessee		Sch. II-V
Texas	In specified practice sites	Sch. III-V (limited to 30-day supply)
Utah		Sch. II-V
Vermont	Formulary	Sch. II-V
Virginia		Sch. II-V
Washington		Sch. II-V
West Virginia	Formulary	Sch. III-V (Sch. III limited to 72-hour supply)
Wisconsin		Sch. II-V
Wyoming		Sch. II-V

[1]Alabama law to authorize physicians to delegate prescriptive authority for Schedule III-V controlled substances to PAs passed in April 2009. Regulations necessary to implement law have not yet been adopted.
[2]In California, PAs may write "drug orders" which, for the purposes of DEA registration, meet the federal definition of a prescription. Controlled medications require a patient-specific order from the supervising physician unless PA has completed a board-approved course on controlled substances.
[3]Illinois law to authorize physicians to delegate prescriptive authority for Sch. II controlled substances to PAs was passed in May 2009. Regulations necessary to implement the law have not yet been adopted.
Source: From http://www.aapa.org/images/stories/Advocacy-state-summaries/Rx_Chart.pdf, accessed Oct. 1, 2009.

Nurse Practitioner Prescribing Summary by State

Jurisdiction	Restrictions	Controlled Substances
Alabama		Not granted
Alaska		Sch. II-V
Arizona		Sch. II-V
Arkansas		Sch. III-V
California		Sch. II-V
Colorado		Sch. II-V
Connecticut		Sch. II-V
Delaware		Sch. II-V
District of Columbia		Sch. II-V
Florida	Legend drugs only	Not granted
Georgia	Legend drugs only	Sch. III-V
Hawaii	Legend drugs only	Pending DEA Approval
Idaho		Sch. II-V
Illinois		Sch. III-V
Indiana		Sch. II-V; no controlled substances for purposes of weight management
Iowa		Sch. II-V
Kansas		Sch. II-V
Kentucky		Sch. II-V; varying limitations on initial length of supply and subsequent refill authority
Louisiana		Sch. III-V; no controlled substances for purposes of weight management or chronic, intractable pain
Maine		Sch. II-V
Maryland		Sch. II-V
Massachusetts		Sch. II-V; varying limitations on initial length of supply and subsequent refill authority
Michigan		Sch. III-V; Sch. II (7-day supply) as discharge meds
Minnesota		Sch. II-V
Mississippi		Sch. II-V
Missouri		Not granted
Montana		Sch. III-V (limited to initial maximum 3-month supply with refills in writing); Sch. II per DEA limitations
Nebraska		Sch. II-V
Nevada		Sch. II-V
New Hampshire		Sch. II-V (certain exclusions apply)
New Jersey	All prescriptions must be written on state-authorized prescription blanks printed with NPI	Sch. II-V (certain conditions apply)
New Mexico		Sch. II-V
New York	Sch. II and benzodiazepines must be written on official prescription forms	Sch. II-V (varying limitations on length of supply and refill authority)
North Carolina		Sch. II-V (varying limitations on length of supply and refill authority)
North Dakota		Sch. II-V
Ohio		Sch. III-V as specified in state formulary
Oklahoma		Sch. III-V (except as excluded by state formulary; limited to 7-day supply)

Continued

Jurisdiction	Restrictions	Controlled Substances
Oregon		Sch. II-V (limitations apply; does not include substances to treat narcotic addiction or Sch. II for weight management)
Pennsylvania		Sch. II-V (varying limitations on length of supply and refill authority)
Rhode Island		Sch. II-V as specified in state formulary
South Carolina		Sch. III-V
South Dakota		Sch. II-V
Tennessee		Sch. II-V
Texas		Sch. III-V (limited to 30-day supply without refill)
Utah		Sch. IV-V; Sch. II-III in accordance with consultation and referral plan; no Sch. II-III for weight management
Vermont	Formulary	Sch. II-V
Virginia		Sch. II-V
Washington		Sch. II-V
West Virginia	Formulary	Sch. III-V (varying limitations on length of supply and refill authority)
Wisconsin		Sch. II-V with limitations in regard to conditions for which certain Sch. II stimulants may be prescribed
Wyoming		Sch. II-V

Bibliography

Chapter 1

American Medical Association. CPT® Code Information and Education. http://www.ama-assn.org/ama/no-index/physician-resources/3884.shtml. Accessed July 17, 2009

Centers for Disease Control and Prevention. International Classification of Diseases, 9th Revision. http://www.cdc.gov/nchs/icd/icd9.htm. Updated September 1, 2009. Accessed June 25, 2009.

Centers for Disease Control and Prevention. HIPAA Privacy Rule and Public Health: Guidance from CDC and the U.S. Department of Health and Human Services. http://www.cdc.gov/mmwr/preview/mmwrhtml/m2e411a1.htm. Updated April 11, 2003. Accessed August 30, 2009.

Center for Medicare and Medicaid Services 1995 Documentation Guidelines for Evaluation and Management Services. http://www.cms.gov/MLNProducts/Downloads/1995dg.pdf. Last updated March 14, 1999. Accessed July 7, 2009.

Center for Medicare and Medicaid Services 1997 Documentation Guidelines for Evaluation and Management Services. http://www.cms.gov/MLNProducts/Downloads/MASTER1.pdf. Last updated December 9, 2009. Accessed June 28, 2009.

Center for Medicare and Medicaid Services. Health Insurance Reform for Consumers. http://www.cms.gov/HealthInsReformforConsume/. Updated May 5, 2010. Accessed July 18, 2009.

Center for Medicare and Medicaid Services. Guidelines for evaluation and management. http://www.cmsgov/MLNProducts/downloads/eval_mgmt_serv_guide.pdf. Updated July 2009. Accessed June 15, 2009.

Center for Medicare and Medicaid Services. Overview ICD-9 Provider and Diagnostic Codes. http://www.cms.gov/ICD9ProviderDiagnosticCodes. Accessed August 2, 2009.

Committee on Data Standards for Patient Safety; Institute of Medicine. Key Capabilities of an Electronic Health Record System. Washington, DC: National Academy Press, 2003.

Dick RS, Steen EB, Detmer DE, Eds. The Computer Based Patient Record: An Essential Technology for Health Care, Revised Edition. Committee on Improving the Patient Record; Division of Health Care Services; Institute of Medicine. Washington, DC: National Academy Press, 1997.

Health Information and Management Systems Society. Basic Facts about Meaningful Use and the American Recovery and Reinvestment Act of 2009. http://www.himss.org/content/files/BasicFactsAboutMeaningfulUseARRA.pdf. Updated January 21, 2010. Accessed July 14, 2009.

Health Information and Management Systems Society. The Legal Electronic Medical Record. http://www.himss.org/content/files/LegalEMR_Flyer3.pdf. Updated 2006. Accessed June 29, 2009.

HITECH Answers: Providing Resources and Independent Analysis of the HITECH Act and EHR adoption. http://hitechanswers.net/about-arra. Accessed July 15, 2009.

U.S. Department of Health and Human Services. Summary of the HIPAA Privacy Rule. http://www.hhs.gov/ocr/privacy/hipaa/understanding/summary/index.html. Updated May 2003. Accessed July 18, 2009.

U.S. Department of Health and Human Services. Summary of the HIPAA Privacy Rule. http://www.hhs.gov/ocr/privacy/hipaa/understanding/srsummary.html. Accessed August 5, 2009.

Chapter 2

Bickley LS. Bates' Guide to Physical Examination and History Taking, 10th Edition. Philadelphia: Lippincott Williams & Wilkins, 2008.

Center for Medicare and Medicaid Services 1995 Documentation Guidelines for Evaluation and Management Services. http://www.cms.gov/MLNProducts/Downloads/1995dg.pdf. Last updated March 14, 1999. Accessed July 7, 2009.

Center for Medicare and Medicaid Services 1997 Documentation Guidelines for Evaluation and Management Services. http://www.cms.gov/MLNProducts/Downloads/MASTER1.pdf. Last updated December 9, 2009. Accessed June 28, 2009.

Coulehan JL, Block ML. The Medical Interview: Mastering Skills for Clinical Practice, 5th Edition. Philadelphia: FA Davis, 2005.

Fontes LA. Interviewing Clients across Cultures: A Practitioner's Guide. New York: The Guilford Press, 2008.

Sullivan DD. Obtaining a cultural history. *Perspective on Physician Assistant Education*, 12(3):197-198; 2001.

U.S. Department of Health and Human Services. Guidance to Federal Financial Assistance Recipients Regarding Title VI and the Prohibition against National Origin Discrimination Affecting Limited English Proficient Persons—Summary. http://www.hhs.gov/ocr/civilrights/resources/laws/summaryguidance.html. Accessed April 16, 2009.

Chapter 3

Adult Preventive Care Timeline. AHRQ Publication No. APPIP06-IP001. Rockville, MD: Agency for Healthcare Research and Quality. http://www.ahrq.gov/ppip/timelinead.htm. June 2006. Accessed January 10, 2010.

Aertgeerts B, Buntinx F, Kester A. The value of the CAGE in screening for alcohol abuse and alcohol dependence in general clinical populations: A diagnostic meta-analysis. *Journal of Clinical Epidemiology*, 57(1):30-39; 2004.

American Congress of Obstetricians and Gynecologists. Screening Tools—Domestic Violence. http://www.acog.org/departments/dept_notice.cfm?recno=17&bulletin=585. Accessed July 14, 2009.

American Urological Association. Prostate Specific Antigen: Best Practice Statement: 2009 Update. http://www.auanet.org/content/guidelines-and-quality-care/clinical-guidelines/main-reports/psa09.pdf. Accessed December 13, 2009.

Babor TF, Higgins-Biddle JC, Saunders JB, Monteiro MG. The Alcohol Use Disorders Identification Test: Guidelines for Use in Primary Care, 2nd Edition. World Health Organization. http://whqlibdoc.who.int/hq/2001/WHO_MSD_MSB_01.6a.pdf. Accessed October 19, 2009.

Berg K, Wood-Dauphinee S, Williams JI, Gayton D. Measuring balance in the elderly: Preliminary development of an instrument. *Physiotherapy Canada*, 41(6):304-311; 1989.

Borson S, Scanlan J, Brush M, Vitaliano P, Dokmak A. The mini-cog: A cognitive "vital signs" measure for dementia screening in multi-lingual elderly. *International Journal of Geriatric Psychiatry*, 15(11):1021-1027; 2000.

California STD/HIV Prevention Training Center. A Guide to Sexual History Taking. http://www.stdhivtraining.org/resource.php?id=3&ret=clinical_resources. Accessed January 10, 2010.

Centers for Disease Control and Prevention. Body Mass Index. http://www.cdc.gov/healthyweight/assessing/bmi/index.html. Accessed October 30, 2009.

Centers for Disease Control and Prevention. Family Health-ware. http://www.cdc.gov/genomics/famhistory/famhx.htm. Accessed December 3, 2009.

Centers for Disease Control and Prevention. Oral Health Resources. http://www.cdc.gov/oralhealth. Accessed November 5, 2009.

Centers for Disease Control and Prevention. Vaccines and Immunizations: Immunization Schedules. http://www.cdc.gov/vaccines/recs/schedules/default.htm. Accessed November 14, 2009.

Cherpitel CJ. Brief screening instruments for alcoholism. *Alcohol Health & Research World*, 21(4):348-351; 1997.

Department of Health and Human Services. About Health Literacy. http://www.hrsa.gov/publichealth/healthliteracy/healthlitabout.html. Accessed June 13, 2010.

Fiellin DA, Reid MC, O'Connor PG. Screening for alcohol problems in primary care. *Archives of Internal Medicine*, 160:1977-1989: 2000.

Guigoz Y. The Mini-Nutritional Assessment (MNA®) Review of the Literature—What does it tell us? *Journal of Nutrition Health and Aging*, 10: 466-487; 2006.

Hidalgo JL, Gras CB, Tellez LJ, et al. The Hearing-Dependent Daily Activities Scale to evaluate impact of hearing loss in older people. *Annals of Family Medicine*, 6(5):441-447; 2008.

Jogerst G. Geriatric Assessment Tools: Functional Assessment. Geriatric Health Questionnaire. http://www.healthcare.uiowa.edu/ igec/tools/function/geriatric_health_questionnaire.pdf. Accessed October 12, 2009.

Katz S, Down TD, Cash HR, Grotz RC. Progress in the development of the index of ADL. *The Gerontologist*, 10(1):20-30; 1970.

Lawton MP, Brody EM. Assessment of older people: Self-maintaining and instrumental activities of daily living. *Gerontologist*, 9:179-186; 1969.

MacMillan HL, Wathen CN, Jamieson E, Boyle M, McNutt LA, Worster A, Lent B, Webb M. The McMaster Violence Against Women Research Group. Approaches to screening for intimate partner violence in health care settings. *Journal of the American Medical Association*, 296:530-536; 2006.

Malnutrition Advisory Group. British Association for Parenteral and Enteral Nutrition. Malnutrition Universal Screening Tool. http://www.bapen.org.uk/pdfs/must/must_explan.pdf. Accessed August 28, 2009.

National Health Statistics Reports, Number 3. National Ambulatory Medical Care Survey 2006 Summary; August 6, 2008. http://www.cdc.gov/nchs/data/nhsr/nhsr003.pdf. Accessed September 10, 2009.

National Institute of Drug Abuse. The Modified Alcohol, Smok-ing and Substance-Involvement Screening Test. Adapted from the World Health Organization Alcohol, Smoking and Substance Involvement Screening Test (ASSIST) Version 3.0. http://www.nida.nih.gov/nidamed/resguide/resourceguide.pdf. Accessed June 30, 2009.

Podsiadlo D, Richardson S. The timed 'Up and Go' test: A test of basic functional mobility for frail elderly persons. *Journal of American Geriatric Society*, 39:142-148; 1991.

Rabin RF, Jennings JM, Campbell JC, Bair-Merritt MH. Intimate partner violence screening tools: A systematic review. *American Journal of Preventive Medicine*, 36(5): 439-445; 2009.

Rubenstein LZ, Harker JO, Salva A, Guigoz Y, Vellas B. Screening for under-nutrition in geriatric practice: Developing the Short-Form Mini Nutritional Assessment (MNA-SF). *Journal of Gerontology*, 56A:M366-377; 2001.

Sheikh JI, Yesavage JA. Geriatric Depression Scale (GDS): Recent evidence and development of a shorter version.

Clinical Gerontology: A Guide to Assessment and Intervention. New York: The Haworth Press, 1986, pp 165-173. http://www.stanford.edu/~yesavage/GDS.html. Accessed August 21, 2009.

Shulman KI, Shedletsky R, Silver IL. The challenge of time: Clock-drawing and cognitive function in the elderly. *International Journal of Geriatric Psychiatry*, 1:135-140; 1986.

Skinner HA. The Drug Abuse Screening Test. *Addictive Behavior*, 7:363-371; 1982.

Sokol RJ, Martier SS, Ager JW. The T-ACE Questions: Practical prenatal detection of risk drinking. *American Journal of Obstetrics and Gynecology*, 60:863-870; 1989.

Tinetti ME. Performance-oriented assessment of mobility problems in elderly patients. *Journal of the American Gerontology Society*, 34:119-126; 1986.

U.S. Department of Health and Human Services. My Family Health Portrait: A Tool from the Surgeon General. https://familyhistory.hhs.gov/fhh-web/home.action. Updated January 2009. Accessed November 11, 2009.

U.S. Department of Labor. Occupational Safety and Health Administration. http://www.osha.gov/index.html. Accessed August 10, 2009.

Vellas B, Villars H, Abellan G, et al. Overview of MNA®—Its history and challenges. *Journal of Nutrition Health and Aging*, 10:456-465; 2006.

Chapter 4

American Academy of Pediatrics. Pediatric Visit Documentation Forms Package. https://www.nfaap.org/netforum/eweb/DynamicPage.aspx?webcode=aapbks_productdetail&key=c8964929-4797-430d-b4b9-8ec1a73e1eed. Accessed January 4, 2010.

Bayley, N. Bayley Scales of Infant and Toddler Development, 3rd Edition. http://www.pearsonassessments.com/HAIWEB/Cultures/en-us/Productdetail.htm?Pid=015-8027-23X&Mode=summary. Accessed January 21, 2010.

Bernstein DP, Fink L, Handelsman L, Foote J. Initial reliability and validity of a new retrospective measure of child abuse and neglect. *American Journal of Psychiatry*, 151(8): 1132-1136; 1994.

Briere J. Child Abuse Trauma: Theory and Treatment of the Lasting Effects. Newbury Park, CA: Sage Publications, 1992. http://www.johnbriere.com/cmis.htm. Accessed January 31, 2010.

Centers for Disease Control and Prevention. CDC Growth Charts. http://www.cdc.gov/growthcharts/. Accessed January 12, 2010.

Centers for Disease Control and Prevention. National Health and Nutrition Examination Survey. http://www.cdc.gov/nchs/nhanes/about_nhanes.htm. Accessed February 1, 2010.

Child Welfare Information Gateway. Recognizing Child Abuse and Neglect: Signs and Symptoms. http://www.childwelfare.gov/pubs/factsheets/signs.pdf. Accessed January 30, 2010.

Department of Adolescent Health, American Medical Associa-tion. Guidelines for Adolescent Preventive Services. Chicago: American Medical Association, 1992. http://www.cdc.gov/mmwr/preview/mmwrhtml/00018165.htm. Accessed January 20, 2010.

Fleming M, Towey K, eds. Education Forum on Adolescent Health: Adolescent Obesity, Nutrition, and Physical Activity. Chicago: American Medical Association, 2003.

Frankenburg WK, Dodds J, Archer P, Shapiro H, Bresnick B. The Denver II: A major revision and restandardization of the Denver Developmental Screening Test. *Pediatrics*, 89:91-97; 1992.

Goldenring JM, Rosen DS. Getting into adolescent heads: An essential update. *Contemporary Pediatrics*, 21:64; 2004.

National Newborn Screening and Genetics Resource Center. State Map Page, Newborn Screening. http://genes-r-us. uthscsa.edu/resources/consumer/statemap.htm. Updated August 2009. Accessed January 9, 2010.

Parents' Evaluation of Developmental Status. http://www. pedstest.com/LearnAboutPEDS/IntroductiontoPEDS.aspx. Accessed February 11, 2010.

Parents' Evaluation of Developmental Status—Developmental Milestones. http://www.pedstest.com/LearnAboutPEDSDM. aspx. Accessed February 11, 2010.

Sege R, Licenziato V, Eds. Recognizing and Preventing Youth Violence: A Guide for Physicians and Other Health Care Professionals. Waltham, MA: Massachusetts Medical Society; 2004.

Squires J, Bricker D, Twombly E. Ages and Stages Question-naires, 3rd Edition. Baltimore: Paul H. Brooks Publishing; 2009. http://www.agesandstages.com/index.html. Accessed February 8, 2010.

U.S. Department of Health and Human Services. Administration for Children and Families. Child Abuse Prevention and Treatment Act. http://www.acf.hhs.gov/programs/cb/laws_policies/cblaws/capta/index.htm. Accessed January 28, 2010.

U.S. Department of Health and Human Services. Early Periodic Screening, Diagnosis, and Treatment (EPSDT) Program. http://www.hrsa.gov/epsdt/. Accessed January 5, 2010.

Youth at Risk Screening Questionnaire. http://www. crisiscounseling.org/Assessments/YouthAtRiskScreen.htm. Accessed February 2, 2010.

Chapter 5

Ballweg R, Sullivan EM, Brown D, Vetrosky D. Physician Assistant: A Guide to Clinical Practice, 4th Edition. Philadelphia: WB Saunders, 2008.

Bardes CL. Essential Skills in Clinical Medicine. Philadelphia: FA Davis, 1996.

Bickley LS. Bates' Guide to Physical Examination and History Taking, 10th Edition. Philadelphia: Lippincott Williams & Wilkins; 2008.

Coulehan JL, Block ML. The Medical Interview: Mastering Skills for Clinical Practice, 5th Edition. Philadelphia: FA Davis, 2005.

Gomella LG, Haist SA. Clinician's Pocket Reference, 11th Edition. San Francisco: McGraw-Hill, 2006.

Hampton JR, Harrison MJG, Mitchell JRA, Prichard JS, Seymour C. Relative contributions of history-takings, physical examination, and laboratory investigation to diagnosis and management of medical outpatients. *British Medical Journal*, 2:486-489; 1975.

Kettenbach G. Writing SOAP Notes, 3rd Edition. Philadelphia: FA Davis, 2003.

Peterson MC, Holbrook JH, Hales DV, Smith NL, Staker LV. Contributions of the history, physical examination, and laboratory investigation in making medical diagnoses. *Western Journal of Medicine*, 156(2):163-165; 1992.

Platt R. Two essays on the practice of medicine. *Manchester University Medical School Gazette*, 27:139-145; 1947.

Roach WH. Medical Records and the Law, 4th Edition. Sudbury, MA: Jones & Bartlett Publishers, 2006.

Roth-Kauffman M. Physician Assistant Business Practice and Legal Guide. Sudbury, MA: Jones & Bartlett Publishers, 2005.

Schwartz MH. Textbook of Physical Diagnosis: History and Examination, 6th Edition. Philadelphia: Saunders Elsevier, 2009.

Seidel HM, Ball JW, Dains JE, Flynn JA, Solomon BS, Stewart RW. Mosby's Physical Examination Handbook, 7th Edition. Philadelphia: Mosby, 2010.

Wasson J, Walsh B, Sox H, Pantell R. The Common Symptom Guide, 6th Edition. San Francisco: McGraw-Hill, 2009.

Chapter 6

American Hospital Association. Put It in Writing: Questions and Answers on Advance Directives. http://www.putitinwriting.org/putitinwriting_app/content/piiwbrochure.pdf. Updated April 2005. Accessed March 27, 2010.

American Medical Association. Guidelines for Physician-Patient Electronic Communications. http://www.ama-assn.org/ama/pub/about-ama/our-people/member-groups-sections/young-physicians-section/advocacy-resources/guidelines-physician-patient-electronic-communications.shtml. Accessed March 10, 2010.

American Medical Informatics Association. Guidelines for the Clinical Use of Electronic Mail with Patients. https://www. amia.org:443/mbrcenter/wg/kim/docs/email_guidelines.html. Last updated February 25, 2003. Accessed March 10, 2010.

American Medical News. Dolan PL. Email means few patient calls and visits. http://www.ama-assn.org/amednews/2007/08/27/bil20827.htm. August 27, 2007. Accessed March 28, 2010.

Bennett E. Over 1,000 Hospital Social Media Sites. http://ebennett.org/over-1000. Last updated January 10, 2010. Accessed April 8, 2010.

Bhargava R. How Doctors Are Using Social Media. http://blog.ogilvypr.com/2009/09/how-doctors-are-using-social-media. September 22, 2009. Accessed March 5, 2010.

Brooks RG, Menachemi N. Physicians' use of email with patients: Factors influencing electronic communication and adherence to best practices. *Journal of Medical Internet Research*, 8(1):e2. http://www.jmir.org/2006/1/e2. Accessed April 1, 2010.

California Health Care Foundation. New Guidelines Help Physicians Choose among Online Patient Communication Options. http://www.chcf.org/media/press-releases/2003/new-guidelines-help-physicians-choose-among-online-patient-communication-options. November 17, 2003. Accessed March 29, 2010.

Chretien KC, Greysen SR, Chretien JP, Kind T. Online posting of unprofessional content by medical students. *Journal of the American Medical Association*, 302(12):1309-1315; 2009. http://jama.ama-assn.org/cgi/reprint/302/12/1309. Accessed April 2, 2010.

Darves B. Social Media and Physicians. http://www.nejmjobs.org/career-resources/social-media-and-physicians.aspx. March 2010. Accessed April 3, 2010.

Dolan PL. Social networking etiquette: Making virtual acquaintances. http://www.ama-assn.org/amednews/2008/06/02/bisa0602.htm. June 2, 2008. Accessed April 6, 2010.

Guadagnino C. Physician websites evolve. *Physician's News Digest*, January, 2008. http://www.physiciansnews.com/cover/108.html. Accessed March 30, 2010.

Hennessy M. How social media can make physicians better doctors. http://www.hcplive.com/primary-care/publications/mdng-primarycare/2009/Oct2009/EdNote. September 28, 2009. Accessed March 31, 2010.

Jain SH. Practicing medicine in the age of Facebook. *New England Journal of Medicine*, 361:7; 2009. Accessed March 3, 2010.

Lowes R. Patient-centered care for better patient adherence. http://www.aafp.org/fpm/980300fm/patient.html. Accessed March 15, 2010.

MAG Mutual Insurance Company. Telephone Encounters and Triage. http://www.magmutual.com/mmic/articles/Telephone-Triage.pdf. Accessed March 20, 2010.

Malamon W. Integrating patient email into your practice. http://www.tmlt.org/newscenter/features/patient_email.html. Accessed March 28, 2010.

Mayo Clinic. Living wills and advance directives for medical decisions. http://www.mayoclinic.com/health/living-wills/HA00014/METHOD=print. July 11, 2000. Accessed March 30, 2010.

Office of the Information & Privacy Commissioner for British Columbia. http://www.oipc.bc.ca/pdfs/Physician_Privacy_Toolkit/UseofEmailbyPhysicians.pdf. Last updated June 25, 2009. Accessed March 28, 2010.

Pho K. Useful Twitter Advice for Doctors. http://www.kevinmd.com/blog/2010/01/twitter-advice-doctors.html. January 7, 2010. Accessed March 29, 2010.

Princeton Insurance. Reducing Risk: Telephone Communication. http://www.pinsco.com/downloads/reducing_risk/Tips.to.reduce.phone.liability.May05.pdf. May 2005. Accessed March 15, 2010.

Quatre T. Email: The New Frontier in Physician-Patient Communication? The Healthcare Entrepreneur Blog. http://www.vantageclinicalsolutions.com/blog/2008/04/23/email-the-new-frontier-in-physician-patient-communication. Accessed March 31, 2010.

Rajecki R. Patients See Benefits of Email and Web Communications—If Free. October 29, 2009. http://www.modernmedicine.com/modernmedicine/article/articleDetail.jsp?id=636485. Accessed March 29, 2010.

Rosen P, Kwoh CK. Patient-physician email: An opportunity to transform pediatric health care delivery. *Pediatrics*, 120(4):701-706; 2007.

Sabatino C. Advance Directives. http://www.merck.com/mmpe/sec22/ch339/ch339f.html. Last updated July 2007. Accessed April 2, 2010.

Schwimmer J. Thoughts on Patient-Physician Email (part 1). http://www.healthline.com/blogs/medical_devices/2007/07/thoughts-on-patient-physician-email.html. July 23, 2007. Accessed March 31, 2010.

Schwimmer J. Thoughts on Patient-Physician Email (part 2). http://www.healthline.com/blogs/medical_devices/2007/07/thoughts-on-patient-physician-email_31.html. July 31, 2007. Accessed March 31, 2010.

Schwimmer J. Thoughts on Patient-Physician Email (part 3). http://www.healthline.com/blogs/medical_devices/2007/08/thoughts-on-patient-physician-email.html. August 8, 2007. Accessed March 31, 2010.

Shafrin J. Physician-patient Email Communication: A Review. http://healthcare-economist.com/2006/08/02/physician-patient-email-communication-a-review. August 2, 2006. Accessed March 30, 2010.

Stouffer R. Doctor use of patient email still low despite benefits. *Pittsburgh Tribune Review*, August 3, 2008. http://www.pittsburghlive.com/x/pittsburghtrib/business/s_580825.html. Accessed March 24, 2010.

Versel N. Doctors and Social Media: Benefits and Dangers. http://www.medscape.com/viewarticle/711717. November 9, 2009. Accessed April 2, 2010.

White CB, Moyer CA, Stern DT, Katz SJ. A content analysis of e-mail communication between patients and their providers: Patients get the message. *Journal of the American Medical Informatics Association*, 11:260-267; 2004. http://www.ncbi.nlm.nih.gov/pmc/articles/PMC436072. Accessed April 3, 2010.

Wynn P. Brave New World of Social Media. http://www.amsa.org/AMSA/Homepage/Publications/TheNewPhysician/2010/0110SocialMedia.aspx. February 2010. Accessed April 8, 2010.

Zhou YY, Garrido T, Chin HL, Wiesenthal AM, Liang LL. Patient access to electronic health records with secure messaging: Impact on primary care utilization. American *Journal of Managed Care*, 13:418-424; 2007.

Chapter 7

Bobb A, Gleason K, Husch M, Geinglass J, Yarnold PR, Noskin GA. The epidemiology of prescribing errors: The potential impact of computerized prescriber order entry. *Archives of Internal Medicine*, 164:785-791; 2004.

California Health Care Foundation. Computerized Physician Order Entry (CPOE) is Succeeding in Community Hospitals. http://www.chcf.org/media/press-releases/2003/computerized-physician-order-entry-cpoe-is-succeeding-in-community-hospitals. Accessed September 2, 2009.

Centers for Disease Control and Prevention. 2006 National Hospital Discharge Survey. National Health Statistics Reports; No. 5, July 30, 2008. http://www.cdc.gov/nchs/data/nhsr/nhsr005.pdf. Accessed September 4, 2009.

Center for Medicare and Medicaid Services. Title 42-Public Health; Chapter 4, Section 482.24. http://edocket.access.gpo.gov/cfr_2004/octqtr/pdf/42cfr482.24.pdf. Accessed September 12, 2009.

Classen DC, Avery AJ, Bates DW. Evaluation and certification of computerized provider order entry systems. *Journal of the American Informatics Association*, 14(1):48-55; 2007.

Institute for Safe Medication Practices. List of Error-Prone Abbreviations, Symbols, and Dose Designations. http://www.ismp.org/tools/errorproneabbreviations.pdf. Accessed August 20, 2009.

Kaushal R, Shojania KG, Bates DW. Effects of computerized physician order entry and clinical decision support systems on medication safety: A systematic review. *Archives of Internal Medicine*, 163:1409-1416; 2003.

Kohn LT, Corrigan JM, Donaldson MS, Eds. Institute of Medicine Report. To Err Is Human: Building a Safer Health System. Washington, DC: National Academy Press, 2000.

OpenClinical. Computer Physician Order Entry Systems. http://www.openclinical.org/cpoe.html. Updated June 5, 2006. Accessed August 30, 2009.

Osheroff JA, Pifer EA, Teich JM, Sittig DF, Jenders RA. Improving Outcomes with Clinical Decision Supports: An Implementer's Guide. Chicago: Health Information and Management Systems Society, 2005. http://www.himss.org/ASP/topics_cds_workbook.asp?faid=108&tid=14. Accessed August 28, 2009.

U.S. Department of Justice. Americans with Disabilities Act, Title II. http://www.ada.gov/t2hlt95.htm. Accessed September 4, 2009.

Chapter 8

American Medical Association. Informed Consent. http://www.ama-assn.org/ama/pub/physician-resources/legal-topics/patient-physician-relationship-topics/informed-consent.shtml. Accessed May 2, 2009.

Gomella LG, Haist SA. Clinician's Pocket Reference, 11th Edition. San Francisco: McGraw-Hill, 2006.

Mersch J. Apgar Score. http://www.medicinenet.com/apgar_score/article.htm. Accessed June 14, 2009.

Moses S. Delivery Note. Family Practice Notebook. http://www.fpnotebook.com/OB/LD/DlvryNt.htm. Updated October 11, 2008. Accessed April 6, 2009.

University of Florida Medical School. Writing an Effective Daily Progress Note. http://www.medicine.ufl.edu/3rd_year_clerkship/documents/Writing_an_Effective_Daily_Progress_Note.pdf. Accessed March 29, 2009.

Chapter 9

American Society of Anesthesiologists. Practice guideline for acute pain management in the perioperative setting: An updated report by the American Society of Anesthesiologists Task Force on Acute Pain Management. *Anesthesiology*, 100:1573-1581; 2004. http://www.asahq.org/publicationsAndServices/pain.pdf. Accessed May 8, 2009.

Cohen MR, Weber RJ, Moss J. Institute of Safe Medication Practices. Patient-Controlled Analgesia: Making it Safer for Patients; 2006. http://www.ismp.org/profdevelopment/PCAMonograph.pdf. Accessed June 1, 2009.

Grass JA. Patient-Controlled Analgesia. *Anesthesia and Analgesia*; 101:S44-61; 2005. http://web.mac.com/bdurkindo/Acute_Pain/Articles_files/PatientControlledAnalgesia%20-%20A&A%20-%202005%20Grass.pdf. Accessed May 15, 2009.

Greenwald J. Improving hospital discharge. *Physician's News Digest*, November, 2008. http://www.physiciansnews.com/cover/1108.html. Accessed May 10, 2009.

Hertz BT. Act Quickly and Listen a Lot: What to do When a Patient Wants to Leave AMA. ACP Hospitalist. http://www.acphospitalist.org/archives/2010/03/against.htm. Accessed April 30, 2010.

Hwang SW, Li J, Gupta R, Chien V, Martin RE. What happens to patients who leave hospital against medical advice? *Canadian Medical Association Journal*, 168(4): 417-420; 2003.

Koo PJS. Balancing Postoperative Analgesia and Management of Side Effects. http://cme.medscape.com/viewarticle/429661_2. Accessed May 22, 2009.

National Patient Safety Foundation. Partnership for Clear Health Communication at the National Patient Safety Foundation. http://www.npsf.org/pchc. Accessed April 28, 2009.

Stranges E, Wier L, Merrill CT, Steiner C. Hospitalizations in which Patients Leave the Hospital against Medical Advice, 2007. Hospital Cost and Utilization Project Statistical Brief #78. Agency for Healthcare Research and Quality; 2009. http://www.hcup-us.ahrq.gov/reports/statbriefs/sb78.pdf. Accessed April 14, 2009.

The Virtual Anesthesia Textbook. Post-operative Pain. http://www.virtual-anaesthesia-textbook.com/vat/pain.html. Updated April 20, 2009. Accessed May 30, 2009.

U. S. Pharmacopeia. Quality Review: Patient-Controlled Analgesia Pumps. http://www.usp.org/pdf/EN/patientSafety/qr812004-09-01.pdf. Accessed June 2, 2009.

Weiss B. Health Literacy and Patient Safety: Help Patients Understand. AMA Foundation. http://www.ama-assn.org/ama1/pub/upload/mm/367/healthlitclinicians.pdf. Accessed May 5, 2009.

Chapter 10

Centers for Medicare and Medicaid Services. http://www.cms.gov/MMAUpdate. Accessed February 1, 2010.

Davis R. Prescription Writing and the PDR. http://www.sh.lsuhsc.edu/fammed/OutpatientManual/PrescripWriting-PDR.htm. Accessed January 20, 2010.

Donyai P, O'Grady K, Jacklin A, Barber N, Franklin BD. The effects of electronic prescribing on the quality of prescribing. *British Journal of Clinical Pharmacology*, 65(2):230-237; 2007. http://www3.interscience.wiley.com/cgi-bin/fulltext/119402893/PDFSTART?CRETRY=1&SRETRY=0. Accessed March 14, 2010.

Families USA. Congress Delivers Help to People with Medicare: An Overview of the Medicare Improvements for Patients and Providers Act of 2008. http://www.familiesusa.org/assets/pdfs/medicare-improvements-act-2008.pdf. Accessed January 25, 2010.

Food and Drug Administration. Medication Errors. http://www.fda.gov/Drugs/DrugSafety/MedicationErrors/default.htm. Updated August 16, 2009. Accessed February 5, 2010.

Hale PL. Electronic Prescribing for the Medical Practice: Everything You Wanted to Know But Were Afraid to Ask. Chicago: Healthcare Information Management and Systems Society, 2007.

IMS Health. IMS Health Reports U. S. Prescription Sales Grew 5.1 Percent in 2009, to $300.3 Billion. http://www.imshealth.com/portal/site/imshealth/menuitem.a46c6d4df3db4b3d88f611019418c22a/?vgnextoid=d690a27e9d5b7210VgnVCM100000ed152ca2RCRD&cpsextcurrchannel=1. Updated April 1, 2010. Accessed June 13, 2010.

Institute of Medicine. Preventing Medication Errors. Report Brief; July, 2006. http://www.iom.edu/~/media/Files/Report%20Files/2006/Preventing-Medication-Errors-Quality-Chasm-Series/medicationerrorsnew.ashx. Accessed December 17, 2010.

Isaac T, Weissman JS, Davis RB, Massagli M, Cyrulik A, Sands DZ, Weingart SN. Overrides of medication alerts in ambulatory care. *Archives of Internal Medicine*, 169(3):305-311; 2009.

Johnston D, Pan E, Walker J, Bates DW, Middleton B. (2004). Patient Safety in the Physician's Office: Assessing the Value of Ambulatory CPOE. The Center for Information Technology Leadership, 2004.

Medicare.gov. Prescription Drug Coverage: Basic Information. http://www.medicare.gov/pdp-basic-information.asp. Accessed January 12, 2010.

National Coordinating Council for Medication Error Reporting and Prevention. Council Recommendations to Enhance Accuracy of Prescription Writing. http://www.nccmerp.org/council/council1996-09-04.html. Accessed February 8, 2010.

National ePrescribing Patient Safety Initiative. The Time for ePrescribing Is Now. http://www.allscripts.com/brochures/EP1_NEPSI_CSv1_10508.pdf. Accessed January 30, 2010.

National Health Statistics Reports, Number 3. National Ambulatory Medical Care Survey 2006 Summary; August 6, 2008. http://www.cdc.gov/nchs/data/nhsr/nhsr003.pdf. Accessed September 10, 2009.

National Institute of Health Policy. The Medicare Modernization Act of 2003. http://www.nihp.org/Reports/NIHPMMA2003Whitepaper.pdf. Accessed January 20, 2010.

National Progress Report on E-prescribing; December, 2007. http://www.surescripts.com/downloads/NPR/national-progress-report.pdf. Accessed November 30, 2009.

OmniMD. Eprescribing. http://www.omnimd.com/html/prescription.html. Accessed November 14, 2009.

OpenClinical. E-prescribing. http://www.openclinical.org/e-prescribing.html. Last updated August 31, 2005. Accessed October 13, 2009.

U.S. Department of Justice. Drug Enforcement Agency. Controlled Substances Schedules. http://www.deadiversion.usdoj.gov/schedules/index.html. Accessed November 16, 2009.

U.S. Department of Justice. Drug Enforcement Agency. Practitioner's Manual. http://www.deadiversion.usdoj.gov/pubs/manuals/pract/pract_manual012508.pdf. Accessed December 3, 2009.

U. S. Food and Drug Administration. Title 21 Code of Federal Regulations. http://www.accessdata.fda.gov/scripts/cdrh/cfdocs/cfcfr/cfrsearch.cfm. Accessed December 20, 2009.

Index